Queer Emergent

**Critical Global Health: Evidence, Efficacy, Ethnography**

A series edited by Vincanne Adams and João Biehl

# Queer Emergent

Scandalous Stories from the Twilight
of AIDS in Peru

JUSTIN PEREZ

DUKE UNIVERSITY PRESS
*Durham and London*
2025

Project Editor: Bird Williams
Designed by A. Mattson Gallagher
Typeset in Minion Pro and Source Sans 3
by Westchester Publishing Services.

Library of Congress Cataloging-in-Publication Data
Names: Perez, Justin, [date] author.
Title: Queer emergent : scandalous stories at the twilight of AIDS / Justin Perez.
Other titles: Scandalous stories at the twilight of AIDS | Critical global health.
Description: Durham : Duke University Press, 2025. | Series: Critical global health:
evidence, efficacy, ethnography | Includes bibliographical references and index.
Identifiers: LCCN 2024047901 (print)
LCCN 2024047902 (ebook)
ISBN 9781478031802 (paperback)
ISBN 9781478028574 (hardcover)
ISBN 9781478060789 (ebook)
Subjects: LCSH: AIDS (Disease)—Social aspects—Peru. | AIDS (Disease)—Peru—
Case studies. | HIV infections—Peru—Case studies. | AIDS (Disease)—Peru—
Prevention. | HIV infections—Peru—Prevention. | Transgender people—Peru—
Social life and customs. | Gay people—Peru—Social life and customs.
Classification: LCC RA643.86.P4 P467 2025 (print)
LCC RA643.86.P4 (ebook)
DDC 306.4/61—dc23/eng/20250218
LC record available at https://lccn.loc.gov/2024047901
LC ebook record available at https://lccn.loc.gov/2024047902

Cover art: The main plaza of Tarapoto. Photograph by Marlon del Aguila Guerrero.

CONTENTS

Acknowledgments                                                vii

Introduction: Scandalous Stories of HIV Prevention              1

1.   Stories That Scandalize: Transactional Sex                 36
     and Postconflict Moral Imaginaries

2.   Collaboration on the *Cancha*: Sustaining and Multiplying  63
     Social Relations through Scandalous Spectacles

3.   Scandal at the Disco: Discrimination, Difference,          89
     and the Cultivation of a Culture of Denouncement

4.   When Projects End: The Fragmentation of Collaboration     119
     and the Afterworlds of HIV Prevention

5.   Stories That Count: The Pathways of                       145
     Discrimination Stories

     Afterword                                                 171
     Notes                                                     179
     References                                                215
     Index                                                     241

## ACKNOWLEDGMENTS

The seeds of this research project were planted while I was an undergraduate anthropology major at the University of Notre Dame. I thank Maurizio Albahari for advising my senior thesis. I am grateful to the Kellogg Institute for International Studies for sponsoring my early research in Peru, with special thanks to Holly Rivers and Sharon Schierling. In graduate school at UC Irvine, I was privileged to have the support of Tom Boellstorff, Susan Bibler Coutin, and Victoria Bernal. Many thanks to Tom Boellstorff, who deftly guided me through coursework, fieldwork, and beyond as an advisor and mentor. Courses and seminars led by Julia Elyachar, Lilith Mahmud, Bill Maurer, Keith Murphy, Valerie Olson, Rachel O'Toole, Kris Peterson, Steve Topik, and Mei Zhan taken alongside Nate Coben, Sean Larabee, Kyrstin Mallon Andrews, Kim McKinson, Simone Popperl, Daina Sanchez, and Natali Valdez made UCI a vibrant intellectual community and helped my scholarship grow in ways I could have never imagined. The opportunity to learn from Kris Peterson as a teaching assistant for the course "HIV/AIDS in a Global Context" was truly transformative. Fieldwork was supported by the Social Science Research Council International Dissertation Research Fellowship, the Inter-American Foundation Grassroots Development Fellowship, and the National Science Foundation Graduate Research Fellowship Program. I am also grateful for the James Harvey Scholar award from the UCI Graduate Division.

This project blossomed during my time at Princeton. It was an honor to hold the Fund for Reunion–Cotsen Fellowship in LGBT Studies at the Princeton University Society of Fellows in the Liberal Arts. I am in awe of João Biehl and truly grateful for the generous support, critical perspective, and mentorship that he has offered me and this project. I extend my gratitude to Elizabeth Armstrong, Wallace Best, Nijah Cunningham, Rhea Dexter, Stefan Eich, Julia Elyachar, Alessandro Giammei, Michael Gordin, Javier Guerrero, Monica Huerta, Regina Kunzel, Maria Papadakis, Bernadette Perez, Carolyn Rouse, Ava Shirazi, Beate Witzler, and Mo Lin Yee. With the additional support of the Princeton Anthropology Department, the Program in Gender and Sexuality Studies, and the Queer Princeton Alumni (formerly BTGALA), I convoked a workshop for an early version of this manuscript. The commentary, feedback, questions, and provocations of Paul Amar, Ulla Berg, João Biehl, Carina Heckert, Amy Krauss, and Natalie Prizel proved invaluable and productively reoriented the trajectory of this book. Follow-up fieldwork and a period of intensive collaboration with the photographer Marlon del Aguila Guerrero was supported by the Princeton University Committee on Research in the Humanities and Social Sciences William Hallam Tuck '12 Memorial Fund Research Grant.

At UC Santa Cruz, I have been lucky to have the support of the wonderful Latin American and Latino Studies Department. I am forever indebted to the inimitable Sylvanna Falcón, who has worn many hats in her endless support of my scholarship, including postdoctoral mentor, retreat organizer extraordinaire, summer writing accountability partner, fierce advocate, and dynamic colleague. I appreciate conversations, encouragement, and advocacy from Gabriela Arredondo, Lily Pearl Balloffet, Saskias Casanova, Nancy Chen, Kent Eaton, Jeff Erbig, Filippo Gianferrari, Phillip Hammack, Fernando Leiva, Carlos Martinez, Mark Massoud, Jaimie Morse, Christina Navarro, Sara Niedzwiecki, Ursula Oberg, Marcia Ochoa, Juan Manuel Pedroza, Patricia Pinho, Catherine Ramirez, Alicia Riley, Cecilia Rivas, Matt Sparke, and Jessica Taft. The Institute for Social Transformation funded undergraduate student support through the Building Belonging program, and I thank the undergraduate students Melanie Renteria, Jesus Najera, and Angelo Claure for their support at different stages of the project. The Dolores Huerta Research Center for the Americas provided grant funding for publication support. The Campus Provost and Executive Vice Chancellor Writing Fellows Program supported my writing with course relief and funding to work with the professional editors Jacqueline Tasch and Mark Woodworth.

I have been able to share drafts, think out loud, workshop ideas, and learn from numerous intellectual communities. The Critical Approaches to Human Rights group, convened and led by Amy Ross and Chandra Sriram through the Social Science Research Council Dissertation Proposal Development Program, was a tremendous resource in the early stages of this project. I am grateful for conversations in Chaska and Cambridge with Samar Al-Bulushi, Jian-Ming Chris Chang, Evelyn Galindo, Alexa Hagerty, Christoph Hanssmann, Grégoire Hervouet-Zeiber, Austin Kocher, Laura Matson, Jaimie Morse, A. Marie Ranjbar, and J Sebastian. Under the guidance of Susan Coutin, members of the UCI Law and Ethnography Lab met on Skype while we were in our respective "fields" around the world to problem-solve and collectively think through the new challenges that we encountered in the process of doing ethnographic fieldwork. I am grateful for the encouragement and feedback of lab-mates Alyse Bertenthal, Josh Clark, Véronique Fortin, and Daina Sanchez. I had the opportunity to participate in the Residential Research Group "Queer Hemisphere/América Queer" at the University of California Humanities Research Institute. Thank you to the group coordinators Kirstie Dorr, Marcia Ochoa, and Deb Vargas for including me, as well as fellow participants Christina León, Ivan Ramos, Jennifer Tyburczy, and Shelley Streeby for convivial cross-disciplinary discussion on hemispheric queer studies and some fabulous karaoke.

Arguments developed throughout the book were expanded, refined, and worked out through the generous and productive engagement I received through talks at seminars, in classrooms, at conferences, and in informal conversations over coffee. I extend my appreciation to Rachel O'Toole, for the invitation to present at the Center for Latin American and Caribbean Studies Seminar at the University of California, Irvine; Javier Fernández Galeano, for the invitation to present at the "Nuevas Perspectivas de Género en Historia de la Medicina en Latinoamérica" seminar at the University of Valencia; Casey James Miller, for the invitation to present at the "40 Years of HIV/AIDS Activism: Perspectives from Around the World" speaker series at Muhlenberg College; Amy Krauss, for the invitation to present at the "Reproductive Justice Beyond Rights" speaker series at the University of Chicago; and Regina Kunzel, for the invitation to present at the Gender and Sexuality Studies Works-in-Progress Series at Princeton University. I am grateful for the insight, recommendations, and feedback of the many colleagues who have engaged my ideas in conference panels, provided feedback on chapter drafts, and helped me think out loud through conversations in Peru and elsewhere: M. Cristina Alcalde, Florence Babb, Sophie Bjork-James, Michael Bosia, Tito Bracamonte, Julio Callo, Giancarlo Cornejo, Amy Cox Hall, Alexandra Cussianovich, Maria del Pilar Ego Aguirre, Joe Feldman, Carl Fischer, Larry La Fountain-Stokes, Carlos Leal Reyes, Silvana Matassini, Javier Muñoz Diaz, Eduardo Romero, Sydney Silverstein, and Salvador Vidal-Ortiz.

The most enduring source of support in my life has been my family and friends. During a very long car ride Natali Valdez convinced me to push send and reminded me that everything will be okay. My comadre Daina Sanchez has been present in just about every day of my life for over a decade, and I am so grateful for our journey. Virtual RPDR watch parties with Monica Huerta and Ava Shirazi lifted my spirits through the depths of the COVID-19 pandemic and have sustained me since. I treasure every memory from volleyball tournaments with Eric Astacaan, Michael Butler, and Ray Mapeso and look forward to more adventures around the globe. Mike and Tina Amerio kept me on track by checking in on my progress. I cherish the love of Mary Perez, Glenny Perez, Charlie Perez, Julia Reimann, Anna Thomas, and Margot Tilly.

I dedicate this book to my parents, Glen and Antoinette Perez. Their infinite love and support make everything possible. Thank you for inspiring me to be an educator and for all the sacrifices you made so that I could dedicate my life to learning.

# Introduction

Scandalous Stories
of HIV Prevention

"*Ay sí, amiga, discriminada total,*" Paula began to explain to me as she vigorously shook her head. I wondered what had happened for her to insist that she had such a clear and total experience of discrimination. Hoping to solicit an effusive and uninhibited recounting of the episode, I replied to her: "What happened, Paula?"

By the time I was ready to listen to and record Paula's story, I knew what had happened. But in that moment I was asking Paula to tell me again. She was a popular and well-known hair stylist in the city of Tarapoto, Peru; her popularity likely came from a combination of being an engaging storyteller and being an excellent stylist. She had recently opened her own salon after years of renting workstations elsewhere. Though small, the salon was always a lively and welcoming space. Throughout the process of conducting ethnographic fieldwork among gay and transgender communities in Tarapoto and other cities of Peru's *selva*, or Amazonian jungle region, I often hung out in Paula's salon to hear her stories about queer social life in the region—stories like the one that she was about to tell.

Paula continued, "It was Christmas night." She and two of her friends had gone out to the popular disco called La Anaconda. Of the handful of large outdoor nightclubs set amid the palm trees and tobacco fields that border the Fernando Belaúnde Terry Highway into the city limits, La Anaconda was perhaps the best-known and certainly the trendiest. Tourists and locals alike flocked there. It was also Paula's favorite. However, on that Christmas night, Paula and her friends arrived to find an uncharacteristically empty disco. Nevertheless, the three of them went straight to the area of the bar where Paula typically hung out.[1] Standing nearby were a security guard and the security boss, and as soon as she and her friends settled into their usual corner of the disco, the security guard approached them. He told Paula that they were impeding the sale of beer at the bar and that they had to go to another area of the disco. "That was a lie," Paula explained to me, "because that was simply where we were standing. The security guard was discriminating against me, no?"

Paula was a clever and engaging storyteller. If you wanted to hear one of her stories, you had to be willing to engage with and reply to her questions. At this point, because she had used this story already to enthrall and entertain her clients, who might be sitting around for hours waiting for their hair color to set or their hair to dry, she needed to *really* convince the hearer that she had experienced discrimination. She knew, with all the evidence that she laid out in the introduction of her story, that a listener might not fully agree that what had occurred to her was *truly* discriminatory. "What if the bartender and security guards really did need you to move?" I said to her, knowing that I was meant to play this role if I wanted the full experience of her story. "But there had been two other groups at the bar as well," she replied, "and the security guard did not say anything to them. So, what does that tell you? It was discrimination for sexual orientation."[2] Now, with the detail that there had been others at the bar, presumably with normative, cisgendered embodiments, Paula was able to win the support of even the most incredulous of listeners. What had happened that night was truly a moment of discrimination.

Of course, Paula was not going to accept the discriminatory treatment: "I got upset, I yelled. I told him, 'Who do you think you are that you are going to tell me to leave the bar? This is discrimination!'" If anyone knew how to argue, it was Paula. For nearly twenty years Paula had been playing volleyball in parks and streets not just in Tarapoto but also throughout the entire San Martín department (a department is the Peruvian equivalent of a state). Volleyball was an important social activity for gay and trans communities there. Every day, from around 3:00 p.m. until dark, Paula could be found at one of the several popular parks and plazas where gay men and transgender women play the game in front of crowds of residents from the neighborhoods where these parks are located. Betting on volleyball was popular, and so because the game carried either the hope of doubling her day's salary with a winning bet if her team came out on top or the risk that her day of playing might be for naught if her team lost, volleyball was an essential and highly significant element of her daily life and income. Paula had perfected the art of arguing on the volleyball court: demanding a replay of a point, persuading the other team that the ball had landed in or out, or insisting on another match with double-or-nothing stakes. I would be nervous if I were the security guard gearing up for an argument with Paula.

"It was the scandal, *amiga, el es-can-da-lo,*" she told me, slowly pronouncing each syllable of the last word to emphasize that she had staged not just *a* scandal but *the* scandal. Right as she had been swearing to the security guard that he would pay for discriminating against her, mimicking the gestures of the wronged protagonist of a telenovela seeking revenge, she noticed the owner of La Anaconda standing in front of her. The owner told Paula there was nothing that could be done about the situation, or at least nothing that would satisfy Paula. Her friends tried to convince her that they should just leave. But Paula vowed she would not let this go, declaring that the logical next step was to march directly to the nightclub's *libro de reclamaciones,* or complaint book.

The complaint book, she explained to me, was there so that the citizens of Peru, whatever issue they might have with a business, can record their complaints right then and there. However, she continued, when she had asked the manager where the book was, he did not want to give it to her: "They were caught between a rock and a hard place." Paula explained that she had demanded the book because she had it in her mind that she was going to write her complaint and that was the only possible solution to the present issue. They reluctantly gave the book to her, but virtually threw it in her face. Nevertheless, she filled out the form, writing what happened; she kept her copy of the form, and the other copy stayed in the book with the disco. At this point in the story, a listener might breathe a sigh of relief.

The sense of catharsis that Paula had felt precisely at that moment, when it was happening, was embedded directly into the experience of hearing her recount the story. That catharsis, however, was fleeting.

Paula continued with the story. With her copy of the form, she explained, she had to go to INDECOPI (National Institute of the Defense of Competition and of the Protection of Intellectual Property), Peru's administrative agency responsible for market regulation, intellectual property, and consumer protection: "INDECOPI, *amiga*, it is a state institution that exists so that no consumer should experience poor treatment or discrimination in a public place like a disco. So that is where I went to file my complaint." A week later, Paula and the owner of the disco were called to a meeting at the regional office. The owner, however, did not show up for the meeting, instead sending a representative in his place. But, she continued telling me triumphantly, she ended up "half victorious." INDECOPI determined that she could file the grievance formally (after paying an administrative fee of 30 soles), and then the office would commit to following the process and fining the disco for the infraction.

"It was a fraud, though," Paula continued, because it took eight months for the grievance to be processed by INDECOPI. Eight months was a very long time, and maybe, Paula hypothesized, the grievance got "lost" in the bureaucratic jumble. But perhaps, she suggested, there was something going on under the table between the disco and INDECOPI. Was it normal, she wondered, "that the bureaucrats of INDECOPI tell you that they forgot about the grievance when you inquire about the status of it?" She even had a friend who worked at INDECOPI. In an exaggerated voice, she reenacted what her friend said to her: "'It is because I forgot about it, Paula. There were other things, things over here, things over there, blah blah blah.'"

"But you said that you ended up 'half victorious,' Paula. Where was the victory?" I asked her, knowing, again, that this was a part I was meant to play if I hoped to get the whole story. It was at this concluding moment of her tale that Paula explicitly announced the lesson of the story and the true consequences of the entire episode:

> Now you see, *amiga*, the staff at La Anaconda now knows that they cannot treat clients this way. They have to give better attention to their clients, whether they are *travesti*, gay, lesbian, Afro-Peruvian, poor.[3] The treatment has to be equal. There are many homosexuals whose rights are run over and they do not even realize it. They do not know how to defend themselves and they do not know what to do when

they suffer discrimination. I suffered this discrimination and made a scandal because no one else would, and now things are better.

Stories like this one were perhaps among the reasons she was so popular. As I hung out with Paula and her friends in her salon, I found that it was not uncommon to hear the same story twice or even more times, fine-tuned with each new iteration. As she was cutting and coloring hair, she knew exactly when to pull away with the clippers and scissors for emphasis as she was approaching the punch lines of the stories. Her choreography was precise and elaborate. Creative license, of course, was part of her process. She embellished aspects, exaggerated encounters, and intensified the emotional stakes of the scandal that she caused in the moment of her experiencing discrimination. For instance, that the *libro de reclamaciones* was "thrown in her face" added a dramatic element to the story, which she recounted with gestures that contributed to making the whole episode such a compelling performance. Over time, as I continued with my research, I came to realize that the kinds of flourishes she added were common in many of the stories I heard circulated across urban Amazonian Peru among communities of gay men and transgender women as they commented on their social world in everyday life.

With its ups and downs, triumphs and failures, Paula's story was entertaining. But the story was not meant just to entertain. It was also pedagogical. While Paula's story was not, on the surface, about HIV prevention, in fact it drew on lessons that she had learned from participating in projects intended to reduce discrimination as a means of improving the social conditions of communities vulnerable to HIV/AIDS. During the 2010s, one of the key communities of these efforts were gay men and transgender women in the cities of Peru's Amazonian region. Over this period, HIV prevention project specialists, community health promoters, and LGBT activists developed and disseminated messages about the importance of contesting and denouncing discrimination. They delivered these lessons to gay and transgender communities through capacity-building workshops, sensitivity trainings, and on-the-ground advocacy and support. As I participated in these activities while also hanging out in the everyday lives of people like Paula, a subject of these interventions in the city of Tarapoto, I came to realize that she was embedding in her story many of the points that she had likely learned along the way: among them, that anyone has the right to demand the complaint book when they experience mistreatment or discrimination at a business, that anyone has the right to go to the offices of INDECOPI and receive help, and, most importantly, that one should never "give up" or leave a situation in the face of discrimination. But she did more than simply reproduce the lessons she had absorbed as a subject of HIV prevention. She dramatized them into a story about her triumphs, persistence, and disappointments as she sought to make widely and publicly known the injustice that she experienced that night at the disco.

*Queer Emergent* takes the stories shared by Paula and other subjects of HIV prevention in Peru as a point of departure to analyze broader social transformations brought about between the late 2000s and the 2010s through the global response to the HIV/AIDS epidemic. On the heels of tremendous global investment in scaling up access to lifesaving antiretroviral therapy (ART) around the world, as well as the emergence of the paradigm that viewed the provision of treatment itself as a form of prevention, a new promise emerged about the possibilities of ending AIDS as a global threat to public health. As a response, transforming the social conditions of populations categorized as key or vulnerable became a newly significant priority. In Peru and elsewhere, the 2010s were a transitional period in the trajectory of the global HIV/AIDS epidemic: after the massive investment in the provision of antiretroviral therapy but also before the notion of the "end of AIDS" materialized. By the 2010s, Peru was no longer eligible for the international funding that had been made available to the country over the prior decade, linked to the scale-up of the provision of antiretroviral therapy. However, the HIV/AIDS epidemic in Peru persisted as a concentrated epidemic, principally affecting gay men, transgender women, and men who have sex with men but do not identify as gay (MSM). The stories collected in *Queer Emergent*—like the one Paula told about her scandalous response to her experience of discrimination at the nightclub—come precisely from this period.

Amid a renewed effort to approximate a post-AIDS future, the sexual practices and social conditions of gay and transgender Peruvians became a newly significant site of social, medical, and scientific scrutiny. In order to contribute to the global effort to end AIDS, those cast as most vulnerable to acquiring HIV—in this case, gay and transgender Peruvians—reoriented how they talked about themselves and their sexual and romantic lives, how they spoke about their experiences of discrimination and marginalization, and how they formed social relations with one another. Through capacity-building workshops, antidiscrimination and sensitivity trainings, and health promotion, individuals were asked to story new aspects of their commitment to living socially responsible and morally correct lives in the name of ending AIDS. Their scandalous stories make uniquely visible not just how they processed these moralizing obligations but also how they collectively challenged and reimagined what it meant to make do in a changing social world and inhabit emergent subjectivities as the ending of AIDS unfolded. In bringing together some of the stories that gay and transgender Peruvians told as they encountered the new impasses, predicaments, and contradictions of HIV prevention, *Queer Emergent* asserts that the "end of AIDS" was not simply a technical project oriented toward ending AIDS but also a project of sexual subjectification and profound social transformation.

As an ethnography of emergent social worlds in urban Amazonian Peru, the research contained herein draws on the long-term ethnographic fieldwork I conducted alongside gay and transgender communities in urban Amazonian Peru from 2012 to 2018 as they encountered efforts to end AIDS. I center the stories and experiences of interlocutors from the city of Tarapoto with whom I conducted a sustained period of fifteen months of fieldwork in 2014–15.[4] Their stories are compared with and complemented by stories I collected from periodic fieldwork conducted in the cities of Iquitos and Pucallpa, two important and large port cities in the Amazonian region, as well as the coastal cities of Lima, Callao, and Chiclayo. These stories are enhanced by the reflections and observations of interlocutors collected through interviews as well as by my own observations.

In emphasizing the unruly, imaginative, and "scandalous" stories they told, I argue that gay and transgender Peruvians challenged the assumptions embedded in the technical project of ending AIDS while also finding ways, from the margins, to make emergent categories of sexual selfhood habitable on their own terms. I develop and sustain this argument throughout *Queer Emergent* by prioritizing three thematic interventions. First, I propose that stories and storytelling are crucial sites of knowledge for building more robust frameworks in HIV prevention and in critical global health that are attentive to social hierarchies and differences. Second, I develop scandal as a genre of storytelling that emphasizes exaggeration, embellishment, and collective authorship. As a cornerstone of the production of the collaborative relationality that characterized gay and transgender communities in urban Amazonian Peru, scandal is thus further rendered as a theory of queer social world-making. And third, I strive to model intersubjectivity as a mode of ethnographic presence and research. Through an intersubjective ethnographic approach, alongside analysis informed by intersectional theories of ethno-racial, gender, and sexual difference, *Queer Emergent* makes uniquely

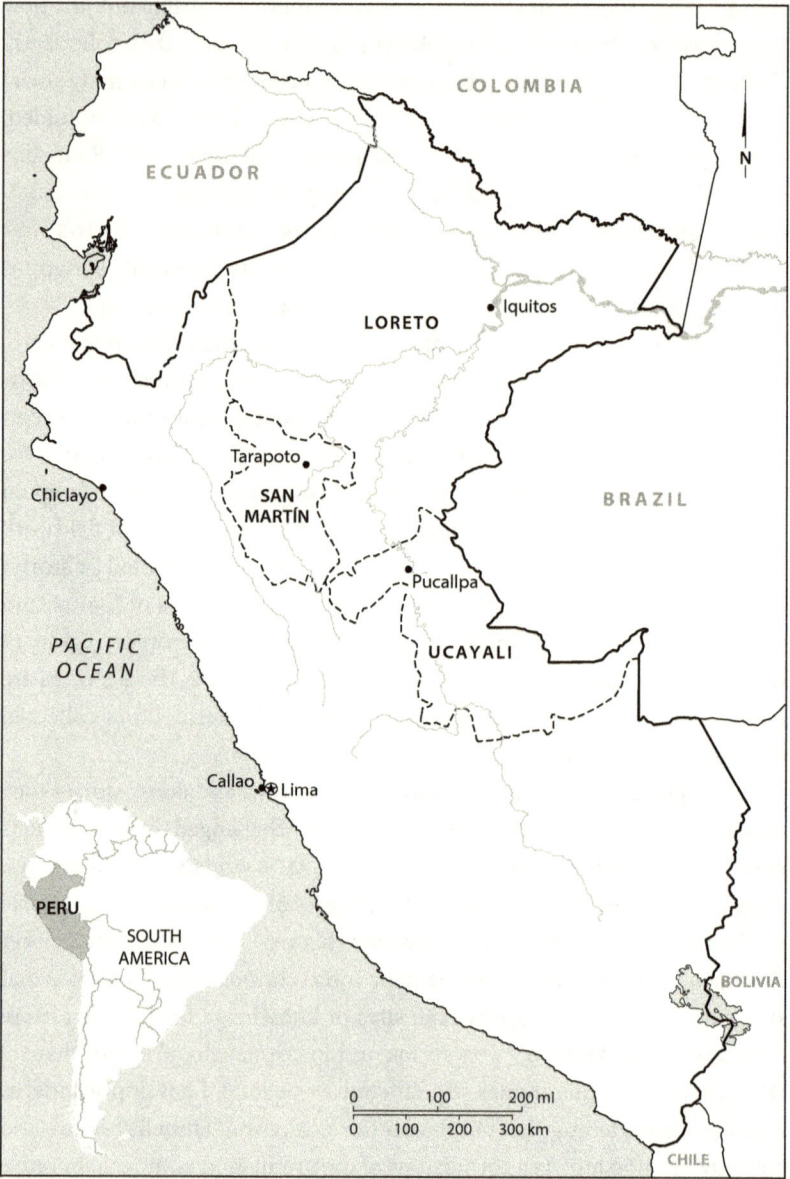

**Map I.1.** Map of Peru. (Cartography by Bill Nelson)

visible the profound social change that occurred as the effort to end AIDS played out in urban Amazonian Peru.

## Queer Social Life within and beyond Categories

The search for the "right" category of sexual subjectivity is ubiquitous and often a site of generative debate in a wide range of scholarly fields, including queer studies and global health sciences, as well as in the regional subfields within these broader scholarly fields. In global queer studies, the tensions between Western terms of sexual and gender dissidence and diversity—*queer, lesbian, gay, transgender*—and non-Western categories can render broader social phenomena like globalization, neoliberalism, and coloniality particularly visible. On the other hand, "traditional" categories of sexual subjectivity can sometimes have a paradoxical effect, either calcifying non-Western sexualities as unchanging or reproducing tropes of non-Western people as exotic Others.[5] In Latin America, the complex space that the categories of "queer" and "LGBT" produce throughout the region has pushed scholars to develop a field of *cuir* theory (Domínguez Ruvalcaba 2016; Falconí Trávez, Castellanos, and Viteri 2013; Reyes 2016; Russo Garrido 2020; Viteri 2014). As a transliterated version of *queer*, the word *cuir* attends to both the historical conditions of colonization shared throughout much of the region as well as the forms of translation, appropriation, negotiation, and subversion that emerge out of the globalization of the categories of LGBTQ.

The health sciences have also been concerned with identifying the "right" categories, especially in relation to HIV/AIDS. Long sensitive to how some categories can reproduce stigma or disincentivize participation in prevention or outreach programs, health science research tends to construct seemingly technical, apolitical categories like "men who have sex with men" as improvements on situated, contextual, and narrower ones. This too, however, can lead to paradoxes. In the case of MSM, the term itself can become an identity; when research data is collected, the category "MSM" can sometimes stand in for self-identified gay men or lead to "ghost populations" in which the subject population at which an intervention is aimed might not exist at all (Boellstorff 2011; Gill 2018; Parker 2019; Wright 2000). The global scale of the epidemic has made the globalization of "gay," "transgender," "men who have sex with men," and other categories of selfhood that originated in the West a fait accompli. It is thus not a particularly novel observation that HIV/AIDS transformed how people came to understand and identify with categories of sexual and gender selfhood.

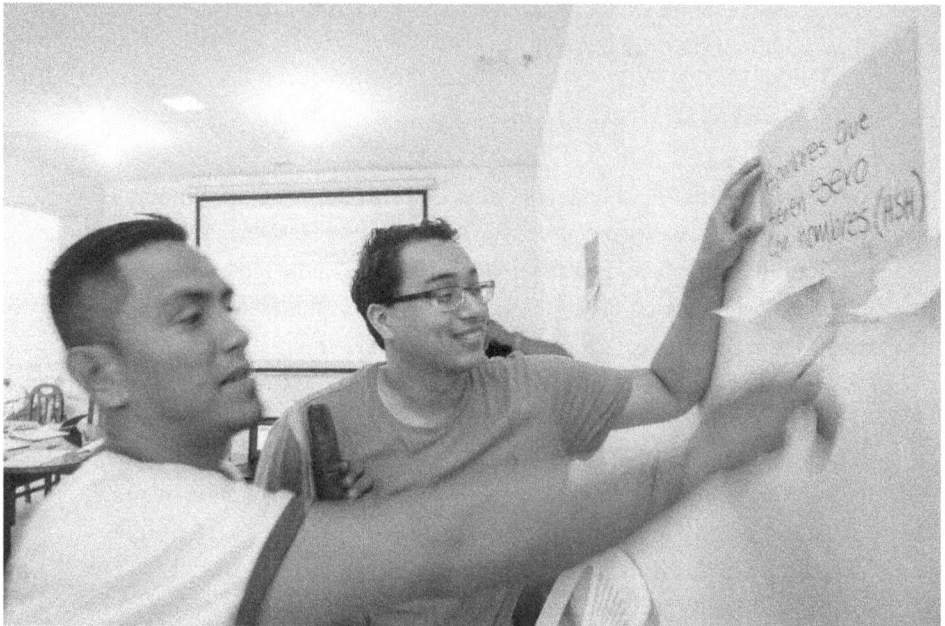

**Figure I.1.** The author (right) and an interlocutor interact at a capacity-building workshop in Tarapoto, Peru. (Photograph by Marlon del Aguila Guerrero)

Categories, though, are always in flux. Throughout *Queer Emergent*, I primarily use the terms *gay* and *transgender* to draw attention to the shared processes of sexual subjectification encountered by the primary interlocutors of the study while also still holding analytical attention on the aspects of their distinct but interconnected social worlds.[6] This is because these were the groups and individuals whose sexual lives and social worlds were targeted by HIV prevention programs. Following anthropological approaches to subjectivity that take health and medicine as sites for the close examination of "hidden processes" of subjectification, I understand sexual subjectification as a system of power through which individuals come to recognize, understand, and speak of themselves as subjects of desire (Biehl, Good, and Kleinman 2007). However, this does not mean these were the only terms that individuals who participated in these programs or whose social worlds were impacted by them used in their lives, or used to make sense of themselves. Some, for example, who were categorized as a "transgender woman" (*una mujer transgénero*) on the part of HIV prevention project specialists or who participated in transgender civic associations, also could have considered themselves *travesti, transexual,* or simply *trans* in other contexts or even in different moments of their life trajectories. Thus, while I use the categories "gay" and "transgender" in the book to reflect the terms of HIV prevention, I also discuss the tensions and differences that arose between how interlocutors inhabited, contested, and exceeded these categories in their everyday lives. To that end, I consider subjectivities to be ongoing and "unfinished." This means that the ethnography attends to the "life-forms, collectives, and new kinds of politics . . . on the horizon, brewing within the leaking excesses of existing force fields and imaginaries" (Biehl and Locke 2017, 9–10). Even though the categories "gay" and "transgender" reached global saturation, particularly via globalization and four decades of AIDS, the project of ending AIDS ushered in a new stage for the ongoing process of inhabiting and contesting the categories of sexual and gender subjectivity. I use the concept "queer emergent" to direct ethnographic attention to the moments in everyday life when interlocutors themselves contended with the limits and potentials of the extant and conventional categories of sexual and gender selfhood. In doing so, I show how they found ways to live with them, without them, and beyond them. Throughout the book, moments of queer emergence occurred, for example, over discussions about whether a soccer team composed of lesbian mothers should compete in the tournament division of gay and transgender players or in the division for cisgender women, or whether beauty contests featuring gay, transgender, and *travesti* contestants should be called "Miss Gay" or "Miss Trans." I employ *queer* not because I observed that all interlocutors were coming to name or see themselves as queer, but rather because the term productively directs analytical attention to the ongoing nature of interlocutors' own debates and discussions around nomenclature and categories.

Moments of queer emergence begat new stories to tell. In constructing this ethnography around scandalous stories—that is, a narrative practice and form collected through long-term ethnographic participant observation—I develop a theoretical agenda that centers the metacommentary that gay and transgender interlocutors themselves engaged in as they experienced ongoing transformations in categories of sexual selfhood. I draw from Boellstorff (2005), who defines subject positions as "extant social categories of selfhood" and subjectivities as "the various senses of self—erotics, assumptions about one's life course, and so forth—that obtain when occupying a subject position, whether partially or completely, temporarily or permanently" (10). This approach poses an alternative theoretical horizon to the descriptive enterprise of enumeration—that is, of adjudicating which categories of sex and gender selfhood "work" and which ones do not (Boellstorff 2007). Instead, it directs social analysis to how people can both make categories work and also exceed, transgress, or transform them. For example, in Figure I.2, a photograph taken at the annual Pride march in Tarapoto, Peru, a contingent of marchers held the international transgender flag. While some interlocutors lived their everyday social life inhabiting a *travesti* subjectivity, in this event they made the globalizing symbol and category of "transgender" both socially meaningful and significant in the context of Tarapoto. There can be many ways to occupy a subject position, and these ways can be mutable and changing.

The scandalous stories explored in this book reveal how the people telling them worked both within and outside new demands and expectations, living with, adjacent to, and beyond the categorical schema imposed on their social and sexual lives. However, the paradoxes and opportunities they encountered were not only the result of the new challenges brought about by HIV prevention; they were, as well, shaped by deeper and more entrenched hierarchies of difference. Formed through the construction of a nation-state founded out of colonial relations, these hierarchies were made particularly visible by the ambition of ending AIDS in Peru. This colonial legacy has persisted in various forms, but most crucially it takes expression through what Quijano (2007) termed the coloniality of power. This was the imposition of racial divisions that emerged from the colonial enterprise and expanded over time to structure postcolonial relations. The myth of *mestizaje*—the myth that racial mixture constituted the newly independent nations of Latin America of the early nineteenth century and onward—persisted to define belonging and citizenship. In Peru, as García (2021) observes, "the logic of mestizaje has been about state-sanctioned exclusions" (7). Drawing on Anderson's (1983) notion of the "imagined" national community, scholars of Peru further point to how the nationalist projects of the state consistently excluded indigenous Andeans as equal members of the "imagined" nation (de la Cadena 2000; Larson 2004; Portocarrero 2007a; Thurner 1995). As Méndez (1996) contends, this legacy further produced an enduring rhetoric that paradoxically exalted the indigenous past while maintaining contempt and disregard for the contemporary indigenous Other. And this process of othering can extend to and shape categories and experiences of sexual and gender diversity in different ways. For example, as theorists of *travesti* social life and history in Latin America demonstrate, *travesti* can signify class and racialized otherness not typically signaled by the English

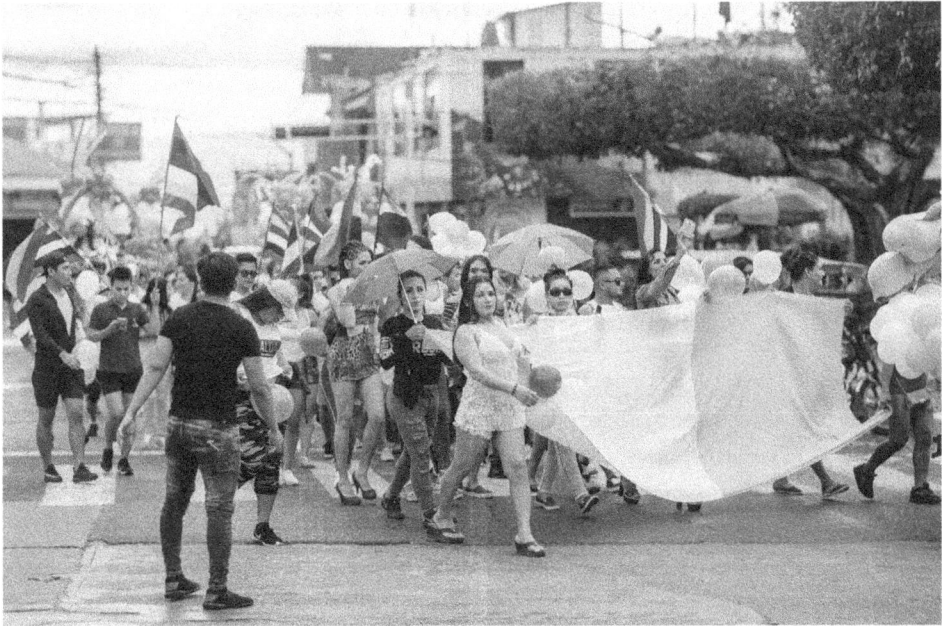

**Figure I.2.** A contingent of trans and *travesti* marchers holds the transgender Pride flag as they participate in the LGBT Pride parade in Tarapoto, Peru. (Photograph by Marlon del Aguila Guerrero)

term "transgender" (Cornejo 2019; Machuca Rose 2019; Rizki 2019; Santana 2022; Silva Santana 2019).

The *selva*, or the Amazonian jungle region of eastern Peru, perhaps even more so than the Andean *sierra*, has figured precariously in the Peruvian national imagination, often only in the short-term boom periods of resource exploitation. The most well known of these booms was Peru's rubber boom of the 1890s–1920s. Since the nineteenth century, different efforts at incorporating the region—such as "whitening" the race by drawing European migrants and selling tracts of land to corporations to pay for debts incurred by wars—have consistently been based on short-term solutions to address the economic and political problems facing the country's coastal and Andean regions (Ludescher 2001; Walker 1987). As a result, interlocutors in the *selva* typically experienced a more indeterminate ethno-racial position within the broader national imaginary compared with those from the Andean or coastal regions of the country. For the most part, interlocutors were non-indigenous and spoke Spanish as a first language, though a few in Tarapoto were from the nearby town of Lamas and either spoke or had some familiarity with the lowland variety of Quechua spoken there. Most interlocutors grew up in and around Tarapoto, though a few had migrated from more distant rural communities. Within Peru, nearly all interlocutors would be considered *charapa*. This is a term that refers to people who come from the eastern region of the country. In a cultural system in which ethno-racial superiority and differentiation tend to be "individualized," meaning established in the context of specific interactions and in reference to specific people, interlocutors' status as *charapa* generally positioned them as "lower" in relation to people from Lima or the coast.[7] However, interlocutors' position as Spanish-speaking city dwellers might also position them as "higher" in relation to people from more remote parts of the region or from indigenous communities. Nevertheless, despite the flexibility of individual encounters of social distinction, interlocutors often contended with entrenched systems of sexual, gender, and ethno-racial differentiation that frequently positioned them outside of privileged hierarchical status.

## Scandal and Scandalous Storytelling

As I spent more time among gay and transgender communities in urban Amazonian Peru, I found they shared distinct narrative practices.[8] Telling compelling, humorous, and engaging stories—like Paula's scandal at the disco—was a cornerstone of their collective sociality and contributed to the complexity of their social lives.[9] Like Paula, several key interlocutors owned, worked at, or managed popular beauty salons at some point in their lives, including while I was conducting fieldwork, and many of the stories I heard likely derived from the social expectations linked to the traditional professional spaces—primarily for hairstyling and event organization—that had been available to elder gay and transgender individuals in the region. Having a repertoire of stories helped clients pass the time as well as entertained those who came to hang out in the salon as a social space. Though I surmise that many of the stories I heard over the course of fieldwork originated in the spaces of the beauty salons, they extended far beyond them, across the diverse sites of gay and transgender social life.

The stories I heard shared a set of characteristics. A typical story tended to follow a similar structure as it dramatized dynamics of social and sexual life that could be considered "scandalous." Scandalousness was a capacious vernacular concept associated with some elements of gay and transgender sociality. In its most conventional sense, scandalousness could be wielded to discriminate against, stereotype, or marginalize people of diverse sexual orientations or gender identities. Broadly speaking, a scandal is often thought to transpire through a patterned epistemic-temporal configuration. In many instances, a scandal results when something previously "unknown," or something not usually publicly vocalized, is revealed about a person. This revelation then transforms perceptions about that person's actions or moral character. Someone assumed to be virtuous or upstanding can be corrupted and rendered disreputable over the course of the scandal. Thus, a scandal often requires a presumption of respect or repute in the first place. A scandal provides a road map, in a sense, for how to know about someone or something and how to feel (e.g., shock, disgust, horror, etc.). If an individual was too loud, caused too much of a commotion in public, or dressed in a way that subverted expected mores, they might be called scandalous.

And yet, within the rich and complex social worlds of gay and transgender interlocutors, the conventional conceptualizations of the term could be played with, re-signified, and transformed. For them, the presumption of repute was typically not applied. In other words, a scandal did not reveal something "new" about an individual or their general behavior and disposition. Rather, a scandal or scandalousness reaffirmed existing notions about their character or person. But more importantly, interlocutors did not always see scandal or scandalousness negatively, even as the term could also sometimes be used that way.[10] To scandalize was, at once, to transgress social norms and expectations and to render the mundane spectacular or make something larger than life.[11] It is in this sense that I use *scandal* in *Queer Emergent*—that is, as an adjective not to describe a person or set of people in a discriminatory way, but rather to describe a habit interlocutors cultivated of telling stories about the world they encountered through the arts of embellishment, exaggeration, and hyperbole.[12]

Scandal, being scandalous, or throwing a scandal was thus an important element of the stories people told. Typically, the protagonist of a scandalous story, who may or may not be the person telling it, finds themself in a desperate or distressed circumstance, often precipitated by their own search for a sexual encounter. As the situation unfolds, the protagonist finds it increasingly hard to escape the situation, until, by a stroke of luck, good fortune, or divine grace, they encounter a resolution to the predicament. Other times the resolution comes thanks to the "collaboration" of others. *La colaboración*, or collaboration, was an idealized social order that emphasized the creation of redistributive relationships and is described in more depth in chapter 2. Ultimately, in a scandalous story, while the protagonist may have learned a lesson, the conclusion comes with a "wink," suggesting that the protagonist may not have changed and may continue to do whatever brought on the distress in the first place. Because of the obvious use of exaggeration and hyperbole, the story is typically entertaining, engaging, and humorous, even when the protagonist is at the lowest of low points or is facing a sensitive or intense personal trauma.

A story can circulate and be retold by any capable narrator. In each retelling, the narrator has the license to exaggerate details and add personalized flourishes. The narrator and the protagonist do not always have to be the same. A story could be retold about someone else, and the narrator can adopt the role of the protagonist while still maintaining the plot and basic details of the preexisting story. New stories can be crafted out of new experiences and thus enter the collective repertoire. Effective narrators can turn a mundane anecdote into a newly embellished, engaging, and exaggerated episode.

One of the most salient and unique characteristics that I observed about the practice of scandalous storytelling in Peru was that any capable gay or transgender narrator could assume the role of the protagonist (the "I"). Although scandalous stories might involve traumatic experiences—such as the experiences of gay and transgender people during the country's internal armed conflict or the pervasive, everyday encounters with stigma and discrimination—the modularity of the "I" enabled a collective expression of shared experiences of discrimination or violence without having to put forward the sensitive details of personal traumas. The same story set in the context of the internal armed conflict (1980–2000), for example, could be recounted from a first-person perspective by many different people, even if during the conflict the narrator had not yet been born. The shared recognition suggested that there was a sense of communal authorship and that stories were intersubjective phenomena for interlocutors. The version of a story that one heard at any moment was likely the result of co-authorship, as new details could always be added along the way. These stories were inherently social, animating collective worlds as they circulated from the beauty salon to the volleyball court to the capacity-building workshop for HIV prevention, or to other sites of social life. Each occasion offers someone the opportunity to embellish and to entertain whoever might be listening while at the same time extending a sense of social connectedness and relationality.

Throughout *Queer Emergent*, I analyze stories that dramatized incidents ranging from sexual encounters with armed insurgents during Peru's internal armed conflict to a story about submitting a proposal on behalf of a community-based organization to administer an HIV prevention program. In deriving source material from the everyday stories that emerged from experiences with new forms of HIV prevention introduced over the decade and transforming that material into new stories, gay and transgender communities in urban Amazonian Peru painted a fuller picture of the lived experiences of efforts to prevent HIV that could not be captured by quantitative measurements and standardized metrics alone.[13] Any retelling of a story opened the possibility for reinvention. As Ochs and Capps (1996) observed, "Everyday narrative practices confront interlocutors with unanticipated emotions and ideas and ultimately with unanticipated selves" (37). Through their scandalous stories, interlocutors responded to the contradictions, challenges, and transformations that transpired as the "end of AIDS" unfolded and, in the process, conceived of new ways to inhabit and to imagine queer social life.

They countered an unequal, discriminatory, and stigmatizing world and rendered these seemingly rigid modes of social differentiation flexible through imagining outcomes that could be conceived only through tales of transgression, excess, and exaggeration.[14] Amid entrenched systems of ethno-racial hierarchy and social differentiation, as well as the obligation to embrace new narrative forms, gay and transgender interlocutors found ways to experience and describe fulfilling moments of pleasure and romance through their scandalous stories, sometimes set in the most unexpected of places and situations. Their stories—about nights out at the disco, beauty contests, soccer tournaments and volleyball games, romantic and sexual encounters amid political violence, the formation of community-based organizations, informal fundraisers organized to prevent the dissolution of community-based organizations, and the ebbs and flows of the unpredictable landscape of international HIV/AIDS funding—came to reveal a rich and robust world of social relations undergoing profound transformation (and even social fragmentation) resulting from their encounter with the global aspiration to end AIDS. To hear these stories as such, however, required work on the part of the listener. The stories exaggerated situations, interchanged protagonists and characters, jumped between time frames and geographic contexts, and obligated listeners to suspend, if only momentarily, any sense of disbelief as to the factuality of the episode and become immersed in the scandalous world of queer social life in urban Amazonian Peru.[15]

Accounts of the global HIV/AIDS epidemic conventionally employ a peri-odization to signal how new technologies and priorities transformed the governance of HIV/AIDS and how communities themselves experienced these shifts. These periods generally correspond to decades or, more aptly, to what Parker (2024) considers "waves." The stories in *Queer Emergent* were collected during a particular period of the global HIV/AIDS epidemic and thus connect to the rich ethnographic study of HIV/AIDS. I offer a brief overview of these periods as a means to briefly situate the Peruvian response to HIV/AIDS within a macro-level chronology and to contextu-alize the research within the deep tradition of the critical anthropology of HIV/AIDS.

The first decade, which often is characterized as beginning in 1981, con-ventionally starts when the US Centers for Disease Control first reported clusters of rare lung infections and cancers among young, sexually active, and previously healthy white gay men in urban New York and California in the *Morbidity and Mortality Weekly Report*.[16] In the middle of the second decade—the 1990s—combination antiretroviral therapy was introduced. This inaugurated a new period in the story of HIV/AIDS. Characterized by the global effort to "scale up" access to antiretroviral therapy, this new pe-riod is generally associated with the third decade, or the 2000s. Following the unprecedented investment in the global HIV/AIDS response over the 2000s, the fourth decade, the 2010s, is characterized by the aspiration to "end AIDS." Despite the triumphalism and optimism of the idea of ending AIDS, the period is generally associated with a "scale-down" of and disin-vestment in the HIV/AIDS response in many countries around the world. *Queer Emergent* chronicles the impasses and contradictions of this period through the stories of gay and transgender communities in Peru.

While the first case of AIDS in Peru was registered in Lima in 1983, the HIV/AIDS epidemic was a low priority for the health sector throughout the 1980s and even into the 1990s. Most of the first registered cases were among gay men who acquired HIV while living outside of the country (Cueto 2001, 47).[17] Over the decade of the 1980s, the epidemic in Peru was mostly confined to the cities on the country's Pacific coast, specifically the capital city, Lima, and was primarily transmitted sexually among those categorized as homosexual. Beyond a comparatively low number of cases, part of the reason the epidemic attracted little notice in Peru at the time was that attention was directed to national crises that were then unfolding.

An internal armed conflict between the state and two armed insurgency groups, the Maoist-inspired Shining Path and the Tupac Amaru Revolutionary Movement (MRTA), began in 1980 and grew as the decade progressed. The conflict lasted until 2000, when Alberto Fujimori resigned from the presidency and fled the country for Japan. Atrocities ranging from torture, kidnappings, and killings by extrajudicial death squads committed by the state and by the armed groups ultimately brought about the death or disappearance of an estimated seventy thousand people (CVR 2003).

As the 1980s came to a close and the new decade began, the country was increasingly consumed by the growing internal armed conflict. And though the violence unequally and disproportionately affected rural, peasant, and indigenous communities of the Andean highlands, violence extended to the capital city, Lima, by the 1990s. Hyperinflation from newly elected President Alberto Fujimori's implementation of a "shock" economic plan at the beginning of his first presidential term was then compounded by a disastrous cholera outbreak in 1991 that appeared nearly out of nowhere. All this, of course, occurred amid an intensifying and ongoing internal armed conflict between the state's armed forces and armed rebels. Chapter 1 more closely explores how stories about sexuality and the intimate relations of gay and transgender Peruvians have been transformed by the overlapping temporal entanglements of the global HIV/AIDS epidemic and the ongoing resonances of the internal armed conflict.

### The Era of Scale-Up

With the introduction and approval of highly active antiretroviral therapy (HAART) in 1996, HIV/AIDS was no longer a "death sentence"; for those with access to healthcare, it could be a treatable and manageable chronic condition. However, by the turn of the century, this lifesaving combination therapy remained out of reach for most of those around the world who needed it. In fact, precisely in the regions of the world where the epidemic was growing most rapidly, access to antiretroviral therapy was the lowest. While combination antiretroviral therapy was saving lives in some parts of the world, its effects were less palpable elsewhere. As a result, the primary ambition of the global response to HIV/AIDS by the 2000s shifted to ensuring access to and equitable distribution of lifesaving antivirals. The Millennium Development Goals, proclaimed by the United Nations in the year 2000, concretized this ambition through targets: (1) achieving universal access to HIV/AIDS treatment for all who needed it by the year 2010 and (2) halting and then reversing the spread of HIV/AIDS by 2015. The challenge was to scale up—that is, to transfer and expand therapies and interventions to communities across the globe. The scale-up of the provision of antiretroviral therapy was a numerical phenomenon, and over the decade it was measured by objectives related to the total number of people receiving therapy.[18] To halt and reverse the spread of HIV, scaling up antiretroviral therapy beyond well-resourced contexts became a key step.

The global transition to the era of scale-up that occurred over the 1990s and 2000s in the global HIV/AIDS response coincided with tremendous political and cultural transition in Peru. By the year 2000, the country was confronting a dire economic outlook—more than half of all Peruvians lived in poverty, and external debt had doubled over the course of the preceding decade. The country also faced a growing HIV/AIDS epidemic. Although then-president Alberto Fujimori had established a national program for control of HIV and sexually transmitted infections (STIs) and increased funding over the latter half of the 1990s in response to the expanding epidemic in the country, it was not nearly enough to guarantee universal access to antiretroviral therapy (Cueto 2001, 112).[19] In 2002, only two years into its postwar transition, Peru established a country coordinating mechanism (La Coordinadora Nacional Multisectorial en Salud, CONAMUSA) and began to work toward submitting its first proposal to the newly established Global Fund to Fight HIV/AIDS, Tuberculosis, and Malaria (the Global Fund).[20] The CONAMUSA was tasked with the coordination of proposal submission and the integration of "vertical," disease-specific interventions funded by the Global Fund into the national health system. When its initial proposal was unsuccessful, the CONAMUSA turned to technical and academic consultants, people living with HIV/AIDS, representatives from affected populations, religious leaders, and relevant government ministries and found more success (Amaya et al. 2014; Sprungli 2007). Over the 2000s, Peru's successful proposals for funding (in the Second, Fifth, Sixth, and Tenth Rounds) ultimately generated over $80 million of HIV/AIDS funding in the country (Cáceres et al. 2013).

As in many low- and middle-income countries around the world, scaling up access to antiretroviral therapy was a primary objective for Peru's initial collaboration with the Global Fund. In fact, a new national HIV treatment program was created. Through Second Round funding, the Global Fund committed to supporting the universal provision of antiretroviral therapy for two years, with the understanding that the state would then assume, by 2007, the costs of treatment for all those living with HIV/AIDS. Once the state covered treatment, subsequent rounds—the Fifth Round (2006–10) and Sixth Round (2007–11)—were increasingly oriented toward prevention activities. This included sex education and syndromic management in the general population, peer health promotion and regular screening and checkups among vulnerable populations, and the promotion of a favorable sociopolitical environment that supported human rights and reduced discrimination and stigma through support of community-based organizations (Cáceres et al. 2013). While funding was intended to build off the precedent of ensuring universal access with robust prevention efforts, published evaluations suggest that the various Global Fund rounds did not always directly build off or even connect with one another.[21] Ultimately, like many low- and middle-income countries around the world, Peru experienced growth in access to funding for HIV/AIDS over the 2000s. However, as the decade came to a close, the funding streams that had made HIV/AIDS "the single most dominant global health issue" in the 2000s began to slow, and they contracted over the 2010s (Parker 2024, 5). It is against the backdrop of this transition period of contraction and defunding that the social transformations explored in *Queer Emergent* transpired.

## The Aspiration to End AIDS

As studies began to show that antiretrovirals could be effective in both treating and preventing HIV, the division between efforts to scale up the treatment of HIV/AIDS with prevention efforts began to collapse and the "treatment as prevention" (TasP) paradigm emerged. TasP was a conceptualization of the prevention of the transmission of HIV as a "secondary effect" of HIV treatment for people living with HIV (Montaner 2011). In other words, since treatment could effectively lower the viral loads of people living with HIV to the point of undetectability, this greatly reduced the risk of transmitting the virus through sex.[22] And as the initial Millennium Development Goals timeline neared its conclusion, in 2011 the United Nations announced a new target for the provision of antiretroviral therapy. Called the "15 by 15" target, the ambitious plan was to provide antiretroviral therapy to fifteen million people by the year 2015, the benchmark year for the Millennium Development Goals. Not only was the 15 by 15 target achieved, but it was achieved ahead of time. The enthusiasm that resulted from distributing ART to fifteen million people by 2015, coupled with the emergent paradigm of TasP, spilled over into the elaboration of one of the United Nations' Sustainable Development Goals: ending AIDS as a global public health threat by 2030.[23]

By 2010, Peru's economic situation had improved according to metrics used to classify country income levels, which meant Peru had reduced eligibility for Global Fund support. This roughly coincided with a wider overall decline in funding streams for HIV/AIDS and a scale-down of the international response. Continued investment was, however, possible because of a particular characteristic of the country's HIV/AIDS epidemic: in Peru, HIV was *concentrated* among vulnerable populations.[24] Specifically, it was concentrated among gay men, transgender women, and MSM in the urban areas along the coast and in the Amazonian region. In the 2010s, it appeared as though the long-term sustainability of Peru's HIV response—which had relied tremendously on investment from the Global Fund over the 2000s— became dependent on the fact that gay, transgender, and MSM communities bore an unequal burden of the country's HIV epidemic in relation to the general population. Continued international support was thus dependent on the inequality of the epidemic in the country. In order to continue receiving international funding, the country's response coalesced around addressing the vulnerability of gay men, transgender women, and MSM in the country. Just as rumblings of an "end of AIDS" era were beginning to take hold at the global level, in Peru the sexual practices and social conditions of gay, transgender, and MSM Peruvians became a newly significant site of research and scrutiny among the health scientists, medical professionals, technical experts, state bureaucrats, and community advocates who played a role in the country's response to AIDS.[25]

### The Tenth Round of the Global Fund in Peru

As Peru began to prepare its application for the Tenth Round of the Global Fund, epidemiological data pointed to an expanding breach between the communities in which HIV/AIDS was most concentrated and the general population. A handful of studies and statistics appear in the documents relating to the country's proposal to the Global Fund that help paint a picture of the epidemiological situation at the time (Global Fund 2017). The National Center for Epidemiology, Prevention, and Disease Control, part of Peru's Ministry of Health, published a monthly epidemiological bulletin regarding the national tally of cases of HIV/AIDS.[26] Its January 2010 bulletin indicated that since 1983, there had been a cumulative total of 40,181 reported cases of HIV and 25,748 cases of AIDS in Peru. A total of 97 percent of the cases were transmitted sexually.[27] At the time, data on HIV prevalence, or the proportion of a specified population affected by HIV at a given time, was derived from two important studies. One was a cross-sectional study conducted in the city of Lima (Tabet et al. 2002). This study determined prevalence among MSM to be 18.5 percent and, crucially, among trans women to be 33.3 percent.[28] Another study, based on HIV sentinel surveillance surveys, determined prevalence among MSM in Lima to be 22.3 percent and an estimated HIV incidence, or the rate of new cases in a given year, among MSM to be 8.3 percent in 2002 (Sanchez et al. 2007).

In light of data that pointed to the high vulnerabilities of gay, transgender, and MSM communities, Peru's proposal for the Global Fund's Tenth Round emphasized efforts to address the social conditions that contributed to this pattern of concentration. The primary sources of vulnerability were discrimination and stigma toward these communities. By mitigating the effects of discrimination and stigma on the basis of sexual orientation and gender identity, it was reasoned, the conditions that produced this vulnerability among gay and transgender populations could be mitigated, and, consequently, new cases of HIV could be prevented. Addressing discrimination and stigma toward gay men and transgender women, in particular, became the primary focus of HIV prevention projects in the ensuing years. The TasP paradigm was circulating at the time of the implementation of the Tenth Round, but because Peru had incrementally inched out of the low-income category, the Global Fund was no longer willing to invest robustly in the provision of treatment as a means of prevention in the country (as the state was by then committed to funding the provision of treatment). Investment for social interventions aimed at mitigating discrimination, it appeared, would have to suffice.

Set to operate from July 2011 until June 2016, the measures proposed in the successful application for Tenth Round funding targeted discrimination and stigma at two levels. At the community level, the intervention aimed to bolster the infrastructure and technical capacities of gay and transgender community-based organizations (CBOs) in places where HIV prevalence was highest. At the individual level, the proposal emphasized teaching gay and transgender individuals how to identify discrimination in their lives and how they might employ formal, legal mechanisms to seek redress. Enculturating the members of community-based organizations into the technical practices of tracking indicators, evaluating projects, and evidencing objectives, the proposal asserted, would ultimately result in a more robust and better-functioning gay and transgender NGO and CBO infrastructure throughout the country and would ultimately lead to a decreased incidence of HIV among the populations in which it was presently most concentrated.

In Peru, and elsewhere, the emergence of "post-AIDS" or "end of AIDS" strategies during the 2010s engendered a significant shift in the global response to HIV/AIDS. For one, the notion of the "end of AIDS" transformed preexisting ideas about HIV exceptionalism—the idea that the experience of living with HIV/AIDS is exceptional (whether due to sociocultural, biological, or political aspects, or a combination of these) and consequently obligates an exceptional public health response (Benton and Sangaramoorthy 2021; Moyer and Hardon 2014).[29] If one reason the HIV crisis was considered exceptional was that it appeared to be never-ending, then the idea of the "end of AIDS" altered this exceptionalism by projecting an expiration date for the epidemic. However, the idea also coincided with a broader defunding of robust, structural HIV prevention and treatment models around the world in favor of narrow, or "vertical," approaches that focused almost exclusively on biomedical treatment for those living with HIV and those vulnerable to acquiring it. This would come at the expense of programming that supported human rights, antidiscrimination efforts, and capacity building. Some scholars have called this shift the re-medicalization of the HIV/AIDS epidemic (Kippax and Stephenson 2016; Nguyen et al. 2011; Parker 2020). Investment in health systems, human rights, and antidiscrimination measures that had been key ingredients for supporting the scale-up of the provision of antiretroviral therapy in the prior decade came to be seen as increasingly costly and unnecessary in the face of new biomedical HIV prevention technologies. And even though experts acknowledged the fundamental need for human rights efforts and antidiscrimination and stigma education, as Kenworthy, Thomann, and Parker (2018) note, the "end of AIDS" discourse came to be endorsed by the entities that stood to gain from privatized, technology-driven HIV interventions.

While in some contexts the reorientation toward the AIDS endgame brought about a re-medicalization of the AIDS epidemic and the dissemination of messages and slogans like "Undetectable = Untransmittable," for those in Peru this was still on the horizon.[30] For some communities, particularly in the Global North, the pharmaceuticalization of HIV prevention was a significant effect during the 2010s. For instance, the development of pre-exposure prophylaxis (PrEP) led to a shift in HIV prevention, transforming the long-dominant paradigm of "safer sex" to one focusing on a pharmaceutical form of prevention. However, in Peru, the re-medicalization of the

AIDS epidemic, as represented, for example, by access to PrEP as a form of prevention, was accessible only to the small number of people who participated in clinical trials.[31] The project to end AIDS in Peru did not emphasize biomedical intervention nor did it meaningfully invest in the continuance of prior efforts to secure universal access to antiretroviral therapy. Rather, the "end of AIDS" was palpably lived and experienced through interventions targeting the social and cultural challenges of discrimination and stigma. Those involved in the everyday and on-the-ground advocacy of HIV prevention shifted their orientation toward the social conditions and individual dispositions that would mitigate discrimination—and, perhaps, clear the way for a future re-medicalization of the AIDS epidemic.

Gay and transgender communities in Peru experienced a rebalancing of emphasis from the provision of antiviral therapy for people living with HIV/AIDS toward increased attention to prevention among vulnerable populations through social interventions. Even as the numbers of those who had access to antiviral therapy slowly rose over the 2000s, access to these resources in contexts around the world remained variegated and unequal.[32] In response, anthropologists studying the experiences, politics, and governance of HIV/AIDS observed how the distribution of treatment, support, and resources often became a function of an individual's capacity to learn and employ certain narrative genres, such as testimony about one's HIV status or the performance of "positive living" (Benton 2015; Benton, Sangaramoorthy, and Kalofonos 2017; Boellstorff 2009; Nguyen 2010). The capacity to speak about one's self came to have direct implications for who lived and who died, and transformed understandings of life, including morality, sexuality, reproduction, and citizenship.[33] Drawing on this insight, but contextualizing it within a new period in the story of HIV/AIDS, *Queer Emergent* tracks how the "end of AIDS" compelled even those who were seronegative to speak about themselves and their social worlds in new ways. As international funding focused on HIV prevention among vulnerable populations in Peru, even seronegative gay and transgender people became subject to new expectations about how to live moral, healthy, and fulfilling lives. Newly cast as key populations in the effort to end AIDS, gay and transgender Peruvians responded to the obligation to reframe how they understood and talked about their sexual relationships and social worlds. Sometimes their stories fit within the new funding requirements disseminated through capacity-building workshops, antidiscrimination and sensitivity trainings, and community health promotion. Their scandalous stories, however, pointed to the new obstacles that came along with the project to end AIDS, and in turn enabled them to draw attention to these predicaments and to collectively make do in a transforming social world.

## Toward an Intersubjective Ethnography

This book draws from the ethnographic fieldwork I conducted in the San Martín department of Peru, principally in the city of Tarapoto, for fifteen months in 2014–15.[34] My primary method of data collection was long-term participation in gay and transgender communities in Tarapoto and surrounding towns, divided between two principal social settings. In the mornings and afternoons, I focused on spaces involving the implementation of HIV prevention programming. This meant hanging out in the community-based and nongovernmental organizations most active in the coordination of HIV prevention projects. Participant observation in these spaces included brainstorming grant proposals, conducting research and translations, and participating in capacity-building workshops and sensitivity trainings. My primary interlocutors in these spaces were project specialists, the gay and trans individuals who worked short-term contracts dealing with various aspects of the implementation of HIV prevention strategies and LGBT human rights issues. This ranged from doing community health outreach to organizing workshops and sensitivity trainings. I attended workshops led by the community-based organizations Diversidad San Martinense (DISAM) and Las Amazonas and the nongovernmental organization Center for Amazonian Development (CEDISA), coordinated in partnership with a range of state entities, including the Ministry of Health, the Ministry of Labor, and the National Ombudsperson (Defensoría del Pueblo), as they implemented activities funded by international donors, including the Global Fund and Hivos.

In the afternoons and evenings, I focused participant observation on the everyday activities of gay and transgender collective social life. The primary space was daily afternoon volleyball games, which took place in parks, on streets, and in empty lots throughout Tarapoto and in surrounding towns. Played by gay men and transgender women, the games were watched by youth and adults from the neighborhood passing by after school or work. Enterprising neighbors sold snacks and drinks to the players and the spectators. While I was sometimes invited to play volleyball in low-stakes games or if there were not enough people to field two teams, I was usually a spectator. I also conducted weekday participant observation at gay- and transgender-

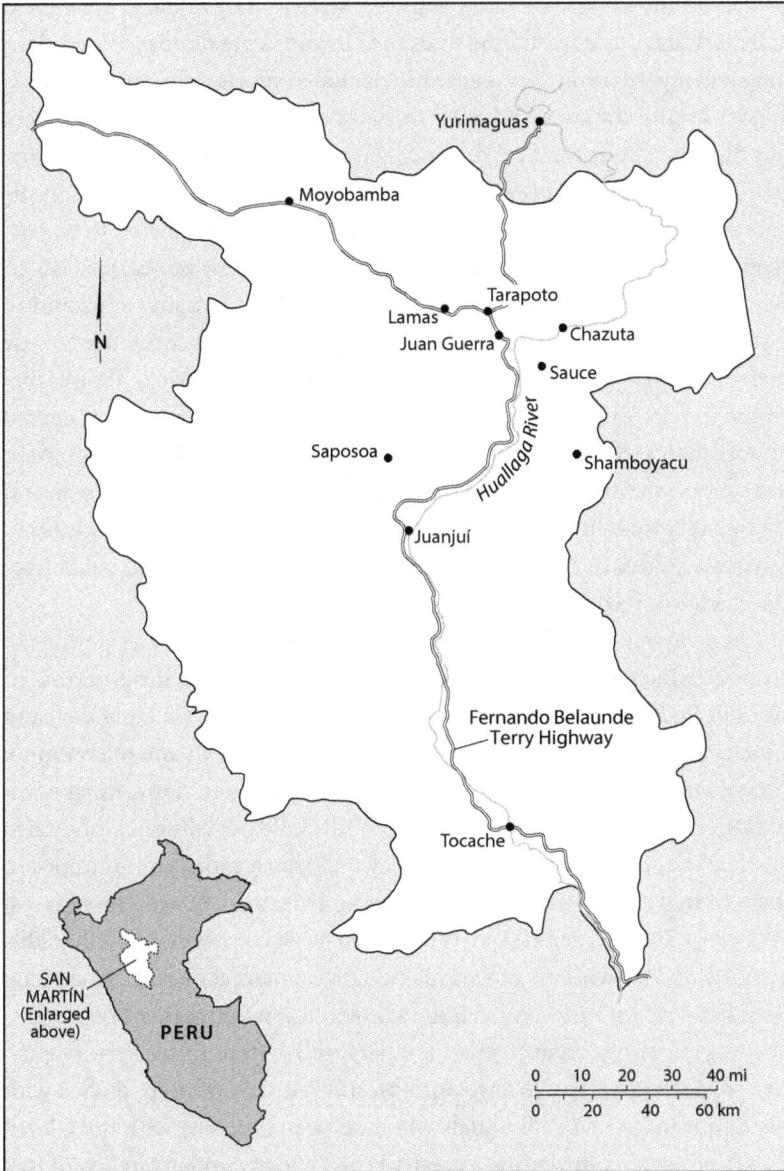

**Map I.2.** Map of San Martín department. (Cartography by Bill Nelson)

owned beauty salons. Weekday activities were loosely organized, whereas activities that occurred on the weekends involved greater degrees of planning and organization. These activities included sports tournaments, transgender beauty contests, and other forms of spectacle-based entertainment like nightclub performances or dance shows. Those with whom I interacted in the afternoons and evenings typically were not directly involved in the coordination of HIV prevention projects, but they were invited to be participants in the workshops and trainings coordinated by project specialists. Because such workshops were intended to bolster human rights and to mitigate the impact of discrimination and stigma in the social lives of gay men and trans women, the HIV status of interlocutors varied, if it was disclosed to me. My presence in activities and informal social spaces offered opportunities to gain insight into everyday dynamics and helped me establish rapport for interviews. I conducted thirty interviews with gay men and transgender women in Tarapoto. In these interviews, I asked interlocutors to renarrate stories that I had heard them tell previously so that I could have the chance to record details I might have missed.

To complement fieldwork in Tarapoto, I conducted shorter periods of ethnographic participant observation and interviews in the Amazonian cities of Pucallpa and Iquitos. I also made brief visits to Callao, Lima, and Chiclayo, cities on the Pacific coast of Peru, for interviews and observation. Global Fund projects for HIV prevention among gay and transgender communities occurred in all of these cities. While I did not carry out long-term participant observation among the gay and transgender communities in these coastal cities, I attended workshops and meetings as well as conducted interviews. In Lima and Callao, I conducted five interviews with LGBT rights activists and/or workers at various nongovernmental organizations who were familiar with the Global Fund's interventions and other LGBT rights projects in Peru in order to provide a perspective from Lima, Peru's capital city. My interviews in Chiclayo, Iquitos, and Pucallpa were conducted with gay and transgender individuals who had been involved with the Global Fund's projects, contributing a greater breadth to my understanding of HIV prevention throughout the country.

Inevitably, over the course of 2012–18, I sometimes became a figure in the very phenomena I was studying. For example, at a capacity-building workshop in Tarapoto in 2013, organizers gave an annual planner to all of the participants. As I opened it and paged through the images accompanying each month, I was surprised to see my picture taken the previous year at a workshop in Iquitos. I often saw photographs of me in social media, frequently in the form of Facebook posts by organizations or interlocutors who were themselves documenting their coordination of or participation in a range of HIV prevention activities. More significant, and perhaps more pertinent to the analysis in this book, was that I unwittingly became a figure in the scandalous stories that circulated in Tarapoto.

Martín, an interlocutor in Tarapoto, dramatized and circulated a story about a special lunch I had with Axel. The background—which many who heard the story would know—was that Axel and I were friends. A fellow volleyball enthusiast, Axel often took me on the back of his motorbike to watch pickup volleyball throughout Tarapoto. The gay and transgender volleyball players, and the spectators, often associated us with arriving together. Martín's story proceeds as follows:

> Axel was leaving Tarapoto for a few months and the *gringa* [me] wanted to do something special. So he invited him to lunch at the Segundo Muelle ceviche restaurant, one of the nicest restaurants in Tarapoto. They ordered a pitcher of *chicha morada* [a sweet beverage brewed from purple corn]. As Justin was drinking a glass, he turned to Axel and asked, "Is it normal for corn kernels to be in the *chicha*?" "No," responded Axel, to which Justin replied, "then what is this?" Sticking out his tongue, he grabbed what he thought was a corn kernel but which turned out to be a fly. He let out a shriek and threw a scandal right there in the restaurant, in front of everyone. Now Axel can never go back to Segundo Muelle because of this fly in the *chicha*.

This story was told at workshops, meetings, informal gatherings, and beauty salons. Martín, in particular, perfected the delivery of this scene: gesticulating the way I might, sticking out his tongue and grabbing a fake fly, imitating my higher-pitched voice and my English-speaker's Spanish accent. Martín was not even at the restaurant—yet he and others told this story so often that, frankly, I remember the details more from how it has been told than from what actually happened. Referring to me as *gringa* or *la Justina*, as Martín and others often did when talking about me in the third person, was in part as a nod to my effeminate mannerisms, but it also signaled that the story was intentionally embellished, as I did not identify as transgender or personally use feminine pronouns. The humor in the story was in the disjuncture between the scandal that was thrown and the fine restaurant where it had occurred: the *gringa* understood that a scandal could be had in the situation, but it was done in an entirely wrong context. While the lunch was intended as a heartfelt farewell, the *gringa* made it funny for almost everyone who heard the story.

The imperative to explicitly situate oneself in the research, known as reflexivity, has become an established practice in ethnographic writing. The reflexive gesture opens space for the ethnographer to author a transparent account of how they arrived in the "field," how they went about conducting research, and the multiple social identities and privileges that are often afforded to participant observers. This story—along with other stories that dramatized me as an ethnographer-in-action, as well as moments when interlocutors conscripted me as a subject of their own research agendas—provides an opportunity to probe the limits of ethnographic reflexivity by drawing attention to the intersubjective dimensions of ethnographic encounters—that is, moments in which the anthropologist and interlocutors co-constructed the anthropologist's position.[35] The openness to explore moments where interlocutors "reversed" the ethnographic gaze furthers both methodological and analytical ends. I bring to the fore the stories and experiences that emerged within ethnographic encounters to situate my own perspective as one that was constituted by the stories, agendas, and projections of interlocutors.[36] And in seeing the disjuncture between their projections of me and my own sense of self, I am able to better sharpen my interpretation of all the scandalous stories contained in *Queer Emergent*.

As I moved back and forth between urban Amazonian Peru and the North American universities that trained, hosted, and funded me as a graduate student, postdoctoral fellow, and faculty member over the course of this project, the person that I understood myself to be did not always coincide with the person interlocutors projected or imagined. I learned this through the difficulties I often encountered in providing compelling or conceivable responses to participants' common questions. Regardless of my response, these questions were often resolved through the frames of reference that made most sense to participants. Many assumed that I was *adinerado*, or excessively and privately wealthy, with a family who simply bankrolled my education and travels to Peru. In reality, I received financial support from the Department of Anthropology at the University of California, Irvine, so I could conduct preliminary fieldwork and then secure grant funding to support fieldwork. The idea that a university would not only support postgraduate studies but further support international travel was simply not a compelling explanation for many interlocutors. A second question was whether I had family from Peru or if I myself was Peruvian. Many wondered why someone who looked like me and had my last name would keep returning to this place. The reality is that I am not Peruvian. I am the grandchild of immigrants to the United States from Mexico and the Philippines. I grew up speaking English and learned Spanish mostly at school and sometimes at home. Generally, I was understood as being both "Latino" and "gringo," most everyone in Peru thought my spoken Spanish sounded funny, and sometimes *motocar* drivers and other people I encountered in the street called me *chino* because of my facial features. This productive tension between how I defined my own position and how interlocutors understood it is ultimately valuable for expanding reflexivity to include the intersubjective dimensions of ethnographic encounters and relationships. At the expense of some embarrassment, I am attentive throughout the book to the way I figured into the scandalous stories that gay and transgender interlocutors circulated, because this magnifies the tremendous capacity of interlocutors' narrative practices to reimagine and rearticulate the globalizing forces that intersected their lives over the decade.

Finally, the combination of a focus on how gay and transgender interlocutors themselves storied their experiences of HIV prevention and an emphasis on intersubjectivity allows ethnographic research to go beyond the limits of traditional techniques of interviewing and data collection in health science research. Anthropologists have long asserted that ethnographic data can "read between the lines" of numerical data as well as reimagine the very forms in which success is conceptualized and measured (Adams 2016; Biehl and Petryna 2013). In their effort to read between the lines of the numerical data of disease and epidemic, anthropologists have found that stories, and the mechanics of how stories are produced and circulate, can have effects on who lives and who dies as real as the effects of pathogens themselves (Briggs and Mantini-Briggs 2003). And while health science research typically implements a "social determinants of health" approach, the "social" is often treated as an unchanging or stable constant (Adams et al. 2019; Yates-Doerr 2020). This has particularly been the case with global HIV/AIDS research: while researchers increasingly recognized that addressing discrimination and stigma was central to ending AIDS, these complex social dynamics are often treated as reified social conditions (Parker and Aggleton 2003). Scandalous stories extend ethnographically informed critiques of the "social determinants of health" framework by putting into sharp focus some of the limits of the methods typically used in that framework. Interviews, for example, can offer tremendous insight into the perspective and experiences of the interviewee, and conducting several interviews can help the interviewer identify trends and patterns across a community. However, structured interviews alone are limited: they exist outside of social context and do not typically lend themselves to improvisation. They are limited by the language and categories of the interviewer's questions, as the interviewee looks back and recalls the world as it was through these categories. Structured interviews do not get at what that world could have been or could be, and they do not allow room for the conditional and the imaginative, which are also an important part of what is "social." Scandalous stories, by contrast, emerged within the social milieu as lived and experienced by interlocutors as they interacted with each other and with me. They thus bring a richer sense of social life and social relations to understandings of the "social"—understandings that have become increasingly imperative to preventing and "ending" HIV/AIDS.

## Outline of the Book

As noted earlier, a fundamental challenge in addressing the concentration of HIV/AIDS through HIV prevention in Peru was to reduce discrimination and stigma toward communities of gay men and transgender women. The ensuing efforts engendered new ways to talk about, document, and measure the sexual and social lives of gay and transgender Peruvians, taking on both imaginative and moralizing dimensions regarding the management of their sexualities and social worlds. In other words, antidiscrimination efforts posited both the social conditions and institutional configurations that would make ending AIDS feasible and the kinds of gay and transgender subjects who would be able to enact this future and be committed to doing so. But they also strove to create and inhabit a social world on their own terms. While the ambition to end AIDS brought about new forms for the management and governance of sexuality, sustained attention to the on-the-ground implementation of HIV prevention efforts illuminates the concomitant forms of contestation that emerged. Amid the failures and disappointments that ultimately transpired as HIV prevention efforts were implemented across urban Amazonian Peru, gay and transgender communities crafted stories that imagined possibilities of what could have been and what could be: what the official records did not capture about experiments in ending AIDS as they developed over the decade, and what could be as the effort to end AIDS continued to unfold.

Chapter 1 situates gay and transgender communities in urban Amazonian Peru at the intersection of two entangled chronologies: the ongoing HIV/AIDS epidemic and the legacies of Peru's internal armed conflict. In Tarapoto, gay and transgender interlocutors themselves brought these distinct historical trajectories together by circulating stories set against the backdrop of the conflict that dramatized their intimate and romantic relationships with men whom they consider to be heterosexual. Central to their stories was the concept of the *peche*, a regional colloquialism referring to the small gifts that interlocutors gave to their romantic and sexual partners. Exhibiting the hallmarks of scandalous storytelling, such as exaggeration and anexactness (being intentionally rather than accidentally inexact), interlocutors evoked the *peche* both as a narrative device to emphasize moral values of discretion and mutual obligation and as a way to participate in ongoing debates about the legacies of political violence. Taking seriously the *peche* as an interpretative device, I then use it as a framework to analyze health science research on "transactional sex," the globalized, technical analogue to the *peche* that has come to be associated with increased vulnerability to HIV. As HIV prevention in Peru shifted toward individualized behavioral interventions among vulnerable populations, reading transactional sex through the lens of the *peche* magnifies some of the moral assumptions undergirding the post-AIDS horizon.

Chapter 2 examines another set of social relations that constituted and sustained the social worlds of gay and transgender interlocutors in Tarapoto: the social relations they cultivated with each other and the strategic relations that some developed with local elected officials. Through the close analysis of a queer soccer tournament co-organized by two interlocutors, as well as the scandalous stories that circulated about the tournament over the month when it occurred, I propose the concept of *la colaboración*, or collaboration, as a theory of queer relationality in urban Amazonian Peru. A theory of collaboration poses two interventions. First, as contrasted with existing theories of redistributive politics in Latin America that emphasize the *mediation* of redistribution between unequal dyads (e.g., clientelism and patronage), collaboration is a triadic system that emphasizes the ongoing *creation* and *multiplication* of redistributive social relationships. Second, a theory of collaboration as a mode of social relatedness requires a reconsideration of the dominant frameworks in global HIV prevention. Instead of positing social and communal cohesion as an *outcome* of HIV prevention, collaboration names an existing condition of queer social life in Peru and, subsequently, can be used to help track the consequences and impacts of HIV prevention projects in the region.

Scandalous stories did not always yield desired social outcomes. Though the cultivation of exaggerated and embellished storytelling helped some interlocutors put forward personal traumas and experiences, the broader association between gay and transgender people and "scandalousness" sometimes limited their ability to counter injustice. This was made evident through the implementation of antidiscrimination components of the Global Fund's Tenth Round project in Tarapoto. Chapter 3 explores a paradox that resulted from the effort to mitigate vulnerability to HIV through antidiscrimination: though intended to improve the social conditions of gay and transgender communities, the obligation to denounce discrimination through formal grievances sometimes intensified existing social hierarchies of race, gender, and class. To illustrate this paradox, I develop a conceptual distinction between *emblematic denouncements* and *scandalous denouncements*. The former were stories of successful discrimination grievances that were circulated through capacity-building workshops and other elements of HIV prevention programs, whereas the latter were stories of discrimination that were never formalized or were dismissed as too scandalous. In giving these scandalous stories what Sara Ahmed (2021) calls "a hearing," I show how the pervasiveness of deeply entrenched hierarchies of race, gender, and class impacted everyday responses to the imperatives of HIV prevention.

Chapter 4 tracks the consequences of the sudden and unexpected closure of the Global Fund's Tenth Round in Peru. It focuses specifically on the fate of project specialists across urban Amazonian Peru. These were the gay and transgender individuals who played pivotal roles in their local communities as organizers of popular social spectacles like sports tournaments and beauty contests and who thus earned reputations as "collaborators." After they were recruited to coordinate the on-the-ground implementation of HIV prevention strategies, however, project specialists experienced tremendous social loss in terms of their reputations when the Global Fund terminated the Tenth Round before it was scheduled to conclude. Even though the Tenth Round turned out to be a brief project in the longer-term effort of ending AIDS, the fragmentation of collaborative social relations that resulted from its early termination continued to resonate in gay and transgender communities long after the program concluded. And yet the crisis of the closure of the Tenth Round became source material for new scandalous stories. Stylized and embellished, these stories were anticipatory lessons in imaging queer social life in the face of the impasses and predicaments they were to encounter as the "end of AIDS" continued to unfold.

A set of numerical benchmarks, known as the 90-90-90 targets, became the key indicators in the latter half of the 2010s for tracking the progress toward ending AIDS by the year 2030. This was both to ensure that countries—especially those receiving international aid—were making progress toward the 2030 target and, more generally, to provide a metric for ongoing evaluation. Following the initiatives and strategies of the 90-90-90 targets would, the story went, fast-track the strategy for ending AIDS by 2030. In Peru, HIV/AIDS advocates confronted the challenge of what Vincanne Adams (2016) calls "data deprivation." As efforts to control HIV/AIDS increasingly turned toward the numerical and quantitative, chapter 5 describes the knowledge practices that emerged when crucial data is inaccessible, unreliable, or inconsistent. The chapter traces a process I term *conversion*; that is, the unanticipated route that stories of discrimination took as they were collected as narratives in the cities of the Amazonian region, sent to LGBT activist collectives and NGOs in the capital city, Lima, and then returned to the Amazonian region in the form of statistical and quantitative data. By drawing on an adjacent field of data centering the human rights of LGBT Peruvians to fill in the gaps when data on HIV/AIDS was unreliable or out of date, advocates in urban Amazonian Peru contributed to the creation of discrimination stories that could be transformed into quantifiable data. That is, stories that counted. In turn, this process transformed queer social relationships and created the space for novel queer subjectivities to emerge.

*Queer Emergent* approaches the unfolding of the technical project to end AIDS during the global AIDS epidemic's fourth decade not just as a straightforward technical effort but more deeply as a moralizing and imaginative project. To do so, the book takes seriously the everyday stories gay and transgender communities in urban Amazonian Peru circulated as they responded to, and even reconfigured, the imperatives and obligations of HIV prevention as it transformed their social worlds. The afterword synthesizes the book's primary interventions and offers insight into what lessons can be learned in anticipation of a new stage of HIV prevention efforts among vulnerable communities in Peru during the 2020s.

# 1

## Stories That Scandalize

Transactional Sex and
Postconflict Moral Imaginaries

Karla was an affable and charming hair stylist who owned and managed a popular beauty salon in Tarapoto. Located on a busy thoroughfare a few blocks west of the city's main plaza, Karla's salon stood next to a handful of other beauty salons. Hair styling was one of the limited professional venues open to many trans women and gay men while they were growing up, and most of the salons located in this area were owned or managed by a trans woman or gay man. In moments during the day when business was slow, it was common for owners and stylists to saunter to one another's salons, hang out, catch up, and share stories. Karla's stories were particularly engaging. In an interview, I asked Karla to recount to me some of the stories that she typically shared when she was hanging out in the salon or when she was entertaining clients as she worked. She recounted a story set about two decades prior about a lover who used to visit her during the period of political violence in Tarapoto, or, as it was colloquially referred to among interlocutors in Tarapoto, *la época de terrorismo* (the era of terrorism). In her story, she referred to her lover as her "*punto,*" one of several colloquialisms used by interlocutors to refer to romantic and sexual partners whom they considered to be heterosexual. Usually this *punto* had stopped by her salon with frequency. However, after a period of about a week in which he didn't come by, Karla explained, he showed up at the salon asking if he could borrow a bicycle. After a couple of hours went by and he didn't return the bicycle, she was resigned to accepting that it was now gone. "This is what happens," she explained to me, "when a *punto* asks to borrow something; it means it is permanent." But then, three days later, he returned with the bike. "What did you do with it?" Karla inquired, to which he briefly replied, "Things." "Listen," he then said to her, "I am sorry, but I am leaving Tarapoto and I am not going to be returning here." She thought that she had heard the last of him. But two weeks later, to her great surprise, she saw him in the newspaper. It turned out that he had been a chauffeur for a high-ranking member of the MRTA, one of the armed insurgency groups operating in the region during the period of political violence, and that he had been captured by the police. This unexpected twist to the story was meant to elicit shock and surprise, and even though I had heard the story several times before, I obliged with a notable jaw drop during our interview.

I often heard stories like Karla's as I hung out in the everyday spaces of gay and trans social life in Tarapoto. Like Karla's bicycle story, the stories that circulated often dramatized another colloquialism that interlocutors called *peches*.[1] *Peche* was a term that some gay men and transgender women in Peru used to refer to the small gifts they shared with some men to incentivize romantic and sexual relationships. The term was used quite broadly to refer to a number of things, including food, money, alcohol, clothing, or even services such as a haircut. In this case, the bicycle Karla lent her lover could be considered a *peche*. The cisgender men who received *peches* were called *maperos* or *puntos*, and interlocutors typically considered *maperos* and *puntos* to be heterosexual.[2] Often set against the backdrop of the period of political violence in the region, their dramatizations of *peches* exhibited the tropes and characteristics of scandalous storytelling: embellishment, exaggeration, and even humor. In their stories, they invoked *peches* to recount or describe the intimate relationships they maintained during the period of political violence in the city.

Gay men and transgender women—the groups most vulnerable to HIV in urban Amazonian Peru over the 2010s—inhabited a social world that was intersected by two entangled chronologies: the global HIV/AIDS epidemic and the ongoing resonances of Peru's internal armed conflict. The starting points for both chronologies have traditionally been located in the early 1980s: Peru's internal armed conflict began in 1980, and the first cases of what would later become known as AIDS were reported in 1981. While Peru's internal armed conflict officially ended in 2000, its resonances persisted decades later and continued to shape the lives and memories of gay men and transgender women in urban Amazonian Peru. Likewise, throughout the 2010s, gay and trans Peruvians encountered the promise of a possible end to HIV/AIDS as a global threat to public health by the year 2030. The overlapping origins and future horizons of these distinct chronologies palpably came together over the decade of the 2010s for gay and trans communities in urban Amazonian Peru. One significant way that gay and trans communities in the city of Tarapoto collectively made sense of these two complex and intertwining histories in their lived experience was through stories about *peches*. Through the ethnographic analysis of their everyday stories about *peches*, this chapter examines how gay and transgender interlocutors defined moral positions about what sexuality should look like, the significance of discretion and mutual obligation with sexual partners, and the privileged and varied perspectives they contribute to postconflict collective memory.

### Transactional Sex

In making both stories about the past and moralizing stories about contemporary affective and romantic relationships, gay and transgender interlocutors further crafted a response and challenge to the introduction of prevailing HIV prevention discourse around responsible sexual practice and the necessary conditions for ending AIDS. As Peru's response to HIV/AIDS shifted from the scale-up of the provision of antiretroviral therapy across the country toward targeted social interventions among key or vulnerable populations, the sexual practices and social lives of gay men and transgender women became a site of increasing scrutiny. In the midst of the triumphalism of a possible "end of AIDS" future, certain social conditions, sexual practices, and general attitudes were framed as barriers to this future. One such barrier was "transactional sex." This was a technical category that circulated globally in HIV prevention research and was the framework through which some health science researchers analyzed and interpreted *peches*. In doing so, research construed *peches* not as a socially meaningful and sexually fulfilling practice but rather as a manifestation of discrimination and broader homo- and transphobia, the result of low self-esteem, and an indicator of a fatalistic attitude toward the future. This disjuncture was more than just a far cry from dominant conceptualizations of *peches* that circulated within gay and transgender communities themselves. The difference also suggested that *peches* were incompatible with the seemingly requisite practices of a post-AIDS future imaginary.

That there existed a gap between a globalized, technical, and presumably value-neutral category like "transactional sex" and the culturally situated, context-dependent analogous category "*peche*" is not surprising.[3] As Pigg and Adams (2005) remind us, "One of the observations made again and again in the sociocultural research literature pertaining to HIV/AIDS is that the categories around which epidemiological and public health reasoning are organized do not map neatly onto existing realities" (18). The *peche* is, again, another reminder that the technical categories around which visions of global HIV prevention inhere are not universal. And yet, I contend that the significance of the *peche* is not solely in its capacity to "veto" transactional sex or enumerate a new concept for the ethnographic record (Boellstorff 2007). Rather, the *peche*, as it was storied and dramatized in Tarapoto, poses a framework to interpret the moral dimensions of its standardized analogue. The moral imaginary that gay and transgender interlocutors collectively projected through stories about *peches*—the shared set of values through which interlocutors positioned themselves and connected to others—enables a reinterpretation of the moral imaginary projected by the framing of transactional sex as a barrier to ending AIDS in the future. Their capacity to render the *peche* metasexual and metasocial suggests that transactional sex, too, is situated in a historical context and embedded with assumptions about gay and transgender sexuality. Just as the *peche* made visible the moral values gay and transgender communities in Tarapoto imagined in the postconflict context, approaching transactional sex like a *peche* can shine a light on the assumptions undergirding broader ideas about the ambition to end AIDS and thereby illuminate aspects of the moral imaginary projected into the post-AIDS horizon.

The Peruvian Communist Party–Shining Path (Sendero Luminoso), a Maoist-influenced insurgency group, began a war with the Peruvian state in 1980.[4] While at first confined to the country's Andean region, political violence extended to the coastal capital city, Lima, by the early 1990s. And while the 1992 capture of Abimael Guzman, the leader of the Shining Path, effectively brought about the group's collapse, the conflict ultimately concluded with the resignation of Alberto Fujimori from the presidency in 2000.[5] In 2001, the Peruvian Truth and Reconciliation Commission (Comisión de la Verdad y Reconciliación, CVR) was tasked with the tremendous assignment of investigating the internal conflict that devasted the country from 1980 to 2000. Over a span of two years, the commission collected more than seventeen thousand testimonies and published its final report in 2003. Throughout the conflict, atrocities committed by armed groups and by the state, including torture, kidnappings, and killings by extrajudicial death squads, ultimately led to the disappearance and death of nearly seventy thousand people, as estimated by the commission's final report (CVR 2003). Importantly, as Feldman (2021) observed, the CVR evidenced the uneven distribution of the war's effects: 75 percent of the dead or disappeared were speakers of Quechua or another indigenous language. As he writes, "In a manner that reflected time-honored tropes of Peru as a failed nation, the historical narrative of the TRC [CVR] emphasized coastal indifference to highland suffering as a key factor in the origins and escalation of the violence" (Feldman 2021, 29–30).[6]

The city of Tarapoto—located at the threshold between the Andean highlands and the jungle lowlands—was, comparatively, spared from the conflict between the Shining Path and the state's counterinsurgency forces. Tarapoto was also largely spared from the violence that emerged at the confluence of the booming cocaine trade and the remnants of the Shining Path that lasted into the late 1990s and convulsed cities further south along the Huallaga River in the Upper Huallaga region, such as Tocache, Aucayacu, and Tingo María (Kernaghan 2009).

However, in the late 1980s, the MRTA established a guerrilla front in the department of San Martín and launched a rural campaign in Tarapoto and smaller cities in its surrounding region.[7] Though in the broader scale of the conflict the MRTA was a minor subversive group in comparison to the Shining Path, its presence was palpable in Tarapoto and its surroundings.[8] As determined by the CVR, the Shining Path was responsible for 54 percent

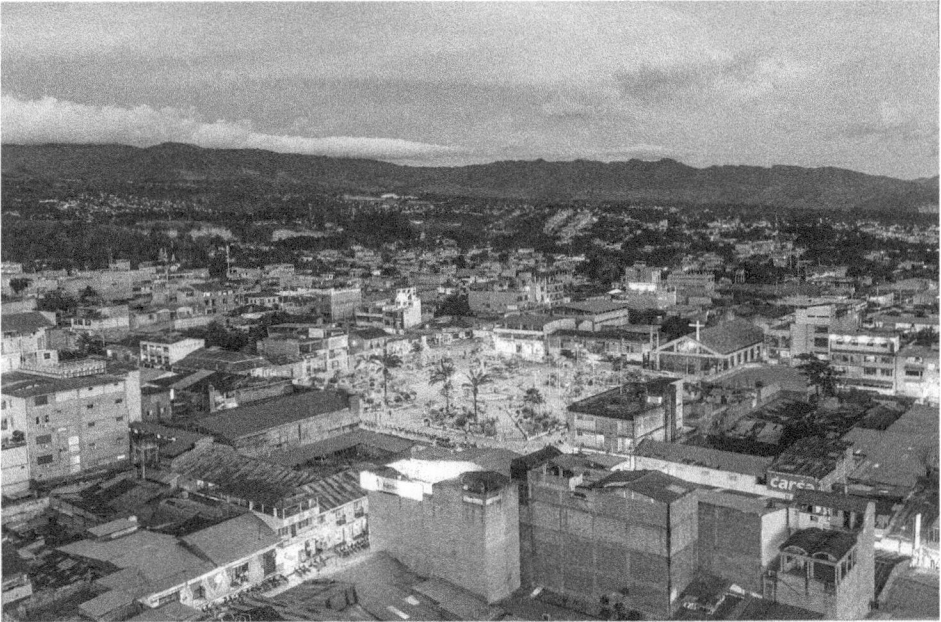

**Figure 1.1.** The main plaza of Tarapoto. (Photograph by Marlon del Aguila Guerrero)

of the total casualties, and the state was responsible for 44.5 percent. The MRTA, on the other hand, was responsible for less than 2 percent of the violence during the conflict.[9] One of the MRTA's characteristic strategies was its insistence on the utilization of political theater: it focused as much on its efforts to win the hearts, minds, and support of the public as on armed actions. The MRTA wielded and reappropriated nationalistic symbols and colors and actively sought out coverage from the media. In line with the analysis of the historian Miguel La Serna (2020) and the anthropologist Bartholomew Dean (2023), the MRTA engaged in symbolic battles meant to construe the Peruvian state as responsible for tearing apart the moral fabric of Peru. The group's violent actions focused on "social cleansing" and the selective assassination of so-called undesirables, including unfaithful spouses, drug addicts, prostitutes, thieves, and homosexuals.[10]

In a section of its final report dedicated to violence toward sexual minorities during the conflict, the CVR described a case from May 31, 1989, when MRTA members stormed the Las Gardenias bar in Tarapoto and assassinated eight *travestis* and other bar patrons (CVR 2003, 432).[11] Though this section of the report was brief, its inclusion in the CVR's report and the handful of cases it contained linked LGBT rights claims to transitional justice and the broader human rights movement (Cornejo 2014). The recognition and commemoration of the Las Gardenias case in particular has since galvanized national LGBT rights movements. For one, the case evidenced the "heteronormative violence" that LGBT communities suffered over the course of the conflict (McCullough 2016). And, as Almenara (2022) observed, the ambivalence of much of the civilian population toward acts of violence against sexual and gender minorities suggested that many approved of the violence as acts of "moral prophylaxis" (97–98). Activists have organized national days of remembrance to commemorate the violence at Las Gardenias, and the case has been editorialized in human rights reports, journalistic accounts, museum exhibits, novels, and documentary film.[12] In 2019, the district attorney's office in Tarapoto began collecting the testimony of former MRTA members about the Las Gardenias case in an effort to extend the prison sentences of the leaders of the MRTA as the authors and indirect perpetrators of the massacre (Anteparra 2019). Through national and international circulation of this emblematic case, a space has opened for LGBT communities—even beyond Tarapoto—to bring to light the experiences of violence during the conflict and the persistence of the violent targeting of queer people even after the war.

Among gay and transgender communities in Tarapoto, stories about the period of the conflict continued to circulate even decades after the period of violence.[13] One of the primary sites of this everyday circulation was beauty salons. Traditionally, hairstyling and other beauty-adjacent activities had been socially acceptable professions for gay and transgender individuals in Tarapoto. The majority of my oldest interlocutors, who were teenagers or young adults in the late 1980s and early 1990s, were hairstylists for most of their lives, and several of them owned and managed salons during the period of my fieldwork. Developing a repertoire of stories for entertaining clients while they cut, dyed, and styled hair was essential to be successful in the profession. And given that the purpose of their stories was entertainment, stories were typically characterized by exaggeration, embellishment, and humor. Even if the subject matter was serious or weighty, like the violence of the armed conflict, there was an underlying wink either at some moment or throughout the story. These stories circulated outside of the beauty salon space and others would repeat them, often changing some details or inserting themselves as the protagonist. While new professional opportunities have since emerged for some younger gay and transgender individuals in

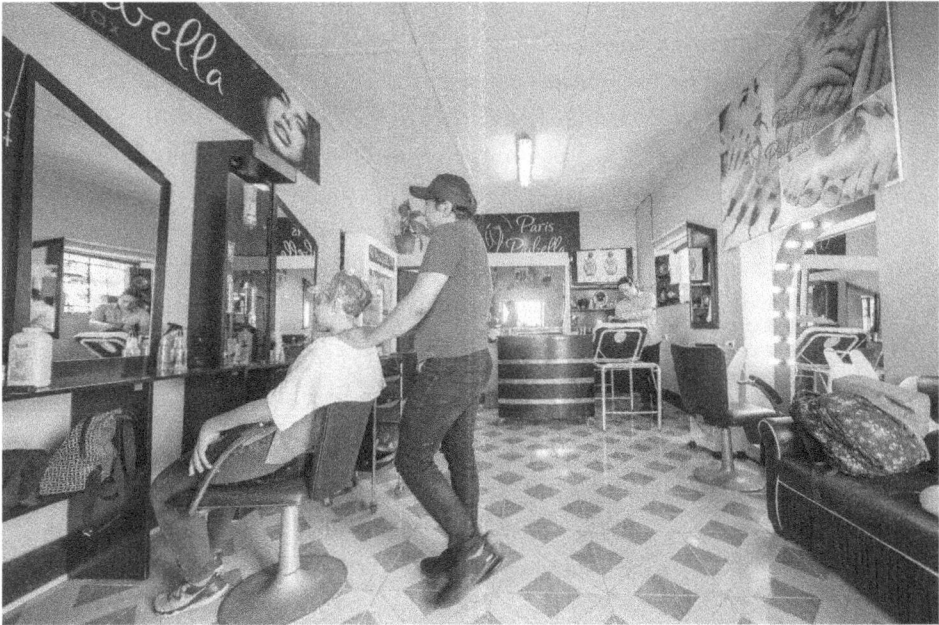

**Figure 1.2.** A typical afternoon in Brenda's beauty salon. (Photograph by Marlon del Aguila Guerrero)

Tarapoto, many apprenticed or worked in beauty salons, and salons were also common places for individuals to simply hang out among friends and socialize even if they did not work there.

Wilmer was a veteran hair stylist and salon owner whose salon offered a place to hang out and catch up on the goings-on of gay and trans social life in the city. One afternoon while I was hanging out with Wilmer in his salon, he began to share stories about his life during the MRTA's occupation of Tarapoto with me and a couple of the young gay and transgender hairstylists who had stations at his salon. He was an effective storyteller, having refined his technique through decades of hair styling. He conveyed the affective force of fear that many collectively felt and experienced during the period. One of the sources of fear was the forced curfew (*toque de queda*) that MRTA militants enforced in the city. Wilmer explained that after 6:00 p.m. one could not enter certain neighborhoods unless one lived there. The Huayco neighborhood, for example, was considered one of these *zonas rojas*. One time a man came into his salon, asking Wilmer to make a house call to the Huayco neighborhood. As Wilmer approached the neighborhood, a man who knew him tried to scare him away so he would not enter. Although he considered walking away, he entered anyway. He thought that being well known would make it okay: "Me, the only hairstylist at the time, everybody knew me." When he arrived at the house, though, he immediately realized that he had been tricked. The woman who needed the haircut actually needed a wig, because the MRTA had cut off her hair as punishment for allegations that she was a *sacavoltera*, or unfaithful spouse. Although the woman was in tears, he told her there was nothing he could do, and left immediately. One week later, two women came into Wilmer's salon. His mother, who worked as the salon's receptionist, greeted them. They asked what her son had been doing in the Huayco neighborhood the week before. His mother explained that he had been tricked and, upon realizing this, had left the neighborhood immediately. This satisfied the women, although they told his mother, "Tell your son to not return to the Huayco again." The *toque de queda* and the temporal and spatial restrictions that it entailed were a salient aspect of how people remember the fear they felt during the conflict in Tarapoto. Though not particularly embellished or exaggerated, Wilmer's story emphasized the cunning, maneuvering, and sometimes pure luck that helped him escape what could have otherwise been a complicated and potentially violent situation. Escaping a "near-miss" was a typical plot point in the stories interlocutors circulated about the conflict; it often came up in stories shared by another interlocutor, Martín.

Martín's stories often epitomized the embellished, scandalous subgenre of stories set during the period of political violence. Back when Martín was a teenager, as one of his stories went, a group of young gay and transgender volleyball players from Tarapoto, himself included, were invited to the town of Saposoa to compete in a volleyball game against a local team of gay and transgender players. Later that night, Martín went to the disco in Saposoa. Since he was not from there, he was getting a lot of attention from the men, who kept coming up to him and inviting him to have a drink. One man who came up to him was inebriated and said that they should go somewhere else. So they left and went to a garden outside the disco, where Martín gave the man *wawis*, a slang term used to refer to oral sex. He noticed the man had a huge wallet in his pocket, so he reached in and grabbed some money out of it. After he took the money, about 100 soles, he left the man there, telling him he had to go back to the disco to find his friends. As soon as he was out of sight, though, he ran directly to the house where he and his teammates were staying that night. But since they were all sharing the same room, the door was locked because someone else was with a *mapero* inside; they told him to come back later. "Ugh," he told himself, then he shrugged and walked back to the disco. As he was walking back down the street, he saw a police patrolman, who also happened to be the husband of one of his friends. The police officer waved to him and called out his name; Martín returned the wave but kept walking. Another man appeared in the distance. As he passed the man, Martín said, "¿*Te hago wawis?*" or "Can I give you *wawis?*" The man replied, "What are you talking about? I don't know what this is." But as Martín prepared himself to go ahead with his plan, the man pulled out a pistol, stuck it in Martín's mouth, and yelled at him to give *wawis* to the gun. Martín pushed the man down and started running for his life, all the way back to the house he was staying at. As soon as he got there, he banged on the door, desperate to be let back in. They opened the door, and just as he made it safely inside, a snake fell from the ceiling and landed right in front of him. He let out a shriek and stepped right over it. After recounting how he narrowly escaped a tragic demise three times that night, Martín concluded the story by saying that after all of that, in the end all he got was 100 soles.

This was a popular and engaging story that often resulted in plenty of laughter at the end thanks to Martín's comedic eloquence and the compelling combination of cunning, bad luck, and sexual maneuverings. He, and others, told it in contexts ranging from everyday social gatherings to the capacity-building workshops and sensitivity trainings carried out for HIV prevention programs in Tarapoto. The story was both serious and lighthearted. It lent itself to moments of improvisational embellishment or exaggeration by Martín or whoever retold the story: the amount of money could change, the specific town in which the story took place could change, and even a new "near-miss" incident could be added. This did not necessarily render the story untrue; rather, it contributed to the fantasy about the conflict that the story projected. With scripted roles for the conflict's main protagonists, whether it was the figure of the policeman (or, in some versions of the story, a soldier), or an armed rebel marked in the story by the man carrying the pistol, all of these actors were cast as potential sexual partners. Regardless of their apparent machismo and the very prominent instances of trans- and homophobic violence perpetrated by state armed forces and the MRTA in the region during the conflict, the story insisted that these very same people were or could also be *maperos*. In fact, it was this very insistence that any heterosexual man could be cast as a *mapero* that precipitated the story's climax. This established a fundamental intertextual tenet. If, as Martín attested, a police officer or a rebel could be a *mapero*, then that person therefore could be a recipient of *peches*.[14]

There are several implications as to the causes of Martín's series of misadventures in the story. It could have been the mistake of stealing the money at the beginning that caused the subsequent events to unfold. It could have been his misrecognition of a *mapero* or the failure to provide a *peche* to him. While set against the backdrop of the internal armed conflict, it was also an examination of the very real risks many contemporary transgender women and gay men encounter. The risk of violence, and even homicide, by intimate partners, municipal security patrols, and the police that many transgender women and some gay men faced in Peru was part of everyday life and was part of the very same conditions that made them vulnerable to HIV (No Tengo Miedo 2016; Silva-Santisteban et al. 2012). These realities could be brought up and openly discussed in ensuing conversations after the telling of this story. Was the money or pleasure worth the risks? The story's resolution opened the space for gay and transgender people themselves to decode and debate the possibilities and contours of their sexuality and assume their own positions toward prevailing moral codes.

Even among the most ardent and effusive storytellers, there was an awareness that stories of such scandalous episodes covered sensitive themes and personal traumas. Over time, as I heard the same stories circulate, I was struck by the coexistence of the humorous and the traumatic. In an interview, I asked Karla about what she made of this coexistence. In our exchange, she specifically mentioned Martín's story, which was perhaps one of the best-known examples within the group:

> Justin I love the stories that you, and everyone else, tell us, and how they make everyone laugh. But they are also very tragic. Well, they are strong histories.
>
> Karla Well, maybe it is because it is our nature. . . . We can laugh at our bad experiences. To the border of death, at the point of being killed, and you save yourself and you tell the story as if it were an adventure. And you laugh and you die laughing, instead of dying from depression. Something like this happens to a normal person, and they die of depression. Imagine [impersonating Martín's voice], "A *piraña* pointed his pistol at me when I was in Saposoa," and everyone in the room laughs.[15] And if you are a normal person who does not know how to deal with this type of event, do you think it will make you laugh? To go through that, you will never smile in your life. But we *maricones* have this gift, I think, of reverting things. To make a comedy out of a tragedy, and you laugh, and it is our strength.[16]

Karla's profound insight speaks to the role that scandalous storytelling can have for making life livable at society's margins. The collective suspension of belief and the recognition of the arts of improvisation, embellishment, exaggeration, and ornamentation not only made possible the continued circulation of the stories but also made the stories resonate with contemporary lived experiences. There was a recognition that while it is hard to put forward one's personal traumas, it can be important for helping others who may encounter similar struggles. Therein lies what Karla conceptualized as "our strength."

## Discretion as a Moral Obligation

*Peche* narratives set during the armed conflict illustrate how interlocutors collectively devised a "charmed circle" within their own historical and social context.[17] In this charmed circle, sexual encounters that involved transaction and discretion were accorded richness and complexity. In fact, sexuality mediated through *peches* was, for some, an ideal, "good," and rewarding sexual practice when conducted with discretion. When time allowed at his popular salon in Tarapoto's Morales district, Wilmer often shared stories that emphasized these qualities. In order to understand the context of the conflict, Wilmer reminded his listeners, one needed to understand that Tarapoto was once not nearly as large as it is now. Because it was small, unknown or new individuals aroused curiosity and suspicion. Wilmer noticed, then, when a mysterious man passed by the front of his salon every day for a week. One day the man decided to walk in. "Do you sell cases of vials of placenta hair treatment?" he asked Wilmer, to which Wilmer replied that he sold them not by the case but by the individual vial, and that he could gift him a couple if he wanted. The man accepted the gift and, as Wilmer recalled, complimented him on his colorful floral-patterned shirts. He then informed Wilmer, "I have been watching you, and I would like to come visit you tonight." That night, when he came over, he told Wilmer, "I am part of the MRTA. I would like to spend the night with you tonight because tomorrow they are sending me off to another city." Before they turned off the lights that night, the man showed Wilmer his pistol. He said Wilmer could take it and hide it wherever he wanted, and he would ask for it in the morning. The next morning, as he was leaving, he asked for his pistol back and for a gift of one of Wilmer's shirts. "Where are you going?" Wilmer asked him, to which he replied, "I don't know, another city."

The two romantic encounters with MRTA members recounted by Wilmer and by Karla at the beginning of the chapter further illustrated the capaciousness and modularity of the *peche*. A *peche* could be a bicycle, a floral-patterned shirt, or hair products. All of the items in this diverse range were identifiable as *peches* through the idioms of gifting or lending them to a hypermasculinized romantic partner. The stories suggested that Wilmer and Karla ameliorated the riskiness of the situation by gifting the vials of hair treatment or lending a bicycle, thereby involving the *mapero* in a set of mutual obligations. Wilmer's unnamed lover set his pistol down, and Karla's lover eventually returned the bicycle she let him borrow. For Wilmer and Karla, there was a normative lesson to be had: discretion and mutual obligations were their strategies for surviving the conflict in the past and for navigating harsh and discriminatory social conditions in the present.

The stories about the armed conflict that Martín, Wilmer, Karla, and others circulated in Tarapoto were met with differing responses. For one, the stories implied that transgressing the code of discretion or failing to give *peches* was a reason other gay and transgender victims might themselves be to blame or at fault for the violence that befell them (i.e., victim blaming). Even if this was not explicitly stated, journalists, activists, and HIV prevention advocates from Lima who encountered these stories while reporting on the Las Gardenias case or leading capacity-building workshops were perplexed by the implicit suggestion that gay and transgender people occupied a complex social position during the conflict.[18] Nevertheless, the emphasis on the value of discretion in their stories and their position of credibility resonated with younger generations of gay and transgender people in Tarapoto. Eduardo, for example, had worked with Karla in her salon before he eventually became involved in LGBT activism and HIV prevention in Tarapoto. In an interview, he explained that while he was not old enough to remember the conflict, Karla, a close friend of his, had lived through it. As he pieced together fragments of stories that Karla, and likely others, shared, he reiterated the significance of the mutual obligation of discretion and secrecy that the *peche* ensured. Because of the *peches* she gave, Karla not only survived the conflict but, from Eduardo's perspective, became a credible witness to the realities of what had happened. He made this clear in an interview: "Karla has very good stories to tell because she has lived the experience. The stories are good because she tells what really happened. So she told me, and I believe her, that it just so happens that she also had boyfriends who carried the pistols for the MRTA, and they walked around with the pistol, like this. 'You know what, my love, today we killed three people.' 'Yes, my love, I will serve you dinner now.' They would come over to rest, too, because they were her boyfriends." Eduardo projected a fantasy about the erotic possibilities open to Karla during the conflict. While this projection coincided with the stories that he heard, it was unlikely that Karla actually lived this scenario exactly as or as nonchalantly as Eduardo described it. But that is what stories and storytelling are for: to explore, imagine, and transmit affective possibilities. And sometimes the stories of everyday life are the only space where certain stories can exist.[19]

In Eduardo's reinterpretation of Karla's story, by serving dinner and providing respite, Karla maintained heterosexual lovers while also ensuring discretion. These lovers and boyfriends came and went—many of the stories end with the lover leaving town—and that was simply the dynamic of *peche*-mediated relationships. Given the assurance of discretion signaled by *peches*, Eduardo surmised that Karla and others likely would have been told secrets about the conflict that no one else could know. While the romance and sexual fulfillment were meaningful, two and three decades later what Karla had gotten in exchange was the position to know privileged truths about the past:

> They told you because they needed to relieve themselves, because they were not going to tell their family, so they told their *maricón*, who was not part of the family, they told them things but they had to be only the receptors of the story, nothing more.[20] The same thing happens today: if they think that you have told your best friend, they are not going to come back [to have sex] with you. Well, before it was a little different, in the time of the conflict, not only did they not come back, but they came back to kill you. Now they just do not come back. That is how it is for *maricones*.

Any cisgender heterosexual man could become a *mapero* through accepting a *peche*. Eduardo collapsed the past and the present to reiterate this point about the enduring predicaments of gay and transgender sexual culture: "This is how it is for *maricones*." Even if the encounter was brief or fleeting, the most unlikely of figures—like strangers with guns—could enter into mutual obligations with a gay or transgender person. At the surface, in exchange for food, money, a place to stay, alcohol, or clothing, a gay or transgender person got a romantic partner and sexual fulfillment. But Eduardo associated *peches* with an even more profound exchange. That is, in exchange for maintaining discretion and providing a confidential space for safeguarding the frustrations, anxieties, and secrets of the conflict, gay and transgender people assumed a credible position from which to remember and recount the past. Karla was, according to Eduardo, a recipient of stories that no one else could possibly know. If discretion ensured that a *mapero* would "come back" or continue a relationship, and if *peches* ensured this discretion, then the lesson of the stories about the conflict, as interpreted by Eduardo, was that *peches* accorded gay and transgender people a place in postconflict Peru.

Broadly speaking, no singular narrative of the conflict ever really congealed. As Degregori (2015) explained, while the Peruvian state may have "won" the internal armed conflict, afterward it found winning battles for memory and justice elusive. Two opposing narratives have persisted over the decades following the official end of the conflict. On the one hand, a "salvation memory" viewed Alberto Fujimori's heavy hand as necessary and justified for ending the conflict and positioned the armed forces as the heroes. A "human rights memory," on the other hand, insisted on recognizing the injustices of the conflict, holding those responsible accountable, and situating "the violence as an extension of ongoing legacies of social and political inequalities of which the Shining Path was a symptom" (Milton 2014, 10). The disjuncture that emerged between the stories circulated among gay and transgender people in Tarapoto about *peches* and the narratives of heteronormative violence in Tarapoto during the conflict collected by the CVR was but one of many arenas of memorialization and cultural production where tensions between these opposing narratives have played out.[21] The exaggerated, embellished, and ironic stories that gay and transgender people told about their sexual encounters with MRTA insurgents during the internal armed conflict may not resolve this tension or offer a unified, ultimate truth about the past, despite Eduardo's insistence on Karla's credibility. Rather, in setting the *peche* against the backdrop of the armed conflict, the everyday questions that gay and transgender people debated and discussed about their sexuality—Was a *peche* really worth it? Was the relationship with a *mapero* authentic? What are the advantages of being with a *mapero?*—were given a role in the most significant event of modern Peruvian history and could come to shape its legacy, even if the historical accuracy was murky. In short, these stories posited that *peches* were of import and of consequence.

**The *Peche* in Practice**

In everyday social spaces in Tarapoto, including beauty salons, pickup volleyball games, and the offices of community-based organizations, gay and transgender interlocutors often spent their time entertaining each other with scandalous stories about sexual adventures and romantic disappointments with *maperos*. While many of these stories dramatized contemporary experiences, this chapter has focused up to this point on a popular subgenre of their stories: stories about sexual encounters set against the backdrop of Peru's internal armed conflict. Apart from this particular temporal setting, another typical characteristic across these stories was that they hinged on a *peche*, the word gay and transgender people used to lexicalize a gift, whether in the form of food, money, clothing, or alcohol, that they gave to their romantic and sexual partners. But what exactly was a *peche* in practice? In other words, how did interlocutors use them outside of the stories and dramatizations that they shared about them? While a truly precise definition of a *peche* is elusive, it was actually through its capaciousness and modularity that the *peche* offered gay and transgender interlocutors a socially meaningful tool for theorizing sexuality.

Who was the intended recipient of a *peche*? As in other cities throughout the Amazonian region, both gay men and transgender women in Tarapoto called these men *maperos*. While gay men and transgender women conceived of their own subjectivities as distinct, both saw *maperos* as potential romantic or sexual partners and *peches* as an incentive for the development of relationships with them. Categorized as "MSM" in the global health sciences, a *mapero* did not assume the latter category as a social identity.[22] Rather, the term was circulated by gay and transgender people among themselves to mark men who otherwise lived their lives unmarked, as normatively cisgender and heterosexual. A *mapero* could be a romantic lover, a boyfriend, or simply a sexual partner. However, they considered *maperos* to be heterosexual and assumed that they also maintained romantic or sexual relationships with cisgender women.[23] Even if a *mapero* was not married or did not have children, gay and transgender interlocutors typically expected a *mapero* to eventually marry and father children even while that was not part of the life trajectory they might have imagined for themselves.

The *peche* dynamic and commercial sex work were not, in practice, mutually exclusive. A gay man or transgender woman might maintain a romantic relationship with a *mapero* through *peches*, while also engaging in commercial sex work.[24] However, payments to sex workers were not considered *peches*. For example, one evening I accompanied Axel, a gay interlocutor, to a late-night food market. As we were walking over, we passed a young man, and Axel whispered to me, "*Buses.*" This was meant to be a warning that what he would say next involved or was related to some element of sexual culture and thus necessitated discretion. He told me that he knew someone who arranged informal sexual encounters with students from the local military and technical colleges. For 20 Peruvian soles, or about $7, he went on, one could pay for a range of sexual encounters with young men like the one we had passed.

This provoked a conversation with Axel about why he continued giving *peches* despite the accessibility of commercial sex work in Tarapoto. "This is much easier and more direct than with a *mapero*. With a *mapero* you have to pay for beer at the disco and buy them the things that they ask for," he explained, and then lamented further that "the men from the military school love going to the disco." If engaging in a commercial sex transaction was so easy, I asked, why would gay and transgender people continue to provide *peches* to *maperos*? He responded by listing off the names of some of our shared gay and transgender acquaintances and then asked me, "How do you think [the acquaintances] can have all of their boyfriends at the disco? It is because they give *peches* so that the rest can see them together with jealousy." In addition to sexual fulfillment, Axel suggested that *peches* had broader social implications. The capacity to give *peches* could win over boyfriends and build popularity. Whether or not others actually were jealous, *peches* shaped intergroup hierarchies.

Beyond shaping the romantic relationship with a *mapero*, or the social relationship with other gay and transgender individuals, *peches* had the potential to extend even further, encompassing mutual obligations with a *mapero*'s family. "I have seen parents who go along with their son being a *mapero*," Axel proclaimed in another conversation. He continued with an example of a man named Carlos, who lived in the town Axel grew up in outside of Tarapoto. When Axel was younger, his father had told him to be careful around Carlos through a vague warning that Carlos "ruins young men." Only as Axel got older did he realize that Carlos was gay and come to understand what his father had been trying to tell him. When Axel was in secondary school, Carlos began dating one of Axel's schoolmates. Because Carlos owned property and had money to spend, Axel reasoned, his schoolmates' parents accepted Carlos because he provided the schoolmate with gifts and bought food for the family. As Axel's schoolmate grew older, he eventually married and had children, though that did not terminate Carlos's involvement with him and his family. Axel then relayed an observation about the configuration between his schoolmate's family and Carlos: "His wife gets uncomfortable when Carlos is around. How could the family be willing to do this because that stage of his life has passed? And sometimes I see that the family prefers Carlos, but I think it is because he gifts *peches*."

*Peches* were circumscribed by varied vectors of power, including age and class. In this case, while the stigmatization of Carlos as gay in the small town may have incited the oft-cited stereotype that gay people influence younger people to become gay, Carlos also wielded his educational and class privileges to incentivize a relationship and enmesh multiple individuals into the *peche* dynamic. While Axel's father may have rejected someone like Carlos had Axel been the recipient, this was not the case for others, who, as Axel recounted in this story, welcomed *peches* as supplements to their household subsistence.

While gay and transgender interlocutors spent considerable time talking about *peches* among themselves, not all shared Axel's perspective on *peches*. In fact, *peches* were the subject of debates over whether they constituted "real" or "authentic" relationships, and interlocutors policed each other over the extent of their use. And while *peches* were generally viewed positively, giving *peches* in excess was criticized. The person who allegedly gifted *peches* without any reciprocal sex from a *mapero* was universally ridiculed. Even if someone gifted *peches* to *maperos*, that person might still criticize another for giving *peches* too frivolously. While the word *peche* could become a subject position—someone who gives *peches* might be called a *pechera*—this was typically used in reference to someone else. Rarely would a person actually assume the identity of *pechera*, even as they openly discussed the gifts they provided to their boyfriend or lover.

Still others assumed resolute stances against *peches*. Walter, a gay interlocutor in Tarapoto, for example, criticized his fellow gay and transgender friends over *peches*. "I do not share the same ideology as my friends," he insisted in our interview, "this mentality that they have of wanting to satisfy oneself with a *macho macho* and give *peches*. I don't understand this mentality, because I think that, at their age, they should be looking for a stable relationship. They are professionals, so they should be looking for an authentic relationship and not have to pay." Walter explained that *peches* indicated a lack of professionalism, sexual maturity, and authenticity. An authentic, mature relationship, for Walter, would instead be one grounded in egalitarianism and monogamy. Walter's position was exceptional in Tarapoto. However, outside of Tarapoto, Walter might find more gay and transgender individuals who shared this position toward *peches*. Gay men from Lima— who typically encountered gay and transgender communities in Tarapoto as a result of HIV prevention programs, national LGBT advocacy work, or tourism—expressed similar positions toward *peches*. So while there was, as could be expected, heterogeneity of sexual practices (and perspectives on these practices) among gay and transgender communities throughout Peru, even at the small, localized scale of Tarapoto, one could also find a diversity of perspectives. Yet Walter's resolute stance, as well as his insistence on his own exceptionality around *peches* in comparison to his friends, ultimately underscored the patterned and prominent role that *peches* occupied in Tarapoto's sexual cultures.

Others transitioned in and out of relationships based on the *peche* dynamic. Late one evening, after I accompanied Martín to a meeting to negotiate the location for an upcoming cultural event he was organizing for the municipal government, we went to one of his favorite restaurants, one that specializes in regional barbecue. Over a heaping portion of *tacacho* (balls of mashed plantain), Martín explained to me that being gay was like being Mary Magdalene from the Bible: "You will always be the other person for a man, weeping and crying like Mary Magdalene because it is impossible for him to truly be with you." He explained that because of this, from that point on he was no longer going to seek out heterosexual men (whom he called *macho machos*), but rather would choose other gays. To be with another gay was to have an equal relationship, but with an *hombre* or *mapero*, the relationship was never equal. Pitching this concept to me as if he needed to convince me, he said that he had not realized this until recently, and that most of his friends do not understand him or why he would want a *gay* boyfriend. When I asked about the impetus for this change, he replied that it was personal experience. The important point to highlight from Martín's explanation was that the dynamic was not rigid or eternal: one moved in and out of it and understood that one could participate in a range of sexual and intimate relationships.

While everyday discussions among gay and transgender interlocutors were consumed by talk about *peches*, it was quite ambiguous what a *peche* actually was. Rarely was the concept invoked in moments when they might have actually given food, money, or alcohol to a *mapero* (e.g., no one would say, "Here, take this *peche!*"). Neither would a *mapero* explicitly solicit a *peche*. Rather, he might ask to borrow money or a particular item, or simply express that he was hungry. The gift—whether food, money, or clothing— was invoked as a *peche* only after the fact. The concept offered a way to describe and make sense of intimate relationships, familial ties, coming of age, and the mutual obligations that a transgender or gay person might have with others. The significance of the *peche* was not just that it named an element of a particular, culturally situated sexual practice but also that interlocutors imbued it with metasexual and metasocial capacities. The *peche* opened space in discussions for reflecting and knowing about the dynamics of gay and transgender sexuality and sociality. And this was why it was left ambiguous what a *peche* actually was. Throughout the constant and ongoing negotiation between what a *mapero* might ask for or expect from a gay or transgender partner, what the partner might be willing to provide, and the point at which either party might move on, there was never any previously defined or mutually agreed upon value for a *peche*. This ambiguity lent the *peche* capaciousness, in that its referents were unfixed and could be any of a changing and wide range of things, and modularity, in that it could be made relevant to diverse social contexts. An effort to conjure a precise definition of the *peche* might evacuate it of its metasexual and metasocial capacities.

## How the *Peche* Became a Problem

The enthusiasm around the global project to end AIDS came together as a result of several biomedical and technological advancements that had occurred over the 2000s and 2010s. For people living with HIV/AIDS, the period witnessed efforts to scale up effective and affordable antiretroviral therapy. For communities vulnerable to HIV, the period saw the introduction of pre-exposure prophylaxis therapy for the prevention of HIV. Access to PrEP as a viable means of HIV prevention, however, was not as globalized as the "end of AIDS" message (which was circulating by the mid-2010s) had suggested. Although Peru had been the site of offshore clinical trials testing the effectiveness of PrEP, it was not commercially available in Peru during my fieldwork. Moreover, beyond the handful of interlocutors who, by coincidence, had mentioned actually having been subjects in clinical trials in Iquitos, most interlocutors were unfamiliar with PrEP as a means of HIV prevention. And though research on vulnerable populations in Peru showed that PrEP could offer a cost-effective method of reducing future cases of HIV transmission, findings emphasized that the possible rollout of PrEP in Peru would be most effective in combination with other HIV prevention measures (Bórquez et al. 2019; Gomez et al. 2012). One of the most significant roadblocks was the problem of those who might be unmotivated to take or adhere to therapy.[25] As HIV prevention initiatives reoriented toward the groups in Peru in which HIV was most concentrated—that is, populations that would need to have the most outsized role in the uptake of PrEP, like urban gay and transgender communities of the Amazonian region—it appeared as though one condition of their sexual culture stood out as necessitating behavioral intervention in order for them to even be considered candidates for effective PrEP intervention in the future. This was a practice termed transactional sex.

Originally, "transactional sex" was a technical category designed to improve HIV prevention. Specifically, transactional sex referred to "noncommercial, nonmarital sexual relationships involving the exchange for money and gifts" (Mojola 2014, 35). It was at first intended to be differentiated from the category "sex work," promising improved HIV prevention messaging and programming by casting a wider net beyond those who self-identified as sex workers. The category has since proven quite adaptable across varying cultural contexts and diverse sexual configurations. It has been used to describe both the vulnerability of heterosexual women in comparison to heterosexual men and the vulnerability of gay men and transgender women in comparison to heterosexual men. It has worked as an effective shorthand to stand in for a range of practices and behaviors that can be shown to be associated with transmitting HIV.[26] That is, what increased HIV risk was not transactional sex per se but rather the dimensions of gender, race, class, and sexuality that have come to make transaction and consumption moral cornerstones of modern subjecthood and can be encapsulated by the category.[27]

Holly Wardlow's (2006) study of *pasinja meri*, or "passenger women," in Papua New Guinea vividly puts into perspective the limits of categories like transactional sex. Passenger women were "women—often married and with children—who run away from their husbands or natal families and engage in extramarital sex, often in exchange for money" (Wardlow 2006, 3). Importantly, Wardlow explains that while Western categories like "transactional sex" increasingly came to describe their sexuality, such discourses "do not by any means explain why the women who come to inhabit this category act in the way they do" (Wardlow 2006, 18). To do so requires historical contextualization and ethnographic attention. In a postcolonial context characterized by increasing male participation in wage labor and in which women found increasing opportunities for mobility, women's agency was "fenced in" and "encompassed" by societal expectations about their labor and their potential value in the form of bridewealth. For passenger women, engaging in transactional sex was not motivated by some intrinsic greed or a laziness around expected forms of women's labor. Rather, it was an act of resistance to being "fenced in" by familial and clan expectations and the system of bridewealth. In other words, it was a form of asserting agency and ownership, even if only temporarily, over their sexuality.

In the case of Peru, the category of "transactional sex" worked to problematize some of the social conditions that contributed to the concentration of HIV among vulnerable populations. Though globally the term has been most associated with cisgender women, in Peru most of the term's use has been around gay men and transgender women. By shifting from identity categories to sexual practice categories, the concept "transactional sex" meaningfully improved to some extent on a prior framework of sexual categorization that had been applied to describe sexual cultures throughout Latin America, the *activo/pasivo* framework. Furthermore, transactional sex offered a compelling script for contextualizing gay and transgender vulnerability within broader social patterns of discrimination and stigma. If ending AIDS pivoted not just on encouraging PrEP uptake but also on instilling individualized affective states and moral values that contributed to adherence, then for some health science and HIV prevention researchers a proclivity toward transactional sex could be empirically identified as a barrier that put this future into question. Thus transactional sex between gay men or transgender women and men they deemed heterosexual came to be framed as a problem.

As noted earlier, the category "transactional sex," and kindred categories like "exchange sex" or "compensated sex," improved upon the descriptive framework known as the *activo/pasivo* distinction. The *activo/pasivo* framework was a set of social scientific categories that had dominated social scientific research on AIDS and homosexuality in Latin America for several decades.[28] Drawing on Freud's distinction between sexual aim and sexual object choice, the ethnographic literature associated with the *activo/pasivo* framework generally posited that throughout Latin America the receptive partner of anal-penetrative sex (the *pasivo*) was stigmatized as gay or homosexual, whereas the penetrative partner (the *activo*) retained the privileges of normative masculinity. By the 2000s, however, the *activo/ pasivo* framework had come to be considered "one among a more diverse set of options available in Latino sexual and homosexual worlds of the early twenty-first century" (Vidal-Ortiz et al. 2010, 254). Another reason the framework lost analytical force was that it did not always hold up empirically: transgender women and gay men often reported performing the penetrative role, even though they, and transgender women in particular, were the most socially stigmatized.

Even as the *activo/pasivo* framework became less conventional in cultural analysis, across Latin American contexts many still used the terms in their everyday lives and as part of a robust vocabulary for talking about sexual culture.[29] In Tarapoto, gay men and transgender women often talked about themselves and each other as *pasivos/as* and might even refer to a *mapero* as an *activo*, even if these categories did not correspond to actual sexual roles. Likewise, the distinction continued to be relevant for HIV prevention because of persistent disparities in HIV incidence between *pasivos* and *activos* (McLean et al. 2016; Peinado et al. 2007). As a category, "transactional sex" could still encompass the dynamics of sexual role, as well as the perceived inequalities that might contribute to this disparity, without fully concretizing *activo* and *pasivo* as rigid social identities. Even if gay men and transgender women did not always perform the passive role in anal-penetrative sex, the sex itself was mediated by an exchange of money or gifts. Much like the concept "MSM," which emerged in an effort to divorce identity from behavior (Boellstorff 2011; Parker 2019; Young and Meyer 2005), the concept "transactional sex" could subsume an ever-expanding list of sex/gender categories and, presumably, transcend cultural differences.

But in order to explain differences in HIV incidence between sexual roles while still eliding imperfect or culturally specific identity categories, research contextualized transactional sex in abstract social imaginaries. One study, for example, pointed to the differences in emotional expectations between *activos* and *pasivos* as an explanation for differences in HIV incidence: "While pasivo participants often hoped for love and intimacy in their relationships with activo partners, the activo MSM interviewed typically considered their sexual contacts with men as incidental events without ties of intimacy or commitment" (Clark et al. 2013, 1325). The authors suggested that a *moderno* sexual role—an egalitarian approach to sexual relationships not mediated by transaction or compensation—could reduce risk. One group of researchers described the dynamics of compensated sex as a "vicious cycle where the homosexual man pays or gives gifts in exchange for company or sexual favors and a heterosexually identified man seeks to obtain something such as money, clothes, food, unconventional sex or alcohol" (Fernández-Dávila et al. 2008, 364). They argued that several factors, including low self-esteem, a fatalistic attitude toward the future, and a pervasive culture of homo- and transphobia, appeared to mislead gay and transgender Peruvians into over-compensating their heterosexual partners: "Their sex with multiple casual partners would serve, for many of them, to fill an emotional vacuum and compensate for the feelings of loneliness and rejection generated by an environment hostile to their way of life" (Fernández-Dávila et al. 2008, 367). For the authors, compensated sex worked as a heuristic for detailing a broader story about gay and transgender sexuality and the sociocultural context in which it was lived. It was a capacious proxy for a range of social dynamics, all of which contributed to an explanation of how transactional sexual behavior could be associated with increased risk for HIV. In the effort to displace individual blame for HIV infection and focus on broader social circumstances, in which transactional sex was the reification of homo- and transphobia and resignation to a future in which HIV was inevitable, then transactional sex was conceivably one site for intervention. But in construing transactional sex as the problem, researchers simultaneously projected a moral imaginary whereby transactional sex stood in contrast to a monogamous, egalitarian, and thus HIV-preventing sexuality. This not only misdirected attention toward individual behavior at the expense of broader social conditions but also foreclosed a conceptualization of *peches* as emotionally fulfilling or socially consequential.

The success of PrEP in Peru was seemingly dependent on converting gay and transgender people into altruistic egalitarians. The exigencies of the post-AIDS future intensified the effort to change gay and transgender people's dispositions toward incentive and transaction. In order for PrEP to be effective, or at least marketed as effective, individuals had to become responsible and consistent adherents to the PrEP regimen, with the will to accept this responsibility and with an underlying commitment to ending AIDS. For example, one study comparing adherence to PrEP across multiple trial sites determined that while trial participants in San Francisco "reported joining the study to give back to their community and help advance HIV prevention science," trial participants in Peru, who were among those with the lowest adherence, "reported socialization, information, and study incentives as key motivations for study participation" (Liu et al. 2014, 532). Instead of being like the San Franciscans concerned about the long-term future of their community, Peruvians and other South Americans were construed by the study as motivated only by the frivolity of socialization and the material goods they received in order to participate. The article suggested that Peruvian participants lacked the altruistic qualities of their northern counterparts and were unable to realize the benefits for the global community that participation in the trial entailed. They were not just practitioners of transactional sex but transactional sexual subjects lacking the requisite commitment to adherence and with a moral viewpoint seemingly incompatible with ending AIDS. In reducing the frequency of transactional sex, HIV prevention initiatives could compel gay and transgender Peruvians to embrace a moral imaginary that would make them ideal future subjects for PrEP and encourage them to do their part toward ending the crisis.

The problem of transactional sex could be summarized as the following: Why would gay and transgender Peruvians allow themselves to be duped out of hard-earned goods when this behavior was associated with contracting HIV and when they had at their disposal more egalitarian sexual practices that would not needlessly squander their already limited resources? For HIV prevention to work, it appeared as though individuals themselves had to become responsible and consistent adherents to PrEP, accepting it as a responsibility and along with that an underlying commitment to ending AIDS. "Transactional sex" worked as a category because it could serve as shorthand for the opposite of these qualities: irresponsible behavior, low self-esteem, and even a fatalism toward the future. In setting transactional sex within the context of efforts to forge an AIDS-free future, research projected moral values like egalitarianism and romance without transaction as necessary requisites for post-AIDS sexualities. This individualization of responsibility, however, elided the structural inequalities within which the very same vulnerable populations found themselves: the ongoing legacies of the internal armed conflict, the social hierarchies and ethno-racial cleavages between the coast and the rest of the country, and the entrenchment of international investment to support the expansion of access to HIV/AIDS treatments. Thus, while the category of transactional sex offered some improvement on preexisting analytical frameworks for studying and representing gay and trans sexual cultures in Peru, it failed to apprehend the rich and dynamic social and historical world in which they practiced and lived their sexuality. The *peche*, on the other hand, did.

### The Imaginative Potential of the *Peche*

Through their embellished and entertaining stories about *peches*, interlocutors held together and made sense of the two distinct chronologies that intersected their lives throughout the 2010s—the legacies of Peru's internal armed conflict and the future of the HIV/AIDS epidemic. For gay and transgender communities in Tarapoto, scandalous stories about *peches* offered a venue for debates about what it meant to live a sexually and romantically fulfilling life, even in the face of two long-term traumas that profoundly affected their communities and friends. Their stories about *peches* stressed the significance of mutual obligation as a site of romantic and social fulfillment, and they suggested that *peches* could positively contribute to the dynamics of sexuality. In contrast, research on transactional sex suggested that relations mediated by *peches* were negative—fatalistic, disempowering, and not based in authentic love. Research that positioned transactional sex as a barrier to desired outcomes or as a problem that could be solved through behavioral intervention presupposed a moral subject and projected this idealized subject into the post-AIDS future. The implication was that it was the duty of vulnerable groups to cease their transactional sexual orientations and commit to a modern, egalitarian ideal for their own good and the good of contributing to the end of AIDS.

In the rapidly changing world of HIV/AIDS science, treatment, and prevention, one in which new technologies and circumstances constantly obligate the creation of new categories to respond to the global epidemic at scale, close ethnographic consideration to the narrative practices interlocutors employed to dramatize *peches* shines a light on the multiple moral imaginaries intertwined with the ambition to end AIDS. As examined in this chapter, gay and transgender Peruvians story *peches* such that they become tremendously meaningful and significant, drawing on them to describe the contours and possibilities of their sexual culture, to assume positions toward moral codes of discretion and mutual obligation, and to carve out a space for themselves in postconflict society. Interpreting the category of transactional sex in the way that gay and transgender interlocutors interpret *peches*—that is, reading transactional sex for the moral imaginaries that make it meaningful and significant for health science and HIV prevention—recasts the persistent tensions that emerge between global categories and their localized and historically conditioned counterparts. This tension appears not just in anthropological responses to the global health sciences but also in other fields equally invested in the varied experiences of globalized categories of sexual practice, sexual orientation, and gender identity. The *peche* does not replace transactional sex as a new and improved operational category, nor does it demand the removal of the category of transactional sex from the global HIV/AIDS lexicon. Rather, it opens avenues for ethnographic interpretation inspired by the scandalous stories of gay and trans communities in urban Amazonian Peru. As the global response to the AIDS epidemic continues to transform, *peches* draw attention to the underlying assumptions and moral values that emerged as new technical categories were introduced and applied to diverse contexts and changing conditions.

The answer is not to excise the *peche*—and other culturally situated concepts that approximate the category "transactional sex"—from the global diversity of sexual configurations. Rather, *peche* stories force a reevaluation of the framing of transactional sex as a problem. Considering the end of AIDS as not just a technical project but also a moralizing one is an opportunity to reimagine the post-AIDS future. Albeit fraught, the *peche* did not represent a fatalistic attitude or resignation about the future for interlocutors, as some research suggested. Rather, it was about surviving in a world of marginalization and exclusion and crafting a place in postconflict society. Positioning transactional sex as a problem designated some communities as incompatible with the demands of certain visions of the post-AIDS future. In expanding these visions and imagining a future that can accommodate gay and transgender pluralities, *peche* stories ultimately invite a consideration of diverse sexual configurations, even those that may, at the surface, seem to be out of sync with assumptions about who belongs in that future.

# 2

## Collaboration on
## the *Cancha*

### Sustaining and Multiplying Social Relations
### through Scandalous Spectacles

As I sat on a street corner one warm evening in Tarapoto, I received a phone call from Ramón. Ramón was an effusive and charismatic gay man who had both grown up in the Morales district of Tarapoto and now lived there. Though he was well into his mid-thirties at the time, he possessed a youthful energy, and virtually anyone he encountered considered him a *joven*, or young adult.[1] He had some experience working as a health promoter on short-term contracts over the past few years and was very public about his status as someone living with HIV—often making posts about it on social media. In fact, because he was so active on social media and often contacted me there, I was surprised to receive a phone call from him. He proceeded to tell me a story of an encounter that had occurred earlier that afternoon. A woman had walked into his family's convenience store looking for the *joven* Ramón. She was a neighbor who, like him, lived in the Morales district of Tarapoto, but she was not someone Ramón knew well. In fact, he could not remember her name. But, he continued, she sought him out for assistance. The woman's sister, Nicole, had recently returned from Lima to their parents' house in the small hamlet of Vista Alegre. She explained that Nicole was *travesti* and that she lived with HIV, but her condition was rapidly deteriorating. She wanted Nicole to come stay with her in Tarapoto, where she would have better access to medical services and the treatment she needed. However, Nicole and the rest of her family were reluctant, and preferred that she stay in Vista Alegre. Nicole's parents had turned to alternative remedies and treatments to help Nicole, but these efforts had not helped. The woman knew that the only thing that would help would be the treatment that Nicole could get at the hospital in Tarapoto. And thus, as Ramón explained, came the request: Would Ramón be willing to collaborate with her by going to Vista Alegre and convincing Nicole to come to Tarapoto?

"Listen, Justin," he explained to me on the phone, "Vista Alegre is in the Shambuyacu district. This is far and I do not know the area. Do you think you could come with me?" I did not know the area either, but I could sense from his voice that he was apprehensive about going alone. I agreed, and the next day at 3:40 a.m. I got a wake-up call from Ramón: "See you at 4:30 a.m. at the car stop!" After a nearly four-hour journey involving three different *colectivo* cars and a *motocar* up an unpaved and muddy hill—the cost totaling around 100 soles for both of us—we finally arrived at the door of Nicole's house in Vista Alegre.

Our arrival was a surprise—while Nicole's sister had informed her family that her friends were coming to chat with Nicole, they did not know if and when we were actually going to come. Ramón introduced himself to Nicole and her family as a friend and neighbor of her sister—and introduced me as an *extranjero* anthropologist who accompanied him from time to time. Though we had arrived unexpectedly, Nicole's parents were warm and hospitable, and they invited us in for a breakfast of rice and fried fish. While we were eating, Ramón presented his case to Nicole and her family. He explained how he had the same condition as she did, that she would be able to have access to the pills she needed in Tarapoto just as he did, and that if she encountered any problems or discrimination at the hospital, he had connections with the National Ombudsperson. Nicole expressed some reluctance at first. She wanted to stay with her parents, but she acknowledged that their alternative treatments were not helping and that she did need to get back on antiretroviral therapy. So she packed a suitcase and was ready to go in no time. We embarked on the long return journey to Tarapoto, this time with Nicole. As soon as we got back, in the early evening, Ramón took Nicole to her sister's house. The next day, Ramón accompanied Nicole to the hospital in Tarapoto to help her navigate reenrolling in Seguro Integral de Salúd (SIS) and accessing ART. And though Ramón was no longer under contract as a health promoter at the time, he brought Nicole to DISAM to consult with the medical professional who specializes in support of vulnerable populations.

At first glance, Ramón performed the classic functions that he had learned as an *agente comunitario* (community health agent) or *promotor de salúd* (health promoter) previously. He was a lay community member who could effectively connect someone to the health services they needed. But deeper reflection on this anecdote brings up a different set of questions that demand a closer and richer depiction of Ramón's social world. What was it about Ramón that compelled someone who barely knew him to seek his assistance and make this request? How did this woman—whose name Ramón could not even recall at the time—know that Ramón would be the right person to share about his experiences and help convince her family that Nicole might be better off in Tarapoto?

The quality that Ramón possessed, and for which he was widely known and recognized throughout Tarapoto, was his propensity and willingness to offer what interlocutors termed *la colaboración*. Collaboration was an ethos that lexicalizes an imagined and idealized social order in which a "collaborator" assumes an important—through frequently underrecognized—role in creating opportunities and inspiring others to direct goods, resources, and/ or opportunities to others deemed to be in need. As opposed to a relational system that privileges the mediation of redistributive processes between unequal dyads (i.e., clientelism and patronage), collaboration is a triadic system that emphasizes the creation of redistributive social relationships.[2] And for some gay and transgender individuals, the route to becoming known as a collaborator involved the organization of large, popular, and spectacular activities like beauty contests, sports tournaments, and informal fundraisers. Thus, when someone from his neighborhood was seeking collaboration— such as the woman who sought to bring her *travesti* sister to Tarapoto for her HIV treatment—someone like Ramón was an obvious person to make or facilitate the connections that could help.

## Interventions in Social Conditions

The idea that specific adverse social conditions—primarily the experience of discrimination and stigma—contributed to the concentration of HIV among key populations was virtually axiomatic for HIV prevention throughout the 2010s. Consequently, HIV prevention efforts in urban Amazonian Peru emphasized the auspicious goal of transforming social conditions and strengthening communities.[3] This approach was certainly not without evidence: improving social conditions and empowering communities could result in effective HIV prevention, especially in combination with other strategies.[4] This translated into a plethora of models, recommendations, and strategies, which in and of itself is laudable and crucially important. And yet despite the universal recognition that the social world was a significant site for intervention, there was often a paucity of recommendations for how to make sense of or understand the existing social conditions that, apparently, necessitated change in the first place.[5] Sometimes it seemed as though notions of what constituted the social and what made a community were thought to be simply self-evident.

Conversely, this chapter considers the idea that what constitutes a community is not always so self-evident or obvious. If one of the central conceits of HIV prevention interventions was to enact social change, this chapter takes a step back and more specifically names, describes, and theorizes how gay and transgender communities in Tarapoto created a robust, communal social life amid and alongside the introduction of HIV prevention projects purporting to strengthen their communities. Drawing inspiration from the classic anthropological insight that communities are constituted by culturally defined forms of social relations, I describe and typify a subset of social relations that constituted gay and transgender social life in urban Amazonian Peru—namely, the social relations that individuals cultivated with one another and the strategic relations they cultivated with local municipal officials. As described in chapter 1, interlocutors spent a considerable amount of time discussing and maintaining their romantic and sexual relations with *maperos* through their stories about *peches*; this chapter's example of Ramón and his soccer tournament emphasizes another set of social relations that constituted their community, focusing specifically on his efforts to organize a gay and transgender soccer tournament that took place over the course of five weekends. Ramón's experiences planning the tournament, recruiting participants and sponsors, and interfacing with the municipal government vividly illustrate the enactment of collaborative social relations and his ambitious trajectory toward assuming a reputation as someone whom interlocutors might call a collaborator. By creating opportunities for collaboration to occur through organizing well-attended and popular activities, and for stories to circulate about them, activity organizers like Ramón transformed potentially scandalous episodes into foundational sites for enacting and multiplying collaborative relations throughout their community.

## Ramón's Trajectory

Ramón had already earned a reputation in the Morales district and throughout Tarapoto as a responsible and popular person who could organize events and bring together a crowd or an audience. Those who sought a favor from the *joven* Ramón—NGO workers who needed seats filled in a capacity-building workshop, municipal politicians who wanted help packing an event, or neighbors who sought to cover unexpected financial burdens through a *pollada* fundraiser or to help mediate communication with a gay or trans family member—often turned to him for support in their efforts. And he was typically easy to find. During the day, he tended the convenience store at the entrance of his family's house just a few blocks from the main plaza of the Morales district. In the afternoons and evenings, he could be found at the empty field three blocks from his house, where gay and transgender volleyball players congregated nearly every day to play volleyball in front of crowds of spectators. Ramón did not play volleyball particularly well, admitting that he played only when the crowds had left and there was less pressure to win, but he loved watching the sport and cheering on his friends. If the mayor, a nightclub owner, or a prospective political candidate showed up at this field, they were probably there to find Ramón and ask a favor. In the meantime, they might also enjoy watching the volleyball, betting on their favorite team, or snacking on a grilled plantain sold by the neighborhood women who set up grills around the periphery of the volleyball court.

Ramón had some experience with the Global Fund's HIV prevention projects in Tarapoto. At one point he had been contracted for a few months as a community health promoter: he received a small stipend to help gay and transgender individuals get tested for HIV and help them access treatment and healthcare (which at this point in the mid-2010s was ensured by the state). However, this gig as a health promoter was intermittent and entirely dependent on factors far outside of his control, such as which nongovernmental organization in Lima was selected as the principal recipient of the funding and who was coordinating the programming in the Amazonian

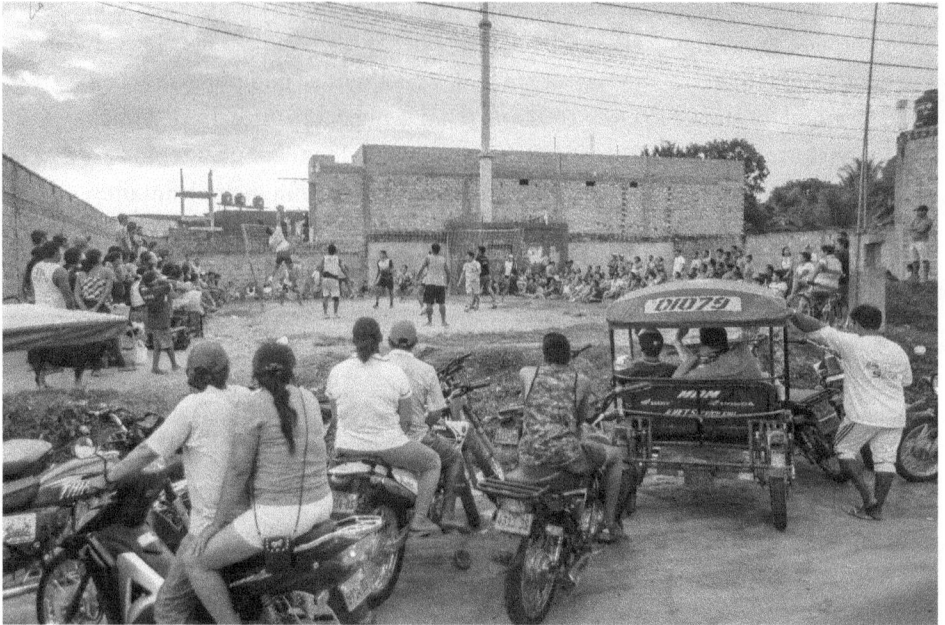

**Figure 2.1.** An empty field near Ramón's house becomes a vibrant volleyball court every afternoon. (Photograph by Marlon del Aguila Guerrero)

region. He did credit this experience as helping him decide to pursue a bachelor's degree in psychology at a local university. As he progressed in his course of study and began to excel among his classmates, he found that this helped him personally come more to terms with his own journey living with HIV. Since he was ten to fifteen years older than most of the other students in his classes, he said it was important as well for him to be a positive role model. For this reason, he was very public about his personal and intimate life—on social media, in the classroom, and to his teachers. He often talked explicitly about his boyfriend, for example, and explained that he wanted young people to see that one could be HIV positive and have a fulfilling romantic life.

The messages he was learning in his studies, alongside what he had been learning in his personal journey through HIV treatment and professional opportunities in HIV prevention, were swirling in his head when he came up with the idea to hold a soccer tournament. While perhaps not specifically referencing studies that show how social support and feelings of communal belonging can reduce risk-taking behavior and increase adherence to antiretroviral therapy among vulnerable or stigmatized populations, Ramón imagined that such an event might foster camaraderie, friendship, and belonging among those vulnerable to HIV in Morales and all of Tarapoto.

## Social Metrics

Ramón's idea of organizing a gay and transgender soccer tournament had precedent in Tarapoto. Before the introduction of large-scale funding for the establishment and formalization of gay and transgender community-based organizations through the Global Fund, popular public spectacles and activities—especially beauty contests and sports tournaments—were central sites of collective social life.[6] While these activities were sometimes put on by formal organizations, they were primarily staged by gay and transgender individuals like Ramón. Many of the well-known and respected figures in the community—those who had "won their name," including Martín and Salomé—had done so by organizing popular spectacles like soccer tournaments, volleyball tournaments, and beauty contests. These individuals also organized LGBT Pride parades or coordinated the participation of LGBT participants in other parades, like those commemorating municipal anniversaries or national holidays (Perez 2020). Salomé, for example, organized Miss Gay Carnival every year.[7] Even during the period when she migrated to Buenos Aires, she continued to be the primary sponsor of the event. But what exactly made an activity popular for gay and transgender people (as well as the broader community), and what expectations would they have for it? What kind of concepts did they use to make sense of and talk about these social spectacles? As Ramón aspired to continue winning a name for himself in the community, what did he need to consider as ingredients for a successful soccer tournament?

The larger, public events put on by well-known gay and transgender organizers—and often featuring gay or transgender participants or competitors—were generally integrated into the local popular entertainment scene, and attendance was not limited to gay or transgender people. However, they typically were the primary audience. And apart from being organized by gay or transgender individuals and mostly featuring gay or transgender competitors, what these activities generally had in common was that they aligned with a set of social expectations generally held about them: *la convocatoria, la colaboración*, and *el escándalo*. These interconnected qualities formed the basis for how any given activity was talked about and perceived, both by other gay or trans individuals and by the broader community, and whether it was considered successful or worth attending again in the future. In other words, these qualities made up the social metrics that were used to evaluate the activity itself and the person who organized it. Consistently organizing activities perceived to possess these qualities was how to "win a name" for oneself.[8]

First and foremost, an activity had to be announced and made public, so that interested parties could sign up to participate, compete, or simply attend. Any given activity could potentially have or lack *la convocatoria*, or convocation, depending on how the turnout for an event was perceived by others. If an activity organizer performed a successful convocation, it meant that they had effectively publicized and promoted the event and the result was high attendance. This special ability to convoke was a positive value, and many gay and transgender activity organizers were seen as being not just able to put on an activity with good convocation but also able to put on an activity that possessed the ineffable quality of *la acogida*, a sense of warmth or welcoming. So while convocation referred to the act of promoting or publicizing an activity, a good or poor convocation reflected both the activity itself and the capacity of the organizer to convoke. The *convocatoria* of a given activity was almost always discussed informally after it happened, becoming a moral value used to determine whether the activity (and any scandal that may or may not have occurred) had been worth the effort.

It was imperative for an activity to be seen as offering opportunities to collaborate, and the activity's organizer had to maintain an image of a "collaborator." The ethos of *la colaboración* entailed not just the distribution of goods or resources to those who were less fortunate; the organizer also had to create opportunities and inspire others to contribute resources. This quality is best illustrated through an informal fundraising activity known as a *pollada*.[9] When someone confronted unexpected healthcare costs or funeral expenses, for example, they might organize, or ask someone to organize for them, a *pollada*. The organizer sells tickets in advance, and people who buy tickets can pick up pieces of grilled chicken on the scheduled date. A well-organized and successful *pollada* provides entertainment and alcohol sales as well, which can greatly contribute to the funds raised. A *pollada* illustrates the two prongs of collaboration: it was not just about channeling resources to the person in need but also about creating opportunities for others to contribute and establish their own relation of collaboration with the person in need. The greater the capacity of the organizer to promote *la convocatoria*, the greater the possibility to proliferate new and more relations of redistributive collaboration. Gay and transgender individuals typically expected that other popular activities like sports tournaments or beauty contests, though not specifically intended to raise money, still generated opportunities to participate in collaboration with others.[10] Connecting a prospective contestant or competitor to a sponsor, for example, was one way in which the organizer created and sustained relations of collaboration through their event. Holding a raffle for baskets of school supplies or food items during an activity was another way an organizer could show their collaborative intentions. Creating opportunities for this particular vision of collaboration was, for all intents and purposes, seen as an ethical obligation for an activity organizer.

And finally, inherent in any successful, compelling, and popular event was the possibility of *el escándalo*—that is, that some scandalous episode might ensue and form the basis for the creation and circulation of a scandalous story. Scandalousness encompassed that which was considered loud, noisy, excessive, or transgressive of the norms of decorum. In taking over and laying claim to public spaces such as a central plaza, a park, or streets, activities like soccer tournaments and beauty contests by their very nature could be seen as scandalous. But that was not all; perhaps the wrong contestant might be crowned winner of the beauty contest, or perhaps something might happen during a soccer game to merit comment and fascination.[11] No one could know exactly what might occur that could become a scandal, but the very possibility of a scandal enticed many to attend these activities and thus contributed to a successful *convocatoria*. Most importantly, scandal was an essential part of the vernacular through which gay and transgender individuals remembered, evaluated, and dramatized an activity through subsequent stories about it. A story about a particular activity was worth telling if it had some element of scandal.

As they animated collective social life through their spectacles and activities, organizers like Ramón prepared to strike a delicate balance between *la convocatoria*, *la colaboración*, and *el escándalo*. As Ramón set out to organize a month-long soccer tournament, he had to keep all of this in mind in order to build on and extend his growing reputation as an effective and responsible activity organizer in the community.

### Multiplying Collaboration through Sponsorship

One of Ramón's first tasks was to find a space to hold the soccer tournament. In the initial stages of his imagining the activity, he envisioned a *cancha*, or field, that could accommodate multiple concurrent soccer games and crowds of spectators in the hundreds. While there were several possible options in Tarapoto for such a spectacle, his ambitions were immediately tempered by several constraints. The ideal option was one of the several large *recreos*, or recreational facilities, located around the western and eastern peripheries of urban Tarapoto. Popular family destinations on the weekends, these *recreos* were multipurpose facilities that had pools, soccer fields, volleyball courts, and restaurants. They could be rented out for events like wedding receptions, wedding anniversary celebrations, school reunions, graduation parties, or quinceañeras. Several of the more popular *recreos* converted into nightclubs in the evenings. Because some gay and transgender individuals had a reputation in the community for organizing quinceañeras or celebrations for others, some activity organizers had established working relationships with the owners of *recreos*. Consequently, these *recreos* were common venues for activities like beauty contests and sports tournaments that were part of collective gay and transgender social life in the region.

Ramón had not yet established a sufficient name and reputation in the community to have the confidence and trust of *recreo* owners. Weekends were the most popular time for the semirural recreational facilities scattered along the edges of Tarapoto; it would present a risk to an owner to allow an organizer to reserve the facility without knowing if the organizer's event could generate a large crowd. So from the outset this option was cost-prohibitive. Ramón did not expect to generate profits from alcohol sales during the daytime soccer tournament to cover the cost of these facilities, nor did he have the down payment necessary to reserve an entire Sunday, let alone the series of Sundays that he was imagining for the tournament. A second, more economical option involved renting a smaller artificial turf soccer field. These privately owned fields were squeezed into residential lots throughout Tarapoto and Morales. Groups could reserve them by the hour, and these fields were particularly attractive because they featured sufficient lighting to play at night. The drawbacks of renting one of these facilities, however, was that they were designed for *fulbito*, a scaled-back version of soccer with fewer players on the field, and did not have the space to accommodate large numbers of spectators. Because the number of spectators was limited, it was uncommon for gay and transgender community activities to occur in one of these facilities.

Faced with these constraints and limits, Ramón turned to his neighbor and mentor Wilmer to think through other ideas. Wilmer owned a popular and successful salon in Morales, located just around the corner from the central plaza of the Morales district. Even if his salon was busy, it was very easy to drop in and hang out there. Keeping clients thoroughly entertained as they were waiting for their hair treatment to finish or simply waiting for their turn was key to the salon's success. And even if Wilmer was occupied, Veronica, a young trans hairstylist who also worked at Wilmer's salon, might be sharing stories, catching up those gathered on the latest gossip, or providing running commentary on whatever was happening on the television.

Wilmer was easily convinced by the idea of holding a soccer tournament to promote solidarity and friendship and came to fully support Ramón's initiative. Wilmer offered his family's *chacra*, or small farm, as the site for the soccer tournament. It needed to be cleaned up and staged in order to be ready for the event, but it had a large, covered patio, plenty of shade, and two large fields that could be used for soccer and volleyball. Even better, Ramón would not have to come up with a down payment to reserve the dates, or even pay for the rental of the space. Rather, they worked out an agreement in which Wilmer's family would oversee the sale of alcohol throughout the days of the tournament and be entitled to the profits. Veronica volunteered to be the announcer throughout the tournament, a role that perfectly aligned with her skills of entertaining clients at the salon with jokes, stories, and gossip.

The agreement that Wilmer and Ramón struck to determine the location of the soccer tournament exemplifies how the concepts of *la colaboración* and *la convocatoria* animated social relations. The agreement hinged on Wilmer's confidence that Ramón could continue to draw a large crowd over each successive date of the soccer tournament. As an organizer, Ramón's capacity to generate *convocatoria* was key for Wilmer and his family to be able to recoup the costs of staging and maintaining the site for the tournament. Likewise, the gesture by Wilmer to open his family's small farm to the rest of the community was generous: it suggested that while Wilmer and his family were comparatively well off, they were still willing to collaborate with those who were not. This is a key component of a collaborative mode of social relations. In multiplying new relations between Wilmer and those who participated in or attended the tournament, Ramón played a key role as a generator of collaborative relations. Rather than mediate the redistribution of resources, as in the case of clientelism or patronage, activity organizers like Ramón sought to multiply relations.

### Recruiting Teams and Sponsors with Hugo

After the initial setbacks as he began planning the soccer tournament, Ramón found his original ambitions reignited by Wilmer's sponsorship. Liberated from constraints of space and the need to accumulate enough money to reserve a location for the tournament, Ramón shifted his attention from basic logistics to strategizing how to draw a large crowd and entertain them. To do so, he extended an invitation to Hugo to co-organize the soccer tournament.

Hugo had already established a reputation in Tarapoto as the organizer of the annual Miss Gay San Juan beauty contest. In his late twenties at the time, Hugo already was known throughout the city to be an effective activity organizer. As he recounted to me in an interview, his trajectory had begun when he was just eighteen and working in a salon as a hair stylist. He used to cut the hair of Carlos Philco, who at the time of my fieldwork was the mayor of the Morales district. However, back in 2010, during Philco's first mayoral campaign, the future mayor invited the young Hugo to join his campaign by running on his ticket as a *regidor*, or city councilperson. After organizing a successful and well-attended Miss Gay beauty contest under the auspices of his campaign, Philco included Hugo on his election ticket as the fifth *regidor*. Though Philco's first campaign was not successful, Hugo found his calling in the process. He realized that he enjoyed organizing Miss Gay San Juan so much that he decided to continue to do it going forward.

At first Hugo was reluctant to join Ramón in this endeavor. For one, they did not know each other that well. Ramón knew of Hugo more from his reputation as the organizer of beauty contests. And Hugo felt that his experience organizing beauty contests was limited. However, once Ramón convinced him that his experience could be applied to organizing a soccer tournament and recruiting participants, he became enthusiastic about it. With Hugo on board, they decided that the soccer tournament would have two different divisions—a "women's division" and the "*machomenos* division."[12] At first the specifics of these divisions were not fully determined, and this became a topic of debate later as the tournament progressed. However, the decision to organize two different divisions was innovative and reflected a vision and commitment to community integration on the part of Ramón and Hugo. While it was common to organize and publicize a so-called *machomenos* soccer tournament, featuring primarily gay and trans participants, the idea of combining such a tournament with a cisgender women's division was novel.

With two different divisions, the next steps—recruiting teams and securing prize sponsorships—required different strategies. To recruit teams for the women's division, Ramón and Hugo approached the Morales municipal office to get a list of the mothers' clubs and Vaso de Leche food-assistance associations that receive support through municipal social services.[13] With the municipal lists, they went door-to-door each morning throughout Morales asking if members of the various associations would be willing to form a team to compete in the soccer tournament. Hugo recalled this recruitment to be a tremendous effort but found it worth the time because they were able to get ten teams to sign up for the women's division. Ramón further explained that including the participants from the mothers' clubs further contributed to his goal of community integration and that, strategically, it would help generate more official support from the municipality for the tournament.

Recruiting teams for the *machomenos* division, however, required a different strategy. The municipality did not have lists of groups and associations of gay and transgender people. Social media and word of mouth, they thought, were more effective in informing people of the opportunity and recruiting them to sign up. The primary strategy, however, was to approach potential "sponsors" for teams. Ideal sponsors were local business owners who would recruit their own players and pay for team uniforms. The team would likely bear the business's name, and throughout the tournament the businesses would receive publicity from announcements over the speakers. Gay and trans beauty salon owners were the majority of the sponsors for this particular event, although a local gym, a dance studio, and a cellphone accessory store also sponsored teams.[14] Hugo's experience recruiting sponsors for Miss Gay San Juan proved to be particularly helpful in this regard. The opportunities created for local business owners to sponsor a team (or, in the case of a beauty contest, to sponsor a contestant) again demonstrated the role that activity organizers like Hugo and Ramón played in creating collaborative relationships between others. In this case, the soccer tournament provided the pretext for better-off business owners to support younger, soccer-playing participants, including housing those who traveled from cities outside of Tarapoto to participate. For Ramón and Hugo, earning a name and reputation in the community meant finding sponsors who would collaborate with the potential participants.

## Collaboration with the Municipality

The qualities associated with gay and transgender organizers and their activities—specifically, being able to convoke large numbers of people and creating opportunities to extend collaborative relationships with them—were qualities that local politicians saw as useful in their campaigns and, once elected, as necessary for maintaining their positions or even sometimes rehabilitating their image with the community. As the story of Hugo's path to organizing the Miss Gay San Juan beauty contest demonstrated, the dynamic could be mutually beneficial: aspiring politicians looked favorably on such large spectacles, and individual organizers could demonstrate their logistical capacities. Municipal governments could be pivotal allies in securing prizes for the event that would incentivize others to participate in the soccer tournament or beauty contest in the first place. However, it required considerable work and advocacy to secure support from municipal offices.

Thanks to Wilmer's foresight, Ramón and Hugo had planned the soccer tournament to align with the municipal anniversary. The municipality always had a budget for community activities, but this budget especially supported activities during the weeks of the municipal anniversary and patron saint celebrations. Rámon and Hugo scheduled a meeting with Felix, a municipal agent in charge of social development, to request sponsorship for a prize in the tournament. This was, at first, an intense conversation. As Ramón and Hugo recounted, Felix expressed several reservations about a *machomenos* soccer tournament during the municipal anniversary celebration. First Felix asked them why they wanted to work only with sexual minorities and not alongside the rest of society. To this point, Ramón and Hugo had an immediate response: they were, in fact, organizing two divisions precisely to integrate the so-called sexual minorities with the "rest of society." In fact, they reminded him, they were working with local mothers' groups to recruit teams for the women's division of the tournament. Then, they recalled, Felix asked why gay and transgender communities focused solely on the fight against preventing HIV/AIDS at the expense of other issues.[15]

At this point, Ramón recounted, he opened up more about his own experience to Felix. It was not the first time Ramón had encountered these viewpoints, and he came prepared to discuss them. He shared details of his experience living with HIV as a gay man and explained that a soccer tournament could have considerable impact for improving the experiences of others who were either living with HIV or vulnerable to it. Even though he was not organizing this activity under the auspices of the Global Fund's project, Ramón's story proved effective, and the municipal government agreed to sponsor a prize for the soccer tournament. In addition to the prize, the winning soccer teams would participate in the parade that culminated the municipal anniversary celebrations.[16]

Ramón and Hugo convinced the municipal administrators that they could be effective organizers, putting on a series of events that could bring together large numbers of people and provide them entertainment over the course of the municipal anniversary celebration. For the municipality, providing financial support for the tournament from the municipal budget was a very small price to pay for the goodwill and public entertainment that a gay and trans soccer tournament could generate, alongside the other activities that were part of the typical anniversary celebrations. And although Ramón and Hugo would still need to seek sponsorship for additional prize money, this was an excellent way to make inroads with the municipality and, as Ramón had desired all along, foster social belonging and camaraderie among the groups most vulnerable to HIV.

## Debating Divisions

With the teams signed up, sponsorship of teams and prizes secured, and the fields on Wilmer's small family farm cleaned up and converted into a *cancha*, or soccer field, Ramón and Hugo were ready for the soccer tournament. It took place over five consecutive Sundays through September and October. Each date was an all-day affair, and as the tournament progressed, the Sunday events became increasingly more popular. *Motocars* lined up along the sidelines to provide families a place to sit in the shade once the palm trees no longer provided enough shaded seating for the spectators. The soccer games began in the morning, and in the afternoon, once they had ended, impromptu volleyball games were organized and played until dark. The mothers' clubs organized food sales, setting up grills with plenty of grilled chicken and fish, plantains, and *juane,* a boiled mixture of rice, egg, and meat. Tasked with offering play-by-play commentary of the games, as well as entertaining the crowds during breaks, Veronica kept everyone's spirits uplifted with her sharp, funny, and completely over-the-top announcements over the loudspeakers. And when Veronica herself was playing, or when she needed a break, the most popular *cumbia* music of the moment was blasting.

The tournament proved to be a massive success. The energy and excitement were palpable, due in large part to the lengths Ramón and Hugo went to in order to create a welcoming environment and draw a large crowd. But another element contributed to the growing success and popularity of the tournament. That is, several scandals erupted, generating enough debate, conversation, and speculation to keep the soccer players, their family and friends, and anyone coming to the spectacle transfixed each week as they waited for the next round of the tournament. These scandalous stories circulated in beauty salons and parks around town and on popular local social media message boards. The stories speak to the dynamism of the scandal concept in communal social life. That is, while scandal could sometimes

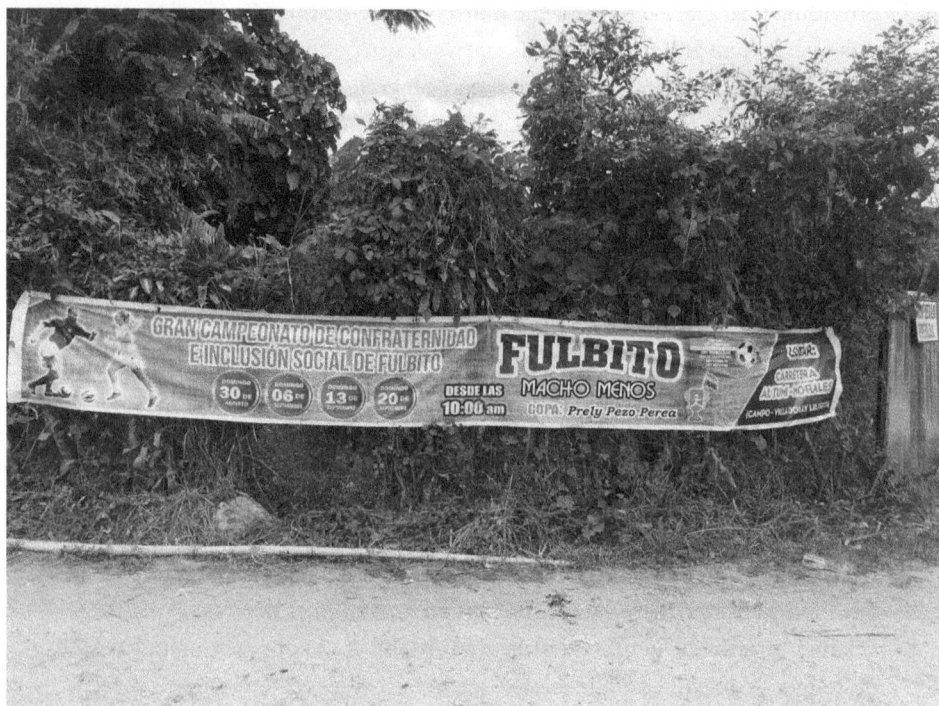

**Figure 2.2.** A banner advertising the *machomenos* soccer tournament.

sully the reputation of an event or activity, it could also animate it and make it feel exciting. During the soccer tournament, scandals became opportunities to bring more people in and integrate them into broader collective discussions about the contours of queer social life and the possibilities and limits of categories of sexual orientation and gender identity.[17] And this is what happened when a controversy ensued in the women's division of the soccer tournament.

After the first Sunday of the tournament, Las Galácticas, a team of lesbian mothers, emerged as a clear favorite to sweep the division. Some of the teams that had formed around the municipal mothers' clubs, however, complained to Ramón that the Las Galácticas team should be competing in the LGBT division. This complaint circulated to social media and became the first scandal to spark debate around the soccer tournament. When I swung by Ramon's store in the middle of the week to chat, he addressed the issue: "We have a scandal on our hands. Surely you have seen the posts about Las

Galácticas." As he workshopped aloud with me his ideas about how he would address the complaints in an announcement that he would make the following Sunday, he concluded that the complaints were lesbophobic. The vision of the soccer tournament was to promote belonging, and the mothers' clubs needed to learn how to integrate homo and hetero societies. And technically, he added, it was not the LGBT division but the *machomenos* division, so on those grounds alone he felt it would not be right to move Las Galácticas to the other division.

The ensuing controversy further revealed how the preoccupation with "right" and "wrong" categories is itself an everyday, lived dilemma.[18] The mothers' clubs that suggested that Las Galácticas play with the gay and transgender teams argued that it made more sense for them to be in the "LGBT division." The players of Las Galácticas, however, wished to continue competing in the "mothers' division," saying that since many of them were also mothers it made more sense for them to compete with the mothers' clubs. In calling the complaints and ensuing debate a "scandal," Ramón effectively made visible some of the nuanced social consequences of a scandal—it became an opportunity to make meaningful interventions on communal understandings of the categories of sexual orientation and gender identity. In this instance, the scandal over Las Galácticas was also a pedagogical opportunity to promote an antidiscrimination message to the large crowds gathered for the tournament. And as the scandal over the appropriate categories and divisions of the soccer tournament unfolded, it provided community members opportunities to articulate their sense of gender identity and sexual orientation, as well as the extent of their relationship to others who shared those identities and orientations or not.

It was also worth noting that there was no controversy about a "gay and transgender" division, or about who would be part of the *machomenos* division. In this instance, the trans players preferred to play on teams with the gay players. They were certainly aware of global debates about gender categories, particularly in sport. For example, nearly everyone was familiar with the transgender Brazilian volleyball player Tiffany Abreu, who came up as a subject of informal conversation and debate in beauty salons or in social media forums whenever Brazilian volleyball was on television.[19] So while some might have expected the terrain of the controversy to revolve around the category of gender (aligning heterosexual mothers, lesbian mothers, and transgender women into one division and gay men in the other), the rubric of motherhood came to determine, at least in Ramón's logic, who would compete in the women's division. Conversely, and likely as a result of the introduction of HIV prevention efforts in the community, the technical framework of "vulnerability to HIV" shaped his logic for the gay and transgender division. As they considered the imperfections of the categories at hand, the soccer tournament organizers, participants, and spectators debated and imagined the ongoing and emergent possibilities of sexual and gender selfhood. And while there continued to be disagreement and ambiguity over the specificities of each division, no team withdrew from the tournament, and the issue felt resolved by the following week. Las Galácticas returned on the second Sunday of the tournament to win their next game and, ultimately, continued their undefeated streak throughout the tournament.

## The War of the Salons

The scandal over which teams were to compete in which division had been virtually forgotten by the second tournament date, when discussion swirled around a new one: the "War of the Salons." Dubbed so by Veronica as she helmed the sonic atmosphere of the tournament through her ongoing commentary that day, the War of the Salons referred to the upcoming game between the team sponsored by Wilmer, Wilmer's Salon, versus the team sponsored by Claudia's salon, Queen Sofia Coiffure. On most tournament days Veronica had several messages to get across throughout the day: safety reminders, updates on what food was being sold and how much was left, and acknowledgments of the sponsors of the tournament prizes, including the municipality of Morales and "the *gringa* anthropologist Justin." However, on this day, she talked at length over the loudspeakers about the War of the Salons and commented that no one would want to miss out on this game. She listed the nicknames of the beloved gay and transgender players on both teams, including herself on this list because she was playing for the Wilmer Salon team. Her exaggerated descriptions of the other players were entertaining, and simply by calling the match the War of the Salons, she communicated that they were meant to be tongue-in-cheek.[20] Of course, there would be superior athleticism on display, but there might also be mishaps or scandals with so many well-known characters on the field at once.

The other games seemed to drag on as I and the rest of the crowd waited with excitement for the War of the Salons to commence. With so much buildup and excitement, Ramón anticipated that a scandal might erupt with this game. As soon as he took over the microphone from Veronica, who had to leave because she was playing in the game, he was quick to counter any potential allegations that the game had been "fixed" or "arranged." He reminded everyone that the match-ups had been drawn randomly and in public: even though the tournament was taking place on fields belonging to Wilmer's family, his team, Ramón assured the crowd, would receive no special treatment. Still, as I sat next to Axel and Norma and watched the game unfold, Axel presciently reminded us that "these things always end in scandal."

As the War of the Salons commenced, the game proved to be thrilling. Yesika, a young trans woman who had grown up in Tarapoto but lived in Lima most of the year, was back in town and had been recruited by Claudia to play for team Queen Sofia Coiffure. In the middle of the game, she decided to take off her shoes. No sooner had she taken her shoes off than the ball was passed her way. When she booted the ball down the field, her toenail came flying off. This forced her to sit out for the rest of the game. With a player down, the War of the Salons became palpably more intense. Wilmer's Salon had started out with more players on their team to begin with, and at this point Queen Sofia Coiffure was left with only four players on the field. As the game continued, Wilmer's Salon increased their lead, with the score 4–2 heading into the final minutes of the game. Wilmer called a time-out for the team, and in their meeting they decided to let Veronica play in the final minutes. Veronica, who had sat on the sidelines for most of the game, ran over to Norma and me, informed us she would be playing, and made a request: "*Gringa*," she said to me, "could you please record the game with your iPhone? In case I score a goal I want a video of it." This request was the result of ethnographic presence—after asking that I record interviews with individuals, that I take notes of meetings, and that I take pictures of events and activities, inevitably interlocutors also requested my recording capacities for the documentation of their own achievements. I got up from my comfortably shaded position on the sidelines, got closer to the field, and proceeded to record the remainder of the game with my phone.

As Axel predicted, the game ended with a scandal. Manuel, playing for Queen Sofia Coiffure, launched the ball toward the goal. Wilmer, who had put himself into the game as goalie for the final moments, moved toward the incoming ball. It ricocheted off his arm, appeared to hit the goalpost, and then went flying into the crowd gathered behind. The referee blew his whistle and signaled a corner kick, indicating that the ball had in fact not gone into the goal but rather had flown out of bounds after hitting Wilmer. With tensions already running high, the field erupted into a frenzy. Manuel ran over to the referee, pleading the case that it had been a goal. The rest

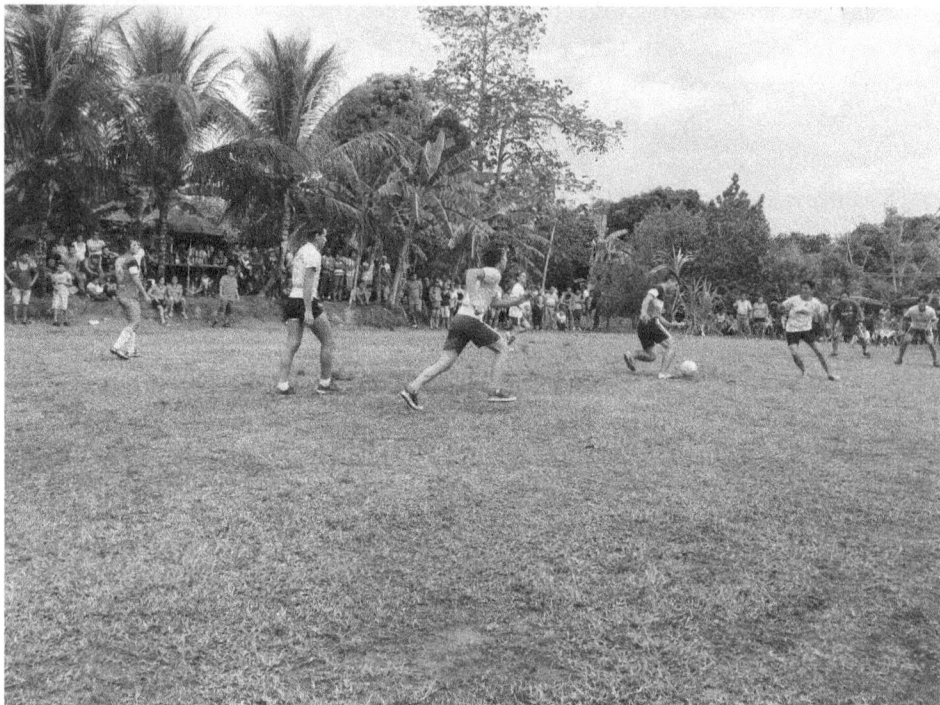

**Figure 2.3.** A crowd surrounds the soccer field to watch the War of the Salons.

of the Queen Sofia Coiffure team began leaving the field in protest over the injustice of the call. Ramon took to the microphone immediately, asking everyone to be patient and reminding them that the referee has the final decision. His entreaties had little effect, and so he continued, "If you leave the field or if you don't respect the referee, you will lose the game or be disqualified." The scandal continued on and on, with players from both teams wagging their fingers at each other, discussing the trajectory of the ball, pointing to where it had hit Wilmer and where it had hit the goalpost, and making their cases to the crowd as to whether or not this was a goal.

Eventually the players returned to the field and the War of the Salons drew to a close, with Wilmer Salon emerging victorious. Even though they ultimately lost, Queen Sofia Coiffure left the field having, in their eyes, saved face. Their on-field performance of indignation at the injustice of the referee's call, of having been robbed of the chance to tie the game and force a penalty kick round, contributed to their own narrative as underdogs for the rest of the tournament. It gave them a reason to come back the next week and prove their resilience and prowess. And it gave those who were following the tournament something to talk about through the upcoming week— whether it was a new reason to cheer for a team or a reason to disdain a team. It gave the spectators an opportunity to relate to the players in a new way—whom to cheer and root for, whom to bet on, and, possibly, whom to sponsor or collaborate with in a future tournament. Most did not disapprove of the scandal thrown by the losing team, again pointing to the dynamism of the concept. A scandal can be justified in the face of an injustice; it can be merited when no other options are available to rectify a perceived wrong. This will be significant in a later chapter for contextualizing why some chose scandal as a strategy for responding to broader societal discrimination.

Having been asked to record the final minutes of the game on my phone, I held in my possession the only video recording of the goal. My ethnographic presence, in this moment, brought another dimension to the tournament, to the breadth of the scandal, and to the dialogue and debate that ensued throughout the following week. As soon as the game concluded, Veronica came over to where I was and asked to see a replay of the goal moment. She proceeded to meticulously inspect the three seconds of video showing the goal, endlessly pausing and inspecting the trajectory of the blurry ball at each moment of the clip. She insisted I send her the clip—which I did—and as soon as I arrived back at my apartment that evening I found that the clip had been plastered all over social media. Veronica democratized the question of whether or not this was a goal by involving her countless followers on social media—and a seemingly endless thread of comments proved that it was truly up for debate. This debate extended into everyday discussion and commentary. When I went to hang out at Wilmer's salon later in the week, my phone was passed around so that people could see for themselves the original clip and determine whether or not Queen Sofia Coiffure had been robbed or if the Wilmer Salon team was the rightful victor. Of course, since I was at Wilmer's salon, opinions tended toward the latter.

The scandal contributed to the persistence of competition in the everyday social life of gay and transgender people in Tarapoto, whether in the form of sports like soccer and volleyball or in the form of beauty contests. At the everyday afternoon volleyball games played throughout the city, disputes over whether a ball landed in or out of bounds occurred weekly. Scenes of players storming off the court until everyone agreed to a replay or shouting over whether the ball hit the net or the opposing player happened all the time. And for this reason, gay and transgender people were sometimes dismissed or stereotyped as scandalous: too loud, too excessive, or too dramatic. But there was always something more going on with a scandal, something that exceeded the idea of a stereotype. Scandals, like the one on the soccer field during the War of the Salons match, make everyday activities continue and help everyone keep playing. Even those who might have lost a particular game can save face and return the next day, the next week, or the next month and still find a crowd to cheer them on. Stories about scandals sustained queer social relations and cohesion. They gave a narrative to compelling moments of collective social life and attracted the attention of the community, thus making possible the expansion of collaboration at activities like Ramón and Hugo's *machomenos* soccer tournament.

### Extending Collaborative Relations

The final day of the tournament was thrilling. The fields were packed full, as word of Ramón and Hugo's tournament continued to spread—no doubt with the help of a few scandals to entice the crowds. In addition to the championship games of both divisions, Ramón and Hugo organized raffles, live music, and performances for this day, and they invited local leaders and politicians to participate in the distribution of awards and prizes. Businesses, entities, and individuals who donated prizes and sponsored teams—including a local gym, several beauty salons, a regional LGBT community-based organization, the mayor of Morales, and *el antropólogo* Justin—received recognition and publicity throughout the day as Veronica continued to animate the sonic atmosphere of the event with her running commentary over the speakers. I focus on the dynamics and aspirations of two collaborators to show how expansive the relations produced through the activity could really be. The first example turns attention inward toward myself to consider how ethnographic relations were produced through the tournament. The second example examines how the mayor of Morales leveraged the opportunities for collaboration to reinvigorate his own image in the community. In both cases, the work of Ramón and Hugo, who organized the tournament, was vitally important.

Reflecting on my own role throughout the soccer tournament illustrates the expansiveness of the possibilities that Ramón and Hugo could create through their activities, even transforming and making new ethnographic relations possible. As Veronica announced the sponsors throughout the day, she consistently mentioned my title of anthropologist as a sign of respect and appreciation. But even those who were accorded respect were fair play for her comedic stylings. So when she outed me over the speakers as the "aficionado" who had recorded the infamous goal from the War of the Salons, or when she implored the crowd to not lose their money by betting on the volleyball team I was playing on later in the day because, she joked, the team I play on always loses, she deftly balanced parody and appreciation. But as she crafted exaggerated, over-the-top details and anecdotes about me, she was making sense for herself and for the community of how the anthropologist somehow could fit as a character into their shared social universe through the genre of scandalous storytelling. My willingness to "collaborate" vis-à-vis the space created by Ramón and Hugo for the tournament was an entry point into how gay and transgender interlocutors themselves had agency over crafting how I could fit into their world. The doors that collaboration opened for me, as an ethnographer, reinforced to me why others would find such social positioning compelling and meaningful.

After a long day of thrilling and emotional soccer games, the winners of the tournament were decided. Las Galácticas won the women's division, and the team La Bella y Las Bestias (Beauty and the Beasts) won the *macho-menos* division. Queen Sofia Coiffure ultimately came in second, followed in third place by their cosmetological rival, Wilmer Salon. As soon as the final soccer games ended, the crowds moved to the opposite end of the field, where a popular cumbia orchestra had set up on a stage and volleyball nets were put up. Over the live music, Ramón took to the stage to announce the final prize ceremony. First up, however, was a raffle. "Thanks to the goodwill of the municipality of Morales and our mayor, Carlos Philco," Ramón explained, "we will raffle school supplies and baskets of basic food items to the *madres de familia* who came to play in the tournament." This appeared to be a crowd-pleasing moment, as different groups cheered wildly when one of their own was selected as a recipient of a new backpack or food basket.

Carlos Philco, the mayor of the district of Morales from 2015 to 2019, was himself an eccentric figure. By the time he became mayor, he was typically perceived as a *figureti*: a person who sought attention at all costs, no matter the mockery that might result. His antics were extensively covered in the local news media, and his tenure as the mayor of Morales had been fraught since the very beginning. One of his debut projects as mayor was to promote a small lake in the district as a tourist destination. In front of a crowd of journalists and media, he stripped off his clothes and jumped into the lake wearing only his underwear, intending to show off the lake's freshness. The scene ended up having an opposite effect, as his portly figure was lampooned by journalists, by local authorities, and on social media.[21] He had a public, ongoing struggle with the popular La Anaconda nightclub, often closing it arbitrarily and upsetting not just the owner but the entire economy of *motocar* drivers and food vendors that orbited the nightclub.[22] And when a group of council members resigned because he refused to attend meetings, he gave a press conference from his bed to address the allegations, which caused one council member to call his mayorship a "clown show."[23]

His eccentricities, however, did not distract the public from denouncing his alleged mismanagement of the district throughout his time as mayor. While he survived a recall campaign in 2016, he was castigated in the local media for allegedly engaging in corruption. Allegations ranged from not fulfilling agreements with unionized municipal employees to robbing social support programs like Vaso de Leche. Many of the campaign promises he had made, such as paving major roads and constructing bridges, never materialized.[24] Most crucially, though, was that in the months leading up to the *machomenos* tournament, it was alleged in popular media that he had used the municipality's petty cash account to pay for personal food costs. While this specific controversy ultimately passed, in 2019 he was found guilty of embezzlement and fraud and sentenced to four years in prison.[25] At any rate, he was confronting an image problem, and it was clear that the anniversary celebrations and the popular *machomenos* soccer tournament could be an opportunity to revitalize it.

After the raffle concluded, the awards were presented to the first-, second-, and third-place winners in each division. Ramón and Hugo had carefully curated a list of individuals to present the awards. Even though no specific instructions were given, each presenter said a few words about the issue of discrimination toward LGBT people and the importance of social inclusion. Because the municipality was one of the primary sources of financial collaboration, representatives from the municipal offices and the mayor were selected to award prizes. The symbolic message from the municipality was made most explicit by one of the representatives who awarded the second-place prize in the *machomenos* division:

> I am proud to be present with each one of you this marvelous afternoon. The second-place prize is for the team representing the salon Queen Sofia Coiffure. It is very well deserved. The mayor of our municipality of Morales, Carlos Philco, would like to recognize this team. As a representative of the municipality, we give this prize to Queen Sofia Coiffure, to communicate to all the members of this community that the municipality is opening its doors for support

and inclusion. It is true that we have been working with every one of them, supporting them in what is necessary. The municipality does not discriminate against anybody and we are here, present, at this sports event.

The mayor showed his collaboration with the local community and displayed a gesture of goodwill through the awarding of prizes. It was not that this was a revisionary, or even radically divergent, image of the mayor, far different from the one often splashed across the pages of the local periodicals or made visible by his antics in viral videos. Rather, just as the tournament was coming to a close and the mayor found himself at the center of swirling allegations of financial mismanagement and corruption, he drew on the opportunities for collaboration created by Ramón and Hugo. Their capacity to create *convocatoria*, a skill that Carlos Philco had long ago recognized and appreciated in Hugo when he asked him to organize a trans beauty contest for his first mayoral campaign, further made possible the gesture of collaboration through the raffles and prizes that Ramón and Hugo staged at the end of the tournament.

### Constituting Community through Collaboration

A fundamental conceit of HIV prevention in the "end of AIDS" era was that social conditions contributed to vulnerability and thus played a significant role in shaping the transmission of HIV. For the groups most vulnerable to HIV in urban Amazonian Peru—men who have sex with men, gay men, and transgender women—the specific social conditions most frequently named as the culprit were discrimination and stigma. Consequently, preventing HIV and ending AIDS obligated fundamental transformations to their social world. But what kind of social world did they inhabit? Were discrimination and stigma all-encompassing? How did gay and trans people make do amid the very conditions that made possible such drastic inequalities with regard to HIV/AIDS? Discrimination and stigma existed alongside a rich relational world for gay and transgender people. This chapter contends that the effort to intervene in the social conditions of a community is strengthened by broadening the conceptual vocabulary for understanding how individuals relate to each other.

To that end, Ramón's journey through organizing and carrying out the *machomenos* soccer tournament made visible an important class of social relations existing among gay and transgender communities in Tarapoto.

Alongside the relations individuals cultivated with potential romantic partners, close analysis of the tournament made visible the varying social relations that not only made the activity possible but also could emerge as a result of it. Tournament organizers, participants, and spectators shared moral, idealized visions of how they related to one another and how they related to their broader community. Through spectacles that could bring together and entice large crowds with the promise of a possible scandal, Ramón and Hugo produced sites for the creation and multiplication of social relations that interlocutors called "collaborative"—that is, an idealized, positive social relation that involved creating opportunities and inspiring others to give goods or resources to those who may be less well-off or in need. And Ramón and Hugo typified the unique role that some gay and transgender activity organizers played in creating a broader relational, redistributive landscape that constantly extended the invitation to others to collaborate.

Following Ramón and Hugo closely through the process of organizing and implementing has exemplified the unique role activity organizers played in animating the vibrant and communal queer social life in and around Tarapoto. This was a world in which relations with romantic partners, with other queer people, with municipal leaders and politicians, and with members of the broader community were forged and reproduced. And it was into this vibrant social world—of collaborating, of scandal-making, of storytelling—that globalized ideas about ending AIDS were ultimately inserted over the decade of the 2010s. In the next chapter, we will continue to follow Ramón as he, alongside Yesika, interfaced more directly with HIV prevention efforts and drew on the tools and strategies learned as a result of the capacity-building workshops funded by HIV prevention efforts. The chapter will follow their efforts to denounce an instance of discrimination that Yesika experienced one night after the soccer tournament at a local nightclub. As a consequence of the new opportunities presented to community leaders and organizers by large-scale, internationally funded HIV prevention projects, some existing social relations based on expectations of collaboration broke down, while new relations emerged.

# 3

## Scandal at the Disco

Discrimination, Difference,
and the Cultivation
of a Culture of Denouncement

The mitigation of discrimination and stigma—especially discrimination on the basis of sexual orientation and gender identity—was an essential strategy for preventing HIV among gay and transgender communities in Peru. This prioritization of discrimination was not unique to Peru's HIV/AIDS response; it was reinforced by a long-acknowledged tenet that discrimination and stigma often emerge as barriers across the HIV prevention and care continuum, and it came from broader emphases on inclusive, rights-based approaches in the global effort to end AIDS.[1] In Peru, the unequal burden of HIV/AIDS affecting primarily gay, transgender, and MSM populations was regarded, to varying degrees, as a consequence of the discrimination and stigma that impacted their lives.[2] As a result, antidiscrimination efforts became a key component of comprehensive HIV prevention. Models about discrimination and stigma among communities living with and vulnerable to HIV/AIDS tend to frame discrimination and stigma as preexisting social conditions that impact, or "determine," the health "outcome" of HIV infection. However, one limit of this overarching model is that the practice of contesting or denouncing discrimination is typically conceptualized almost exclusively as an after-the-fact "intervention" introduced in vulnerable communities as a result of externally funded global health or international development projects. In this chapter, I proceed from a fundamentally different assumption: that antidiscrimination itself was as intrinsically a part of everyday queer life in urban Amazonian Peru as the conditions and experiences of discrimination and stigma. Co-authoring and circulating dramatized—sometimes scandalous—stories about their experiences of discrimination underscored the determination, zeal, and agency that gay and transgender communities in urban Amazonian Peru possessed to make widely and publicly known (that is, to denounce) the discrimination and injustice they encountered in their lives. At its core, this chapter is about how gay and trans interlocutors experienced and storied discrimination *and* antidiscrimination simultaneously.

This is not to contend that HIV prevention programs did not have profound material effects in the region in terms of advancing antidiscrimination. Initiatives associated with the Global Fund spurred passage in the region of several municipal and regional antidiscrimination ordinances that included protections for sexual orientation and gender identity, mandated the development of a technical system for documenting and tracking instances of discrimination, and were supplemented by trainings to help gay and transgender people to identify instances of discrimination in their everyday lives and to file formal grievances with the appropriate authorities. One of the most significant measures was the introduction and dissemination of a protocol for filing formal discrimination grievances called the Sistema de Defensorías Comunitarias, or the System of Community Protection.[3] Colloquially, project organizers, technical assistants, and community health promotors referred to these collective antidiscrimination efforts as an abstract project in cultivating *una cultura de denuncia*, or a culture of denouncement. In other words, the goal of preventing new cases of HIV among gay and trans communities pivoted on the capacity of individuals to narrate their specific experiences of discrimination through the administrative and bureaucratic process of filing formal discrimination grievances. Doing so meant having or possessing a culture of denouncement, and, regardless of the context or space of the incident, this notion was central to imaginings about the future possibility of ending AIDS. Embedded in the idea of cultivating a culture of denouncement as a means of preventing HIV was, importantly, the assumption that a shared and collective contestation of discrimination (i.e., the culture of denouncement) could become manifest in vulnerable populations only through an external intervention.

Gay and transgender communities in Tarapoto circulated and shared compelling and dynamic stories about their everyday experiences of discrimination that sometimes transcended the formal administrative procedures that HIV prevention programs intended for them to use. In fact, in their stories, the very process of filing a formal grievance about discrimination became an extension to their ongoing stories about seeking justice and redress. To analyze these stories, I first describe how the System of Community Protection was developed in urban Amazonian Peru and offer a close reading of the phrase that was most associated with the system's central ambition: the "culture of denouncement" among the gay and transgender communities across the region. Crucially, I interpret the concept of "culture" within a longer, colonial history of ethno-racial hierarchies and modes of creating and sustaining social differences. As I listened to the stories of and accompanied several interlocutors engaging in the process of responding to their experiences of discrimination and attempting to take action and denounce injustice, I show how the obligation to denounce discrimination through formal grievances—though intended to improve the lives of gay and transgender people—in practice paradoxically intensified entrenched forms of social hierarchy and differentiation.

I found that many stories about everyday experiences of discrimination centered around episodes in which an individual (typically a trans individual) was denied entry into a popular nightclub or disco. These stories circulated both among interlocutors themselves as well as in popular media, possessing what anthropologist Ellen Moodie terms the "double quality" of being "both about the world and part of it" (2010, 9). Stories about discrimination at the disco resonated because they spoke to the everyday experiences of gay and transgender people in urban Amazonian Peru, reflecting how discrimination was a widely lived experience and part of their world. But they were also powerfully about that world. The very circulation of these stories through informal means was also a way of contesting and denouncing discrimination, even if the stories were not administratively formalized or collected. To describe this double quality, I develop a theoretical distinction between "emblematic denouncement" and "scandalous denouncement."

Some stories were invoked in HIV prevention settings as exemplary cases of denouncement that ought to be modeled by gay and transgender people in their day-to-day lives. The story of Godfrey, a trans woman who was denied entry into a popular, upscale nightclub in Lima and successfully filed a formal grievance, was one well-known case that circulated in Tarapoto as an emblematic example. On the other hand, I also heard stories and examples of discrimination—many not too different from the version of discrimination encountered by Godfrey—that never became formal discrimination grievances. Following feminist and queer theorist Sara Ahmed, I give these complaints "a hearing" (Ahmed 2021, 3). Through a framework attentive to intersectional forms of difference—including ethno-racial hierarchies, gendered difference between gay men and transgender women, and class-based distinctions—I analyze the varying axes of social differentiation that impacted how some gay and transgender people responded to the imperative to identify discrimination and seek redress.[4] As interlocutors like Yesika, Pamela, Norma, and Martín animated abstract ideas about discrimination and HIV prevention in their everyday lives, their scandalous stories reveal not just the pervasiveness of the multiple forms of difference that they encountered but also how they reconfigured the directives of HIV prevention on their own terms. In doing so, discrimination and antidiscrimination are rendered not simply as static "conditions" and "outcomes" but rather as synchronous experiences lived within profoundly entrenched social hierarchies and modes of differentiation.[5]

### The System of Community Protection

Even before the introduction of Global Fund projects in the region, the effects of HIV/AIDS-related discrimination and stigma were long palpable for gay and transgender communities. The first LGBT collective in Tarapoto, the Movimiento Homosexual de Tarapoto (MHOTA), was formalized in 1998 as a peer health organization providing HIV prevention services in coordination with the Peruvian Ministry of Health.[6] Well into the second decade of the global HIV/AIDS epidemic, and after the introduction of lifesaving combination therapies, elder interlocutors typically recalled that the first cases of HIV/AIDS they remembered in Tarapoto emerged in the late 1990s, *after* the more intense period of violence in the region associated with the armed conflict had subsided.[7] Anderson, who was just beginning his career in activism and advocacy then, recalled that many of the first cases in Tarapoto were of gay and trans migrants who left Tarapoto during the period of political violence to live in Lima or abroad and returned as they began to confront AIDS-related health complications. He recalled participating in and helping organize *polladas* and other fundraisers to help pay funeral and medical costs for the *compañeros* and *compañeras* who returned, especially for those who experienced rejection by their families and discrimination from healthcare services.

When projects supported by the Global Fund to Fight AIDS, Tuberculosis, and Malaria began to be carried out in urban Amazonian Peru in the late 2000s, MHOTA assumed new responsibilities as a regional coordinator of HIV/AIDS-related programming. Continuing to provide community-based programming to the city of Tarapoto, the organization expanded its technical capacities and carried out projects that included broader LGBT and human rights issues and partnered with LGBT organizations in the cities of Pucallpa and Iquitos. To reflect this new role, the organization changed its name briefly to the Movimiento Homosexual de San Martín before settling on the name Diversidad San Martinense (DISAM).[8]

Throughout the 2010s, DISAM established a reputation across the country for capably coordinating HIV/AIDS-related projects and was, in fact, considered exemplary in producing "deliverables." In 2008, working with programming objectives coming from the Global Fund's Fifth and Sixth Rounds, DISAM proposed a project that ultimately resulted two years later in a municipal and regional antidiscrimination ordinance that included the prohibition of discrimination on the basis of sexual orientation and gender identity.[9] In 2013, with the support of the Tenth Round, a tripartite agreement was signed between the Ministry of Health, the Municipal Government of Tarapoto, and DISAM to fund a health clinic and community space specializing in attention toward LGBT people. In 2014, Manuel Nieves was elected to the position of lieutenant mayor of the Municipal Government of Tarapoto and subsequently assumed the position of mayor in 2018 when the preceding mayor, Walter Grundel, resigned his post to run for mayor of the regional government. Nieves, who had long collaborated with DISAM and was a key factor in establishing the tripartite agreement, became the first openly gay man to be a mayor in Peru and was recognized around the country for this.

The System of Community Protection was a major component of the implementation of the Tenth Round's HIV prevention programming in the Amazonian region. It was planned and executed across the three major cities of the region (Iquitos, Pucallpa, and Tarapoto) and was the product of tremendous coordination between three technical assistants: Jefferson in Tarapoto, Arturo in Iquitos, and Gisela in Pucallpa. They collaborated with consultants based in Lima, though they assumed authorship of the project and its execution in each of their respective cities. The Tenth Round funded each technical assistant, who was then tasked with implementing three main objectives: (1) orchestrating capacity-building workshops with gay and trans community-based organizations on the topic of discrimination and how to file a formal grievance, (2) coordinating the System of Community Protection with state entities like the Defensoría del Pueblo (National Ombudsperson) and INDECOPI (National Institute of the Defense of Competition and of the Protection of Intellectual Property), and (3) accompanying individuals who sought to utilize the formal grievance process to report discrimination. The technical assistants worked with community-based organizations throughout their region to run capacity-building workshops that would train individuals on the process of filing a formal discrimination grievance. Jefferson, Arturo, and Gisela were each already associated with a community-based organization in their cities, though they also coordinated with other organizations in their cities and in the surrounding region. For example, Jefferson implemented the project with two community-based organizations in Tarapoto (DISAM and Las Amazonas, a transfeminine community-based organization), as well as with organizations in the surrounding towns of Juanjuí, Bella Vista, and Sauce.

The three main technical assistants imagined the System of Community Protection as an early warning system and a systematized registry of discrimination. To that end, they developed two major administrative technologies: a flowchart and a standardized grievance form. The flowchart served as a strategic route for linking antidiscrimination efforts aimed at HIV prevention with state and municipal institutions and authorities. The grievance form asked for pertinent information from the victim of discrimination, and its standardization contributed to its ability to be shared across organizations and entities. The overarching idea was that community-based organizations could be rapidly and effectively mobilized when an incident of discrimination occurred. They also emphasized the system's significance as a database of rights violations toward LGBT people, beyond the key populations specifically targeted by the Tenth Round, and as something that would be accessible across the Amazonian region.

Jefferson described the notion of *el seguimiento*, or following up, to be an integral aspect of the role of the technical assistant. If someone voiced an instance of discrimination, then following up with them would be the encouragement that they often needed to proceed with a formal grievance.

However, he also expressed a realistic concern about the longevity of the project, so it was important to develop the administrative procedures into something that would be able to persist beyond the eventual closure of the Tenth Round. That is, even if the technical assistants were ultimately unable to see a specific grievance through the entire administrative process, it was still important to raise awareness of how to file a discrimination grievance by using the flowchart and grievance form. *El seguimiento*, however, was a challenging process, especially given the funding constraints of the Tenth Round. It meant more than just holding one capacity-building workshop about the System of Community Protection; it also meant following up with community members at monthly meetings to check in on progress or to identify new cases of discrimination. In conversations that I had with Jefferson while the Tenth Round was in progress and after it was abruptly frozen (an episode further explored in chapter 4), he described being frustrated that he was not able to follow up because, justifiably, he was only one person and there was not enough funding to hire more technical support. He also expressed that because advocates in Tarapoto had made significant achievements like the antidiscrimination ordinances, there was pressure from Lima to bring forward emblematic cases of discrimination in Tarapoto.[10] At the time, only a handful of jurisdictions in Peru had passed antidiscrimination ordinances that explicitly included sexual orientation and gender identity, and such protections did not exist at the national level.[11] And, as Jefferson explained, part of the reason the proposal put forward by the three of them was selected was that it would be implemented in jurisdictions that already had antidiscrimination ordinances including protections for sexual orientation and gender identity. Jefferson explained that technical assistants in the Amazonian region were under pressure to somehow produce exemplary cases because others, especially in Lima, viewed the region as having governments that were more "favorable" to the needs of gay and transgender people.

Yet, despite limits on funding, Jefferson insisted that the most significant challenge for bringing the System of Community Protection into operation was the general ambivalence toward discrimination that he felt among many of his peers. In an interview, he described this ambivalence as a lack of a culture of denouncement: "The personal situation is that one does not have the habit of denouncing. . . . In the moment we might help someone go to the police commissary or the public ombudsman to file the grievance, but they do not carry out the follow-up, they are not interested in resolving it. . . . It's that the culture of denouncement does not yet exist in Tarapoto."

Part of carrying out *el seguimiento* meant holding monthly meetings and workshops with different organizations to identify potential cases of discrimination. However, despite Jefferson's efforts, many times either no one reported a case, an individual's experience did not constitute discrimination, or an individual did not uphold their part of following through with the grievance. To meet the demands of project monitoring and evaluation, Jefferson explained, he needed to document and collect cases of discrimination grievances—formal grievances that were filed officially with the national police, the auxiliary municipal police, the Defensoría del Pueblo, INDECOPI, and other state entities—to demonstrate the impacts of HIV prevention programming in Tarapoto. Although he had tried through a variety of initiatives to compel individuals in the city to file discrimination grievances through the System of Community Protection, he felt that individuals and the community as a whole lacked the will to follow through. After making a trip to Juanjuí one month, for example, he described how members from the partnering organization there reported that they had not found one case of discrimination in the entire city. For Jefferson, this indicated not that there was no discrimination in Juanjuí but rather that he needed to continue "sensitizing members of the LGBT community so that a behavior and culture of denouncement is generated." Likewise, after he held a meeting with Las Amazonas, the group reported that they had not found even one case of rights violations or discrimination toward trans women in Tarapoto that month. Jefferson felt that instead of being able to devote time to following up with specific cases of discrimination, he spent most of his time explaining over and over again how the System of Community Protection worked and why it was important to denounce discrimination.

While he was frustrated with what appeared to be a lack of a culture of denouncement, he saw the process of instilling a culture of denouncement as a long one. "Regarding Las Amazonas," he concluded, "they find themselves in the process of learning and accepting that they are citizens who possess the same rights and obligations as anyone else." Ultimately, he saw the embrace and practice of a culture of denouncement as something that simply had not emerged yet in Tarapoto.

### Culture, Denouncement, and Ethno-Racial Difference

I was struck by the frequency of the phrase "culture of denouncement" in my interactions with Jefferson, Anderson, and other project organizers and health promoters involved in HIV prevention. Though it typically operated as a shorthand for describing the intentions and objectives of broader anti-discrimination efforts, a closer reading of the phrase's two constitutive elements, "culture" and "denouncement," make visible some of the underlying social structures that shaped the implementation of HIV prevention efforts beyond the dictates of the Global Fund. For one, the fact that Jefferson (and others) fixated on a *culture* of denouncement was significant given the history of the "culture" concept in Peruvian society.[12]

Cultural difference, Marisol de la Cadena contends, has been "the social convention . . . at the heart of the Peruvian racial formation" (2000, 1). While the hierarchies of ethnic and racial difference in Peru are deeply rooted in colonial formations, persistent and long-standing ethno-racial categories such as "*cholo/a*," "*mestizo/a*," and "*indio/a*" have come to take on a dynamic nature. First, these categories have shifted over time. The term *cholo/a*, for instance, no longer refers to its colonial administrative definition as a category between the categories of "Indian" and "white," but now marks Andean migrants in Lima or serves as a general pejorative denoting low ethno-racial and class status.[13] And while categories have gone through significant transformations, "past and present remain inextricably intertwined, with remnants of colonial logics inflecting discourses believed to be thoroughly modern" (Leinius 2022, 52). Second, these categories are often individualized. This means they can shift from one interaction to the next; an individual's relative superiority vis-à-vis these categories can change in different circumstances and in reference to different people (Huayhua 2014; Portocarrero 2007a). Over the twentieth century, as large-scale migrations brought about explosive urban growth and new possibilities for social interaction and difference-making in Peru, these colonial categories lost their strict genealogical, or "blood," definitions and instead came to be defined through indicators and attributes, such as clothing, language, education, occupation, and other cultural markers. Consequently, notions of decency, educatedness, and civility—though they might not at first appear to be explicitly "racial"—have become surrogates for traditional racial categories (Cuenca 2014; de la Cadena 2000; Dorr 2018; Ewig 2010; Mendoza 2000; Poole 1997; Quijano 2007; Weismantel 2001; Zavala and Zariquiey 2009). To maintain the strtatification of existing hierarchies, ethnic, cultural, and class differences came to displace race as a dominant vocabulary for claiming superiority or justifying subordination in broader society.

While categories such as "*mestizo*" and "*cholo*" have a clear connection to the ways in which racial and ethnic hierarchy has persisted in the Andean and coastal regions of Peru, the vocabulary for articulating gradients of racial differentiation (both in everyday interaction and in scholarly analysis) is less explicit in the urban spaces of the Amazonian region. The term *charapa*, for example, can be used to refer to and describe a person from the region, though it does not occupy as significant or central a place in national imaginaries as the term *cholo* does. In her ethnographic account of gender and technical schools in Tarapoto, Silverstein (2017) describes the ethno-racial makeup of her interlocutors as "a regional form of *mestizaje* distinct from that of Peru's coastal or Andean regions" (586). Besides long-standing stereotypes of hypersexualization, the ethno-racial lexicon of or about monolingual, Spanish-speaking urban Amazonians was much more indeterminate than for their Andean or coastal counterparts (Motta 2011). Thus, because the concept of "culture" already operated as a shorthand for social stratification and classification, it worked in the context of understanding and differentiating the gay and transgender communities of urban Amazonian Peru. Given the transformation of ethno-racial categories into understandings of "culture," some cited culture to make sense of why some gay and transgender individuals appeared ambivalent to antidiscrimination and HIV prevention efforts that obligated them to formalize their experiences of exclusion and marginalization through discrimination grievances. Through the language of culture, HIV prevention initiatives made visible how racialization intersected with sexual and gender differences. Even though racial categories were not explicitly invoked to talk about the status of gay and transgender communities in Tarapoto and other cities of the Amazon, the idea that those communities lacked a *culture* of denouncement coalesced broader notions about discrimination with a more contextualized form of explaining and naturalizing otherness and difference. While the original intention of the "culture of denouncement" concept was to decrease discrimination and stigma toward gay and trans communities as a means to mitigate HIV transmission, the idea of cultivating a culture of denouncement invoked a vocabulary that was consistent with theories of race and social hierarchy in Peru.

The concept of "*la denuncia*," which I translate as "denouncement," further intersects with a particular configuration of Peruvian social life. In his seminal essay "El silencio, la queja y la acción," the eminent Peruvian sociologist Gonzalo Portocarrero (2007b) outlines three culturally sanctioned responses that characterize the development of the strategies used by the most marginalized communities in Peruvian society to ameliorate and confront injustice: silence, complaint, and action. Portocarrero argues that the widespread notion that silence is an appropriate response to suffering is a colonial inheritance that stems from a religiosity promising future salvation in exchange for sacrifice and pain in the present. As a result of secularization and expanding opportunities and rights, silence was later replaced by complaint as a mode of responding to continued poverty and oppression. Complaint, however, was limited—it indicates a resignation toward suffering, and the lack of tools to elaborate a full-fledged response. Action, as Portocarrero points out, means assuming control over the conditions that bring suffering into one's life. Action involves the recognition that one's circumstances could change if confronted through individual will. In this framework, denouncement—making widely known an experience of injustice and discrimination—came to be seen as exemplifying the liberatory possibilities of responding to social exclusion by taking action. Portocarrero's framework offers an important reference point to help explain why program coordinators, technical assistants, and others involved in the implementation of antidiscrimination efforts aspired to cultivate a culture of denouncement as a means of mitigating the effects of discrimination on gay and transgender communities and promoting their rights. Because program coordinators in Lima typically assumed that the regional governments were more "favorable" to gay and transgender communities in the Amazonian region, they were often surprised at how few individuals from Tarapoto seemed willing to put forward formal discrimination grievances. From their perspective, it appeared as though the conditions were ideal in Tarapoto for an exemplary case of discrimination to emerge that could then inspire others to file formal discrimination grievances. Denouncement was important because it was seen not just as a way to mitigate the effects of discrimination and stigma on the transmission of HIV but also as a mode of making a place for oneself in society along the lines of taking "action" in the Portocarreran sense.

**Emblematic Denouncement**

There were a few stories that circulated about successful instances of denouncement. These stories became emblematic because the denouncements they described featured one or more of the following elements: they set a legal or institutional precedent, they were covered on the national news, they were cited in capacity-building workshops as exemplary and inspirational models to follow, or they were brought up in everyday conversations. During my time in Tarapoto, the story that was most often cited was the emblematic case of Godfrey.[14] In 2012, Godfrey, a well-known trans makeup artist and entertainer, was denied entry into the then-popular Gotica nightclub in the exclusive Larcomar shopping center in Lima.[15] Arriving with a larger group, Godfrey was told by security guards to pay a cover charge to get into the nightclub that was double what everyone else had paid, and that Godfrey would have to go in through a different entrance. Godfrey denounced the nightclub informally through appearances in the news media and submitted a formal discrimination grievance to INDECOPI. With assistance from activists and lawyers associated with nongovernmental organizations working on sexual rights, Godfrey was able to present evidence of discrimination, including video recordings from cellphones and security camera footage. Godfrey was eventually awarded 370,000 soles (approximately $130,000) through a fine imposed on the nightclub by INDECOPI in a ruling that confirmed that Godfrey had been discriminated against on the basis of sexual orientation and gender identity.[16]

Part of the reason this story circulated so widely was the national media coverage of the case. A voiceover at the beginning of a report on the important and influential weekly Sunday evening Peruvian news program *Cuarto Poder* that aired in 2013 proclaimed, "It is not an exaggeration to say that Godfrey Arbulú has made history in our country."[17] As the *Cuarto Poder* news report explained, Godfrey's case set a precedent: in the two decades of INDECOPI's existence, this was the first time that discrimination on the basis of sexual orientation and gender identity had been effectively demonstrated in a commercial space.

Premised on the conceptual distinction between silence, complaint, and action as three possible responses to injustice, Portocarrero's framework offers a starting point for an analysis of Godfrey's emblematic story of denouncement and some of the consequences of its widespread circulation. Despite the idea that silence was the normalized, compulsory response to suffering, Godfrey's narrative was not one of martyrdom and undue suffering. This is significant; in many contexts throughout Latin America, such as Chile (Perez 2017) or Nicaragua (Howe 2009), trans- and homophobic violence and martyrdom have been preconditions for demands for anti-hate-crime or antidiscrimination laws that include protection for diverse sexual orientations and gender identities. Rather, as editorialized in the *Cuarto Poder* news report, the story concluded with footage of Godfrey being crowned Miss Evolution at a beauty contest in New York. Drawing on a cultural idiom about what it means to get ahead (*salir adelante*), this conclusion evoked the moral obligations that Berg (2015) observes in connection with Peruvian stories of international migration: when one gets ahead, one has a moral obligation to bring others along with one. In ending with a *triunfo en el exterior* (success abroad), the report resolved the story of discrimination with a distinctly triumphant tone intended to inspire.

Godfrey's case became a practical example for explaining how and why it might be important to record and denounce discrimination when it occurred. Although Godfrey's case was independent of the Tenth Round, its popularization across national media allowed it to become a clear and relatable example to include in capacity-building workshops and community-based organization meetings about contesting social exclusion, advocating for rights, and, for the purposes of the Tenth Round, alleviating the impacts of discrimination on HIV transmission. In short, it effectively became an emblematic story, in the sense that it was a story that was used to tell myriad other stories. As Portocarrero (2007b) insightfully suggested with his tripartite framework, Godfrey's story was compelling because it exemplified the notion of action: in the story, discrimination was overcome not through suffering and silence with the hope of future recompense, but through active denouncement and strategic circulation of the message in as many channels as possible. As gay and transgender communities across the Amazonian region attended workshops aimed at teaching them to identify discrimination in their everyday lives and seek redress, workshop leaders cited Godfrey to inspire participants to identify discrimination and advocate for redress. Here, the idea of possessing or lacking a culture of denouncement was invoked as a theory for explaining why some, like Godfrey, have been able to successfully resolve discriminatory experiences while others have not. For the purposes of the implementation of the System of Community Protection, Godfrey's case stood as a practical example of what possessing a culture of denouncement might look like, and Godfrey was the idealized protagonist of an emblematic denouncement and a model of a fully capacitated and self-actualized HIV-preventing subject.

## Scandalous Denouncement

One warm Sunday evening in August 2015, after a long day of cheering on teams playing in the *machomenos* soccer tournament, I noticed that Ramón had posted a note across social media about an incident that had just occurred at the La Mega disco. "Listen, listen, ladies, gentlemen, and the security guards at La Mega. A young trans woman Yesika wants to enter and they tell her no because her shorts were too short. She tells them that there are young women inside already with shorts just as short. And the security guard answers her, 'She is a woman and you are not.'" Ramón's post spread rapidly across social media as his friends and acquaintances liked, shared, and commented on it. Others posted it to popular group pages devoted to news and gossip about Tarapoto and the surrounding region. While some encouraged Yesika to file a formal grievance, others encouraged her to continue to make noise and publicize the incident on social media, in local periodicals, and on regional television stations. "Publish it everywhere," wrote one of Ramón's friends, "make the disco be embarrassed." Many voiced their opinions on social media, but the story resonated particularly among gay and transgender people, who offered their perspectives about discrimination and nightclubs as they hung out at their friends' beauty salons or in the parks where they typically spent their afternoons playing volleyball. Conversations that week often mentioned not just what had happened in the ongoing soccer tournament but also what had happened to Yesika at La Mega. It was clear that the experience of being discriminated against at the nightclub was resonating across Tarapoto.

Eager for any suggestions on how to proceed, Ramón requested that I visit him one afternoon at the store he tended, located on the first floor of his family's house. He explained to me that Yesika was contemplating filing a formal discrimination grievance with INDECOPI, though she was still unsure whether to proceed. Both Ramón and Yesika were familiar with the System of Community Protection because they had participated in workshops or meetings led by Jefferson about the protocol. Though she had grown up in Tarapoto and returned several times a year to visit her family, Yesika lived most of the year in Lima. For that reason, they wondered whether the grievance process might take so long that it wouldn't make sense to initiate it. Her other option, which felt more useful in the circumstances, was to confront the owner of La Mega directly, with the aim of resolving the issue and compelling the owner to stop discriminating against trans women at the door.

As I began to follow Yesika's and Ramón's efforts more closely, and realized that the incident had become a popular topic of conversation among other gay and trans people in Tarapoto, I asked others how they perceived what had happened. Several days after Ramón's original post, I brought up the case with Anderson. Educated as a lawyer and established in the community as a dedicated LGBT rights activist, Anderson had long been involved in coordinating and implementing Global Fund programming throughout the Amazonian region. Anderson was aware of what had happened and had even met with Yesika and Ramón. However, while Yesika had received support and encouragement on social media to file a complaint, Anderson

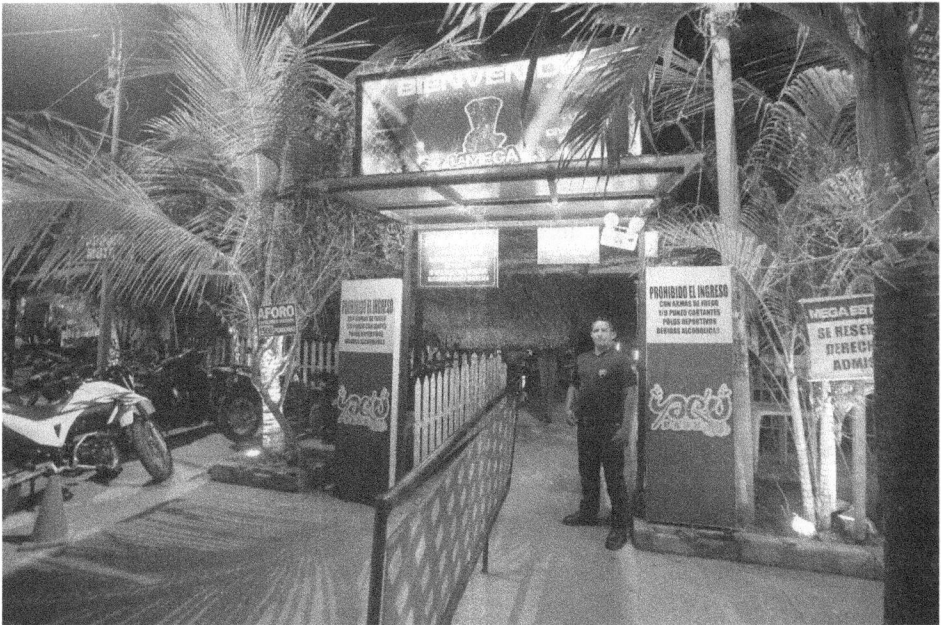

Figure 3.1. A security guard at the entrance to the La Mega nightclub. (Photograph by Marlon del Aguila Guerrero)

offered a franker assessment of the situation. "The problem is that they do not have any evidence," he explained to me. "They did not write in the *libro de reclamaciones* [complaint book] that night, and there is no video evidence of what the security guard did."

If they could not file a formal grievance, Ramón suggested another option to Anderson: circulating an informal denouncement of the La Mega nightclub among the local newspapers, to the local television stations, and on social media. After all, the obligation to denounce discrimination was habitually reinforced by Global Fund activities and workshops, and Yesika still felt that she should call attention to the broader issue of discrimination toward trans women at the doors of the nightclubs in Tarapoto.

Anderson strongly advised against this strategy. "You do not want to create scandal or, worse, slander the owner," he explained to me later. He believed that what happened to Yesika could not plausibly turn into a successful discrimination case and, therefore, could not become an emblematic case of discrimination. He was preoccupied with the broader social consequences of publicizing what had occurred and summarized this preoccupation with the concept of scandal. When I asked him to explain what he meant, he described scandal as "the typical stereotype that other people have about us, that we are uneducated, that we are laughable because of the noise we make, because they want us to stay quiet." Since the possibility of converting the instance of discrimination into an emblematic denouncement appeared to be off the table, any commotion or publicity created by Yesika or Ramón, was, effectively, a scandalous denouncement.

The posts that Ramón, Yesika, and others had circulated on social media did in fact draw the attention of the owner of the disco, who contacted them and invited them to a meeting to discuss and resolve the incident. Yesika and Ramón later recounted this episode to a group gathered at a DISAM meeting. When they arrived, they explained, they were surprised to find that the owner had also brought a lawyer and the nightclub's manager. The management offered Yesika the opportunity to come back to the disco. She would not have to pay any cover charge and would be given *barra libre*, or open bar, the whole night. They also offered to fire the offending security guard who had prohibited her entry. Yesika was dissatisfied with this offer and requested a public apology from the owner of the La Mega disco himself. She wanted this apology to be directed to all the transgender women in Tarapoto, assuring the community that they would not be prohibited from entering La Mega for arbitrary reasons.

As the members of the group discussed the new development in the story, the conversation turned to a comparison with the case of Godfrey. There were many parallels between how the group gathered at DISAM understood Godfrey's story and how they interpreted what they were hearing from Yesika and Ramón. Reminding the group about what had happened with Godfrey, Yesika asked aloud, "Can't we sue La Mega for discrimination? One time, at the Gotica club in Lima, in Larcomar, they discriminated against a *travesti* and she was compensated for the discrimination." Godfrey's story was, in essence, doing the work of an emblematic case of denouncement. It became widely known and inspired Yesika to denounce a similar experience of discrimination that she lived. However, one of the limits of the emblematic case was that many details were elided. As the story circulated through national media, social media, word of mouth, and, even in the process of HIV prevention, the logistical support and advocacy that went into turning Godfrey's case into a formal grievance were often left out of the recounting.[18] Given his experience as a lawyer, Anderson again reiterated to Yesika and others that, in fact, the cases were different: "They had charged [Godfrey] double for the entry to the disco, and then they made her walk in the back entrance, and they had the proof of it, the receipt and the video. You do not have the evidence." With that, discussion on the topic ended, and the meeting turned to other issues. Yesika eventually left Tarapoto again, and new topics and incidents emerged, consuming communal discussion and debate.

## Scandal as a Form of Individualized Discrimination

Yesika and Ramón were ambitious and committed in their efforts to denounce what had occurred at the disco. Their actions challenge the widespread theory that the lack of a culture of denouncement explained why they were unable to produce a discrimination grievance. It was not that Yesika lacked the individual disposition to take action or to learn the tools to become a denouncing subject; she learned from the story of Godfrey and was set on circulating a denouncement of her own experience. However, because she did not possess the kind of evidence that could convert her experience into an emblematic case of denouncement, she and Ramón were unable to convince the network of community-based and nongovernmental organizations implementing the System of Community Protection and other projects promoting human rights to support their advocacy. Yesika's efforts to circulate the story, to demand an apology, and to rectify the situation were, ultimately, viewed as causing noise and being "scandalous."

"Scandal" was a capacious category in gay and transgender social life. Sometimes it could be a strategic tool, a "weapon of the weak" to draw attention to injustice. Paula's story about discrimination at Anaconda (described in the introduction), for example, transformed her encounter into a pedagogical story about how to counter injustice. But scandal could also be unwieldy and unruly, and it was sometimes applied unevenly, even among gay and transgender people themselves.[19] As the story of Yesika's discrimination at La Mega persisted, the act of having embraced the culture of denouncement paradoxically intensified allegations toward Yesika that she was scandalous. In other words, though efforts to denounce discrimination were intended to mitigate its impacts, sometimes they produced the opposite result and amplified discriminatory attitudes toward those who sought to denounce.[20]

Several months after the initial incident, the Defensoría del Pueblo arranged for a workshop in coordination with DISAM, Las Amazonas, and other community-based organizations throughout the region. A group of ombudspersons from Lima were compiling a systematic, nationwide report about the status of LGBT discrimination across Peru. Building on the momentum of the antidiscrimination ordinances and the implementation of the System of Community Protection, staff from the Defensoría del Pueblo came to Tarapoto to solicit specific examples of discrimination to include in the report. Dr. Leguía, the ombudsperson from Lima who led the workshop, explained to all of those gathered that they would be asking for specific examples of discrimination to include in the report.[21] He was asking the gay and transgender community members gathered to collaborate on the report by coming forward with and sharing the details of specific cases of discrimination that they had experienced. To explain what he meant, he emphatically proclaimed, "Surely you have all followed the emblematic case of Godfrey." Again, in this instance, comparison to Godfrey's story of discrimination became an ethnographic phenomenon. It was invoked as the example of the kinds of stories that the ombudsperson was expecting to hear in this workshop. And he was right—virtually all those at the workshop had heard of Godfrey and knew the story of discrimination at the disco.

While Yesika was no longer in Tarapoto and so did not attend this workshop, Ramón brought up her case of discrimination. From Ramón's perspective, Yesika's story ought to have been ideal for the report and the communal discussion that the workshop intended to generate. After describing the details of the incident to Dr. Leguía, his team, and the gay and transgender individuals gathered at the workshop, Ramón revealed even more of the story than what I had heard previously. He explained how he had contacted a reporter from a local television station and they produced a short report on the incident. Just as Yesika and Ramón had seen in the report about Godfrey, they thought this would be one strategy for making the denouncement heard and amplifying the story of Yesika's experience. However, Ramón alleged the segment was later canned by the television station because the owner of the television station was friends with the owner of the disco.

Ramón's recounting of Yesika's story was cut short by the other workshop participants. They claimed that Yesika had been too scandalous. She had created too much noise, they said, and this did not help the situation of transgender people in the region. Yesika's experience, and its legibility as an instance of discrimination that merited inclusion in this report, was devalued because others described her and her claims as scandalous. Dr. Leguía ultimately concluded that this was why it was important to have a culture of denouncement. According to Dr. Leguía, if only Yesika and Ramón had turned the incident into a recognizable case of discrimination, rather than creating scandal, things might have been different and the case could have

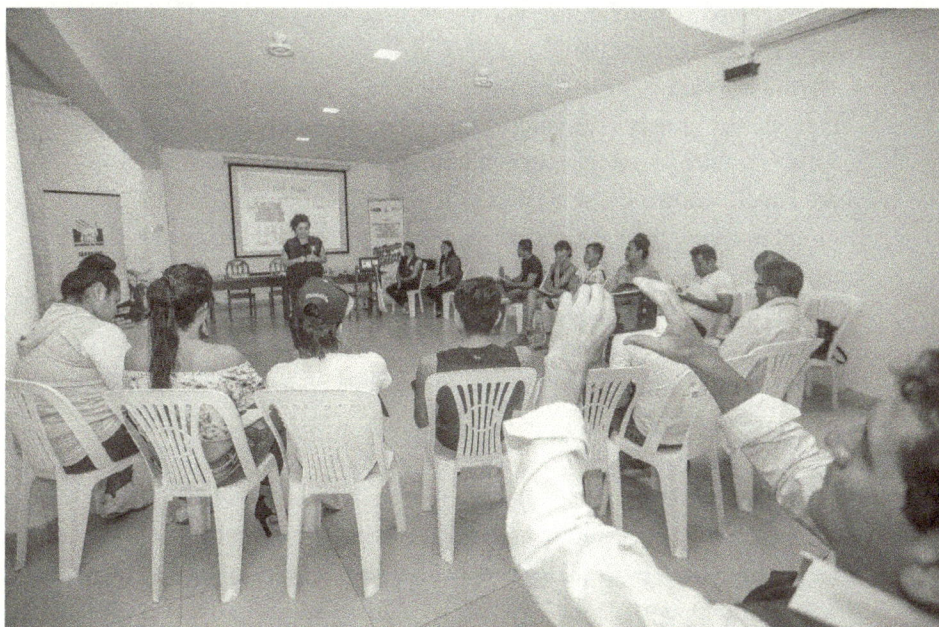

**Figure 3.2.** A capacity-building workshop led by the Defensoría del Pueblo for gay and transgender communities in Tarapoto, Peru. (Photograph by Marlon del Aguila Guerrero)

been included in the report. In this encounter, the idea of scandal worked against Yesika and her story. In fact, it paralleled a concept that scholars of Peruvian society such as Portocarrero (2007a) have termed "individualized discrimination." This is the idea that, because of the country's history of *mestizaje*, ethno-racial hierarchies are constantly established and reestablished at individualized, person-to-person levels in everyday interactions, in comparison to others. In other words, a person establishes an ethno-racial status perceived to be "higher" or "superior" by subjecting another to a lower category in the perceived ethno-racial hierarchy. The same individual can assume a "higher" ethno-racial position (e.g., "white" or "coastal") at one moment in one interaction, but also, in another moment and in another interaction, be subjected to the categories of lower positioning in the ethno-racial hierarchy (e.g., "*cholo*," "*mestizo*," or "*indio*"). As the interaction at the workshop showed, scandal could work in a parallel fashion: individuals who in other instances might have been dismissed as scandalous established a sense of differentiation from Yesika by categorizing her story and her efforts to seek redress as scandalous.

In the years following its conclusion, Godfrey's case provided a pedagogical tool for the project of expanding the technical capacities of individuals. Godfrey's emblematic story of denouncement was frequently circulated and shared in the workshops associated with HIV prevention and human rights promotion throughout the Amazonian region. Ramón and Yesika picked up on the message and were attentive to elements that made Godfrey's case of discrimination legitimate, compelling, and ultimately, emblematic. They consulted and connected with community-based organizations. They turned to the media to amplify the story. In essence, they understood deeply what it meant to take action and practice a culture of denouncement. Even if they did not have the right evidence to file a successful grievance, they still persisted in denouncing the injustice that Yesika experienced. Yet while Godfrey exemplified a culture of denouncement, Yesika and Ramón were unable to convince even their peers to see the merits in calling attention to the discrimination Yesika experienced. Rather, her story was dismissed as scandalous.

The process of converting Godfrey's case of discrimination into an emblematic story of denouncement meant that some of the conditions that made the case successful—such as having the support of lawyers and dedicated advocates to publicize the case and working with investigative journalists who had a national platform—were elided. This was, of course, to make the story inspiring and easy to circulate. Yesika and Ramón did not have the legal resources to propel her discrimination grievance forward, nor did they have access to the journalistic resources needed to editorialize the story and disseminate it on local (or national) television or radio. But in day-to-day interactions, it was not just about the legal or journalistic resources; the deployment of scandal also impeded Yesika's ability to transform her experience at La Mega into an emblematic story of denouncement. With the local television journalist who produced a segment about Yesika that never aired, with the other gay and transgender individuals who dismissed her efforts, and with the representatives from the Defensoría del Pueblo, Yesika and Ramón encountered an everyday deployment of scandal by others, even by some who may have at other times been considered or called scandalous themselves.

Yesika and Ramón ultimately acknowledged that they did not have the evidence to pursue a formal discrimination grievance to the same extent as Godfrey. However, the circumstances were similar enough for, at the very least, her denouncement of the experience to be seen as justified and legitimate by others. The wielding of the "scandal" concept to describe her efforts ultimately foreclosed the possibility of converting her case into an emblematic story of denouncement. Even though she and Ramón persisted in circulating what had happened, it appeared as though Yesika lacked a culture of denouncement because her story was never ultimately converted into a successful formal discrimination grievance, catalogued in a human rights report, or editorialized as an injustice in a news report. Paying attention to her efforts dispels the assumption that communities vulnerable to HIV—like gay and transgender communities in Tarapoto—were ambivalent about antidiscrimination efforts because they did not produce formal discrimination grievances. Nothing could be further from the truth: Yesika and Ramón persisted in circulating the denouncement and strove to take action against the injustice she experienced at the nightclub.

## Tarapoto's Nightscape

The disco, or the nightclub, carries an important cultural significance in the social life of Tarapoto. Yesika's demand to take part in the city's nightlife was no trivial matter, and her experience at the club was a potent example of the exclusion that she and others faced in society. Nightlife was a key draw of the tourism economy, it was a source of regional pride, and it was even accorded significance in the national imaginary. Besides the more self-evident reason of the mere fact that discrimination persistently occurs, part of the reason that stories about discrimination at the entry into discos circulate is that they resonate powerfully as an unjust exclusion from social life. Therefore, understanding the weight of Yesika's denouncement requires a thicker description of the city's nightscape.[22] This contextualization also, in part, explains why Yesika's story was met with distrust by some of the other gay and trans people in the community.

First, the spatial elements of the discos lend themselves to a connection with general ideas about regional and national economic growth and development. Arriving eastbound into Tarapoto along the Fernando Belaúnde Terry Highway, one is welcomed at the edges of the city limits by palm trees, tobacco fields, coffee-processing facilities, bordellos, the campuses of a handful of universities and technical schools, and the large, open-air nightclubs that have become known throughout the country.[23] Visitors and tourists, many coming from Lima, might see Tarapoto as an affordable weekend getaway that offers a milder taste of the jungle climate and a bustling nightlife. Reality television stars, popular musicians and orchestras, and other members of the Peruvian *farándula* (the world of popular entertainment) made frequent appearances at the discos, both as featured performers and as visitors.[24] Traveling west out to the far edges of the city, those living in Tarapoto saw the scattering of nightclubs as an opportunity to be part of the new patterns of consumption that transformed the emergent Peruvian middle class in the 1990s and 2000s. Previously, during the period of political violence in the country, particularly at its height in Tarapoto in the late 1980s and early 1990s, nighttime curfews were enforced. Those who might have otherwise enjoyed nightlife during their younger years were deprived of this opportunity; thus it was common for multiple generations of a family to go out together to the discos in Tarapoto. For some, the large and popular discos like La Anaconda, La Pachanga, and La Mega offered a chance to engage in a ritual of consumption that had been inaccessible during the years of violence, hyperinflation, and curfews that characterized a prior period. Arriving in a pickup truck instead of a *motocar* or motorcycle, ordering bottle service at a private table, and milling in the VIP zones indexed an entrepreneurial spirit and business savvy, some of the key values of the regional middle class and elite. Being and consuming in the disco marked membership in this success story. The denial of entry to a disco was a potent and symbolic form of exclusion, an exclusion both from the disco itself and from a broader sense of belonging.

Second, the discos were not generally divided between "gay" and "straight" discos. Unlike in other cities in Peru, where the collection of bars and nightclubs that catered to different segments of LGBT communities constituted an *ambiente*, there was a general sense that, in theory, anyone could go to the discos in Tarapoto.[25] Rather, LGBT people crafted a space for themselves within the domains of local diversions and entertainment. Not only that, they were integral in animating the city's nightlife, often through performing and choreographing official entertainment and shows. However, this did not mean that nightlife was not stratified. Rather, class and gender played important roles in shaping where people went out. The regional elite and middle class often went to the discos closer to the city, while the clubs farther out of town, such as La Mega, were associated with working-class patrons. These differences were further accentuated by gender: gay men, for example, were more likely to gain access to the middle-class and elite nightclubs, whereas lesbians and transgender women tended to frequent the working-class ones. Likewise, while an upscale nightclub might hire a gay

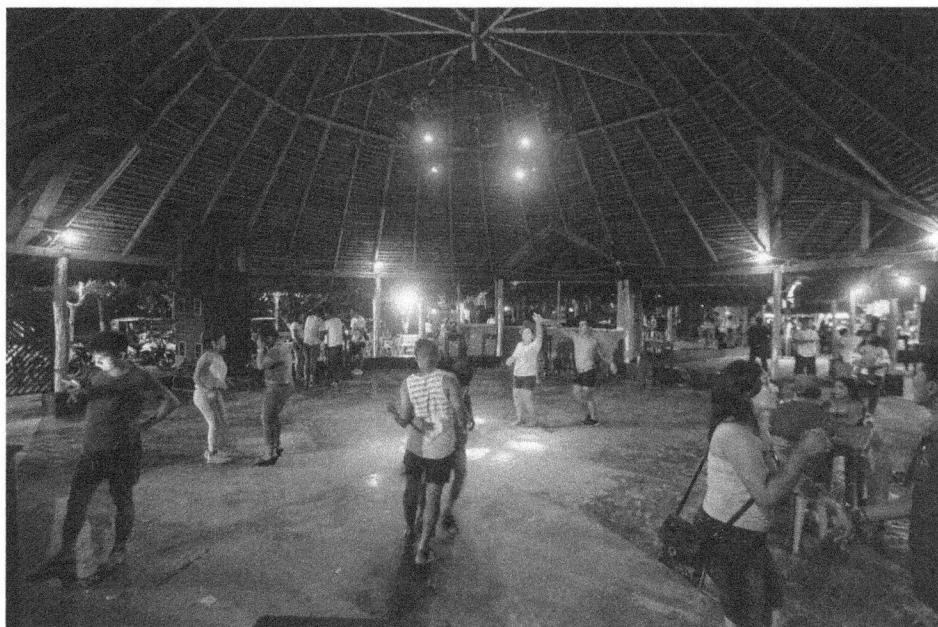

**Figure 3.3.** A typical open-air disco under a traditional thatched roof, or *maloca*. (Photograph by Marlon del Aguila Guerrero)

choreographer or feature a performance by a gay drag queen, events such as transgender beauty contests typically took place in the discos and open-air plazas farther from the center of town. Finally, there were key temporal differences that also shaped nightlife. Whereas Friday and Saturday nights were most popular for the regional elite and middle class, the busiest times for La Mega were Sunday afternoons and evenings. Locals who worked weekends might rest on Mondays and thus enjoyed the discos on Sunday nights after work. Gay men, who typically had more access to education and professional opportunities, were more likely to be able to go out on Friday and Saturday. Transgender women, who typically had significantly less access to education and white-collar employment, were more likely to go out on Sunday. Thus, for some in Tarapoto, Yesika's story was surprising because many would have expected her to encounter few problems going to La Mega on a Sunday night. In fact, that might have contributed to why other gay and trans people dismissed her story as scandalous—*because* it challenged some of the assumptions and patterns of the Tarapoto nightscape at the time.

## Martín's Sandal Scandal

Though both gay men and transgender women were categorized as "vulnerable" and "key" populations for the purposes of HIV prevention, and though they shared aspects of collective social life (e.g., the soccer tournament profiled in chapter 2), their differing experiences with discrimination and denouncement illustrate some of the important differences in their lives in Tarapoto. Gender thus played an important role in how individuals recounted their experiences of discrimination and in shaping whose stories were determined to be reliable and whose denouncements were considered worth pursuing and publicizing.

In Tarapoto, stories about discrimination at the entrance to discos often revolved around clothing. While Tarapoto is not as hot and humid as the other major cities of the Amazonian region, the city still has a warm climate. It stays hot, even into the night, and shorts, sandals, and T-shirts are the standard apparel both for the daytime and for nightlife. Conventional dress for going out was, overall, considerably casual. But the question of clothing was an important part of the convention of stories about discrimination at the disco: because it did not make sense to overdress given the heat and humidity, it was generally understood by any listener in Tarapoto that exclusions over casual clothing would be a clear instance of unequal treatment and differentiation.

Martín, an ebullient and impassioned storyteller, included in his repertoire of stories an encounter of discrimination he had experienced at the entrance of the nightclub La Anaconda. In an interview, I asked him to recount a version of the story. He began by explaining that his nephew had been visiting Tarapoto and suggested they meet at La Anaconda. However, he was surprised when he got there and the security guards denied him entry because, they said, he was dressed in shorts and sandals. He called his nephew to tell him he was having trouble getting inside. His nephew, who was already inside the disco, was also dressed in shorts and sandals. He came out to the front and learned that Martín was being denied entry because of what he was wearing. When the nephew realized that it was over the sandals, he began to throw a scandal right there. It was his nephew who drew attention to the inconsistent application of the dress code. Altering his voice to signal it was his nephew talking, Martín quoted him: "'How is it that my uncle cannot come in when he is wearing shorts and sandals, and I am allowed in before?'" As his nephew caused more and more noise, the rest of the security team came over, and they started pushing Martín and his nephew. It was at this point, Martín explained, that despite his best efforts to minimize the encounter, the episode turned into a scandal. In front of the crowd waiting to get in and the scowling security guards, Martín sat and waited for a friend of his to arrive with an extra pair of shoes so that Martín could change and then finally get into the disco. However, even after he had changed his footwear, the security guards still did not let him in. Martín explained why he had left the disco at that point: "I went to enjoy myself, not to fight and make a scandal. It made me uncomfortable because everyone there knew me and then this scandal happened and I did not like it. I did not like it at all. Since I would have been a paying customer and I would have consumed something, I decided that I should publicly denounce what happened." So he contacted journalists to explain what had happened at the disco and see if they would be willing to publish a story denouncing the disco. In the process of sharing the story with journalists, he realized that what had occurred to him was indeed discrimination:

> Eventually with the journalists we came to the conclusion, since the journalists also did not understand why my nephew was allowed in and I was not, and they said, "Well, you changed out of the sandals and they still did not let you in? Well, maybe it was not because of the sandals, but because you are gay and that was why they did not let you in!" And the journalists asked me again, "What was the problem? The sandals? But you changed the sandals and they still did not let you enter. Or was it something else?" I myself did not even realize that it was discrimination until I began to talk to the journalists.

While it was clear that exclusion itself was a common experience for gay men and transgender women in Tarapoto, the stories about such encounters shared a number of common elements. First, the stories center on entry into the disco and the requirements for entry. In the moment when entry is prohibited, the denial appears to be over a particular article of clothing. In Yesika's case, it was over her shorts. For Martín, it was over a pair of sandals. However, as the story progresses, we come to find out that these rules are inconsistently applied by the security guards. Yesika peered inside the disco and saw other women with shorts just as short; Martín's nephew had already entered the disco with sandals on his feet. Like the stories about *peches* discussed in chapter 1, the modularity and collective authorship of these encounters at the nightclub enabled interlocutors to express and affirm the shared experience of discrimination. And although the stories were told from a first-person point of view, a listener understood the possibility that the storyteller added embellishment to the story, as a way to express an embarrassing episode without having to put forward so much of oneself.

Despite these similarities, there were significant differences between Martín's story and Yesika's story. For one, the disco itself played an important role. La Anaconda was the most prominent nightclub in town and branded itself as modern and high-end. Part of why journalists might have encouraged Martín would have been that, in general, there was a lot of public interest in the image of La Anaconda, and this episode would have revealed a different face of the club. But it also shows how gay men were sometimes encouraged to come forward and publicize a denouncement, whereas transgender women who told a similar story were actively discouraged from making a public denouncement and dismissed as scandalous. In his retelling, Martín explicitly emphasizes that he did not want a scandal. In fact, in his dramatization of the incident it was his nephew who caused the scandal at the entrance. And it was the journalists who encouraged him to denounce La Anaconda. Some gay men were able to elude the allegation of being "scandalous" if they wanted to, whereas transgender women did not have that option. Transgender women encountered more obstacles to getting others to circulate their stories of discrimination and were typically assumed, at the start, to be scandalous. Norma's experiences with her transfeminine community-based organization Las Amazonas further shows this gendered difference.

### The Culture of Denouncement at Las Amazonas

Norma, a trans woman from Tarapoto, had long been involved in trans, transgender, and *travesti* advocacy through her connection with prior iterations of the organization DISAM. However, as a response to changes in the Global Fund's allocation model for community-based organizations throughout Peru, in 2013 she decided to establish a transfeminine community-based organization, named Las Amazonas. Some of the efforts to implement the System of Community Protection and cultivate a culture of denouncement through HIV prevention efforts with members of Las Amazonas further show how the circumstances surrounding the denunciation of discrimination varied between gay men and transgender women.

Las Amazonas operated out of Norma's house. She was an expert at converting her space and using it for multiple purposes. The large, open courtyard could operate as a studio for the aerobics and step classes she taught in the afternoons; by evening, the fitness equipment had been cleared out and replaced with tables and chairs for a workshop or meeting with Las Amazonas. Norma said she had long insisted that the decision to hold capacity-building workshops or other HIV prevention activities in the morning or as all-day events effectively excluded many transgender women, who found it difficult to attend because they often worked at night and rested in the mornings or even into the early afternoon. Norma credited the support from the Global Fund for helping her establish a space exclusively for trans women that could be available in the early evenings as an important innovation that helped more equitably distribute HIV prevention resources.

Despite the new funding opportunities dedicated exclusively toward antidiscrimination capacity-building for trans women, she still encountered many difficulties formalizing discrimination grievances. Norma and other members of Las Amazonas, for example, consistently denounced the persistent harassment they experienced from the *serenazgo* (auxiliary municipal police) in Tarapoto. Though sex work is legal in Peru, members of Las Amazonas reported that the *serenazgo* often detained them arbitrarily and called them inappropriate names when they were in areas associated with commercial sex work. In collaboration with coordinators for the System of Community Protection and the Tenth Round projects, a municipal official who oversaw the *serenazgo* agreed to a meeting with Las Amazonas one evening.

During the meeting, which I attended as a participant observer, individuals offered the municipal official several concrete examples of discrimination they had experienced. One group member, Pamela, nearly choking back tears, recounted how just the week prior, members of the *serenazgo* had detained her late at night and driven her to the small town of Juan Guerra, nearly thirty kilometers away. They kicked her out of the truck and told her that if she wanted to return to Tarapoto, she would have to walk back. Noticeably moved by the testimonies and experiences of the women gathered that evening, the municipal official proposed that the municipality, with support from Tenth Round funding, hold a sensitivity training workshop with the *serenazgo*. However, the official continued, Las Amazonas would also have to do their part. He could not do anything if transgender women did not take action by filing grievances and denouncing discrimination. "The compromise is for you to embrace a culture of denouncement. Anything that you can denounce, you have to begin to denounce," he emphasized to those who were present. Even state representatives invoked the "culture of denouncement" concept as the recommendation for effectively reducing state-sanctioned harassment, violence, and discrimination.

Both the municipal official and the project coordinators assumed that Pamela was responding to discrimination with silence. From the standpoint of the System of Community Protection, since she did not file a formal grievance at the *comisaria* (police station), there was nothing that could be done regarding this particular incident. If only she had embraced a culture of denouncement, the logic followed, then they might have been able to advocate for formalization of the grievance. This assumption reflected Portocarrero's observations about suffering in Peru: silence was long considered an appropriate response to suffering, in that it stood in as an investment for future recompense. Instead of silently suffering discrimination, Pamela and others should take action. Eliding the willful inaction on the part of the auxiliary municipal police in responding to complaints and the preexisting assumptions about trans women as "scandalous," the representatives focused on what they perceived as a lack of a culture of denouncement among the women of Las Amazonas themselves. Norma, though, contested this vision. "'Maybe it appears that we are silent, that we silence ourselves,'" she responded, "but our grievances are not taken seriously.'" She explained that she and others had gone to the *comisaria* and filed grievances, but their files were deliberately misplaced, closed, or lost. They were told that regardless of what had happened, they had probably brought it on themselves by being scandalous.

In insisting that members of Las Amazonas consistently filed discrimination grievances, Norma drew attention to the systematic administrative practice of ignoring or rejecting claims of discrimination by transgender women. And yet, because emblematic discrimination grievances were directly linked to HIV prevention efforts and the System of Community Protection, the municipal official and the project coordinators gathered at this meeting continued to see discrimination grievances as a proxy for ascertaining the collective capacities of transgender women in Tarapoto. As Norma herself observed, the idea that they lacked a culture of denouncement effectively pardoned law enforcement for their unwillingness to seriously consider the claims of transgender women by displacing widespread institutional disregard onto the individuals themselves. As shown by the stories that Norma, Pamela, Yesika, and others shared, it was not actually the case that they lacked a culture of denouncement. Rather, it was that the broader mechanisms did not take their denouncements seriously.

## The Terms of Denouncement

A crucial element of HIV prevention efforts revolves around the alleviation of discrimination and stigma toward people living with HIV/AIDS *and* toward communities vulnerable to it. Though antidiscrimination efforts broadly characterized HIV/AIDS interventions around the world, how interventions were experienced was also profoundly a function of local, regional, and national histories. In urban Amazonian Peru, deeply entrenched modes of maintaining and reproducing difference—entangled in long-standing hierarchies of race, ethnicity, and gender, and in a particular lexicon around the notion of scandal—shaped how interlocutors lived the moralizing imperative to denounce discrimination as a form of HIV prevention.

Project specialists and health promotors in Tarapoto contended with external pressures to identify and formalize discrimination grievances in the region. This pressure stemmed from broader assumptions about the Amazonian region in the national imaginary. Because antidiscrimination ordinances that included protections for sexual orientation and gender identity had been established in municipalities throughout the urban Amazonian region, there was an assumption that conditions there were more favorable for formalizing discrimination grievances. Another assumption was that, culturally, the Amazonian region was more open to sexual and gender difference than the Andean or coastal regions of the country. Amid these assumptions, the notion of cultivating a culture of denouncement emerged and circulated among project coordinators to make sense of why it was so challenging to produce formal grievances. This abstract concept referred to the objective of alleviating the negative impacts of discrimination and stigma on control of the HIV/AIDS epidemic by compelling individuals to come forward with and pursue formal discrimination grievances with a range of state entities. However, in using the "culture" concept to describe why some gay and transgender communities experienced injustice and exclusion, the idea of a culture of denouncement invoked long-standing forms of creating and maintaining ethno-racial hierarchy and difference.

Many responded to the call to take action against discrimination. However, because of the overlapping forces that silenced individuals or stymied their efforts, their experiences were most often not transformed into formal grievances. Through an analysis of a range of stories—all revolving around the exclusion of an individual from a disco—I introduced a distinction between "emblematic denouncement" and "scandalous denouncement." In the effort to cultivate a culture of denouncement, some of the project specialists involved in HIV prevention circulated emblematic stories of denouncement to inspire and incentivize individuals to come forward and take action when they experienced injustice. However, these emblematic cases sometimes elided the overlapping hierarchies and social barriers that transgender women and gay men encountered in urban Amazonian Peru. From the willful ignorance of the auxiliary municipal police to allegations that a person was being too scandalous in their denunciation of discrimination, the effort to cultivate a culture of denouncement paradoxically intensified the experiences of social stratification and discrimination already impacting gay and transgender communities.

Instead of foregrounding the emblematic denouncements of discrimination, this chapter dwelled on the stories interlocutors told of their scandalous denouncements. These were the stories of discrimination that never became legible, formal, or successful discrimination grievances. In these stories, scandal emerged as an unpredictable and dynamic social force with which they had to contend. Scandal was wielded against transgender women much more forcefully than against gay men. It could be used to dismiss or delegitimize an individual's allegations of discrimination, as was the case for Yesika and the members of the Las Amazonas organization. Alternately, scandal could be a strategy to amplify one's own account of discrimination. But ultimately, the scandalous denouncements showed that there was, in fact, a robust and vibrant culture of denouncement in Tarapoto. There was an existing, collective narrative about discrimination that many could inhabit and animate as a way to make sense of and make publicly and widely known their experiences of social exclusion. The fact that there were no emblematic cases of denouncement from Tarapoto did not mean that gay and transgender communities were ambivalent about or uninterested in the project of taking action and collectively contesting injustice in their lives; rather, the scandalous denouncements show how they did so on their own terms.

# 4

## When Projects End

The Fragmentation of Collaboration
and the Afterworlds of HIV Prevention

The ethos of collaboration, or *la colaboración*, was a constitutive element of gay and trans sociality throughout urban Amazonian Peru. As explored in previous chapters, the concept named a collective idealization of social life that most palpably emerged in the moments when someone assumed the important role of compelling and inspiring others to direct goods, resources, and opportunities, however small, to those considered to be in need. As opposed to a redistributive system that privileges the mediation of redistribution between unequal dyads, collaboration stressed the multiplication of ephemeral redistributive social relationships. Typically, the reproduction of these small moments of collective redistribution occurred in popular spectacles, such as beauty contests or soccer tournaments, but also through smaller fundraising activities. The enterprising and effusive individuals who successfully organized these events created the space for moments of small acts of redistribution to occur. As a result, they "won their names" as effective and responsible organizers. While they could be called *colaboradores*, or collaborators, this was not a widely recognized or typically lexicalized subject position. In other words, in Tarapoto, I never heard Anderson, Norma, or Martín—individuals who all had, at some point in their lives, "won their name" for effectively organizing redistributive activities—actively assume or name themselves as "collaborators." And yet I often heard comments and remarks about individuals over the course of fieldwork about the extent to which they were perceived to collaborate or not with the wider communities.

When projects addressing HIV/AIDS among key populations were introduced into the cities of Amazonian Peru in the late 2000s and early 2010s, it was the gay and trans individuals who had won reputations for organizing events, for collaborating with others in the community, and for being able to bring together large crowds and inspire them to engage in small acts of redistribution who transitioned into the new opportunities that came with the introduction of Global Fund projects. Some of these individuals, like Olaf in Pucallpa and Norma in Tarapoto, went through the long administrative process of formalizing their existing collectives as community-based organizations with *personaria juridica*, or legal personhood. Others earned short-term contracts to support the implementation of HIV prevention. As they reoriented themselves to the new tasks of HIV prevention in the 2010s—recruiting participants to attend capacity-building workshops, encouraging individuals to file formal discrimination grievances, and collecting and compiling the signatures and reports that evidenced that activities occurred and benchmarks were met—project specialists refracted the ethos of collaboration through the demands and obligations of HIV prevention projects. In the process, collaborators came to assume a newly introduced subject position: the project specialist.[1]

The category of "project specialist," in fact, became so widespread that even local newspapers began to use the term. *Diario Hoy*, a periodical of the San Martín region that covers regional governmental affairs, printed an announcement in 2013 with the headline "A Proposal on Sexual Orientation and Gender Identity Is Presented."[2] The brief article reported on a meeting that had taken place the day before between the members of the Homosexual Association of Mariscal Cáceres (Asociación Homosexual Mariscalence, AHOMA) and the director and civil servants of the Mariscal

Cáceres provincial education management sector.[3] In the meeting, AHOMA presented a proposal for an official directive in the provincial educational sector that would prohibit discrimination on the basis of sexual orientation and gender identity in primary and secondary schools. One of the most striking elements of the article is the photograph that accompanied it, directly under the headline. For a periodical that typically features droll updates, announcements, and ordinances regarding the municipal and provincial governments throughout the region, the fierce poses, contoured body positioning, and affectionate interlocking hands among the gay and trans members of AHOMA depicted in the photograph brought some pizazz to the day's news. In the article was a description of one of the members of the collective as an *especialista en proyectos*, or project specialist. By the early 2010s, some of the gay and trans collaborators who had long been known for organizing the activities that enabled collaboration now inhabited this new—and lexicalized—position and were broadly recognized as such.

However, the ambition to end AIDS—manifested in urban Amazonian Peru over the 2010s through the Global Fund's efforts to bolster the social conditions of key populations—paradoxically brought about new impasses that ultimately transformed the texture of the existing social fabric. This transformation was made evident in the stories of project specialists over the course of the Global Fund's Tenth Round and, more significantly, during the intense period of crisis that developed in 2014–15 when the Tenth Round was frozen and, subsequently, closed. While the decision to terminate the Tenth Round was the result of structural shifts in the provision and implementation of HIV prevention and determined by a governing board in Lima, located beyond the immediate social worlds of interlocutors, the closure of the Tenth Round was most palpably felt and lived through the transformation of social relations between project specialists and their communities.

Paradoxically, the sudden and abrupt closure of the Global Fund's Tenth Round precipitated social fragmentation among the communities that it sought to bolster. This paradox was symptomatic of the temporal limits that can emerge amid what Meinert and Whyte (2014) term "projectified landscapes." Building on the contradictory temporal entanglements of HIV/AIDS projects in which limited-time projects with predetermined ending points have been implemented to address a long-term epidemic, this chapter extends the concept to name and examine the enduring social consequences of a short-term project even years after it ended.

Despite the new predicaments that came along with the global ambition to end AIDS, project specialists imagined ways for queer social life to persist.

With the early termination of the Tenth Round they experienced tremendous loss to their names and the reputations they earned as collaborators prior to the introduction of the projects. Yet while the crisis of the ending of the Tenth Round brought intense periods of social fragmentation and, for the project specialists, a loss of their reputation as collaborators in their communities, it also generated productive moments of debate as well as source material for new stories. Stories about the Tenth Round insisted on alternative configurations for how queer social life might persist, most immediately after the Tenth Round's untimely ending but also in anticipation of the inevitable setbacks and failures that might emerge over the long-term effort to end AIDS in the future.

**The Freezing of the Tenth Round**

To receive funding, the Global Fund obligates countries to implement a model of multisectoral health governance. In theory, this means that the administration of health-related interventions is overseen by both the state and civil society. Most importantly, representatives of affected populations (e.g., people living with HIV/AIDS, sex workers, trans women) are supposed to have a seat at the decision-making table.[4] However, the hierarchical organization of the system created a considerable gap between the project specialists who interfaced with the vulnerable communities targeted for intervention and the CONAMUSA, or country coordinating mechanism, responsible for major decisions related to the implementation of Global Fund projects. For example, the CONAMUSA was responsible for the selection of the "principal recipient" of funding and the monitoring of the principal recipient's progress toward accomplishing the proposed objectives.[5] Nongovernmental organizations submit proposals to the CONAMUSA to administer Global Fund projects as the principal recipient. In Peru, this involves administering any given project across multiple regions throughout the country, and thus a significant amount of infrastructure, staff, and technical capacity. As a result, the NGOs typically eligible for this role are based in the country's capital city, Lima. In the case of the Tenth Round, the principal recipient then subcontracts the grant to smaller NGOs located in the regions of the country where the program is to be implemented. These NGOs are called sub-recipients. The Tarapoto-based Center for Amazonian Development (CEDISA) was the NGO selected as sub-recipient for the Amazonian portion of the Tenth Round, which operated in the cities of Tarapoto, Pucallpa, and Iquitos. Located in and around each of these cities were the community-based organizations (CBOs) that organized and implemented the on-the-ground, everyday activities associated with the Tenth Round. Project specialists assumed administrative and technical roles at the level of community-based organizations.

Over the course of 2014, a series of events transpired that ultimately brought about an untimely and unexpected end to the Tenth Round. INPPARES, the NGO that was originally selected to coordinate the first phase of the Tenth Round, renounced its continuation as principal recipient. The CONAMUSA thus terminated the contract with INPPARES and published a call for proposals for a new NGO to oversee the second phase of the Tenth Round. The Support Program for Health Sector Reform (PARSALUD) was selected to administer the second phase of the Tenth Round. PARSALUD was initiated in 2009 as a "project of public investment" managed by the Ministry of Health and financed by the Inter-American Development Bank, the World Bank, the Global Fund, and the National Treasury. Originally, the program focused on addressing infant and maternal health in the poorest regions of the country, as well as the Eighth Round of the Global Fund for a tuberculosis component in 2010. The CONAMUSA selected PARSALUD as the new principal recipient for the second phase of the Tenth Round's HIV/AIDS component.

Regional NGOs and CBOs across the country encountered a new set of problems, though, once PARSALUD assumed the coordinating responsibilities for the Tenth Round. PARSALUD was technically an agency of the Ministry of Health and, as a result, was subject to a different set of restrictions regarding acquisitions and contracts than INPPARES.[6] The way these restrictions most immediately impacted community-based organizations implementing HIV prevention was a shift in how operating costs and payments for rent would be funded. Instead of transferring money for rent— the largest and most significant cost encountered by the twenty-seven community-based organizations around the country involved in the Tenth Round—community-based organizations would have to pay rent up front and then wait to be reimbursed by PARSALUD. Until a solution to this administrative issue was solved, the Tenth Round was "frozen." In other words, project specialists were encouraged to continue their everyday operations related to HIV prevention and maintain their spaces, and they were assured that once the Tenth Round funds were unfrozen, operating costs for community-based organizations would eventually be reimbursed. However, in the meantime, they reported that they were responsible for either self-financing their spaces or going into debt with landlords.

By December 2014, the problems involved in the selection of a state entity as a principal recipient became insurmountable. PARSALUD renounced its role as the principal recipient and terminated the contract with the Global Fund.[7] Faced with the decision of whether to circulate another call for another NGO to become principal recipient of the Tenth Round or to terminate the Tenth Round entirely and elaborate a new "concept note" to the Global Fund, the CONAMUSA opted for the latter and effectively terminated the program as of January 2015.

## The Discrimination Archive

Several months after the closure of the Tenth Round, I asked Anderson to reflect on the impacts of the project. He suggested we have an informal conversation while we went through the records of the project in Tarapoto. He took me to a small room in the basement of CEDISA, where he had meticulously maintained the documents and reports relating to the implementation of the Tenth Round. There were about fifteen banker's boxes in the room, all carefully organized and labeled, and each tightly wrapped with clear plastic wrap. The boxes held the records of the Tenth Round for the entire Amazonian region, thus encompassing reports from Tarapoto, Iquitos, and Pucallpa. The majority of the documents detailed specific capacity-building workshops and trainings, each with an accompanying list of participant signatures, photographs of the event, and, sometimes, newspaper clippings that covered the activity. As a project specialist, Anderson was responsible not just for carrying out and implementing the goals of HIV prevention but also for being the project's principal archivist.

Anderson directed me toward the emblematic cases of discrimination that had been collected and archived through the System of Community Protection. He explained how, in coordination with other project specialists, they had been able to begin to cultivate a culture of denouncement by documenting these episodes of discrimination. There were three cases in total; each was documented on a technical form that had been specifically created for the purpose. Though only three pages long, the form contained a wealth of information that not only helped the victim of discrimination identify appropriate resources but also helped orient the project specialist through the process of supporting the formalization of the grievance. The first page of the form was straightforward, giving space for personal information about the victim, the *agresor* (the perpetrator of the discrimination), and any witnesses to the incident. It also had space for indicating

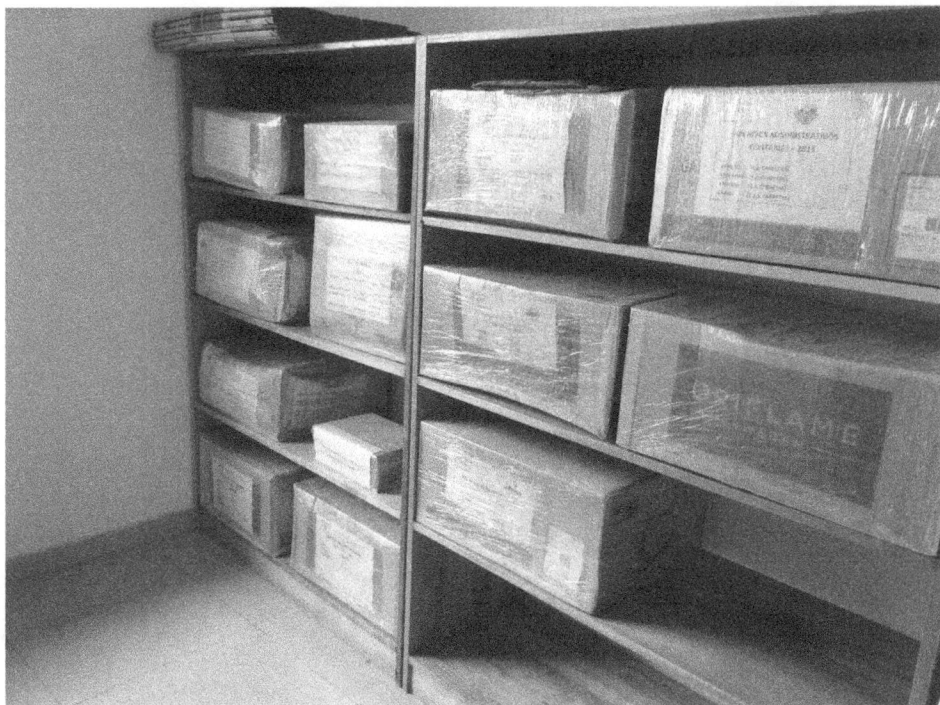

**Figure 4.1.** The administrative archive of CEDISA, storing documents pertaining to the System of Community Protection.

the context of how the story was collected (e.g., by which project specialist and at which community-based organization). The second page was more open-ended, asking the victim to describe the incident. After the space for description, the rest of the page contained a table outlining the procedures for formalizing the grievance (*el seguimiento*), such as filing a formal grievance with the police, with the Defensoría del Pueblo, or with INDECOPI. For each of these actions, there was space for the project specialist to document when the action was taken, pertinent file numbers, and the name of the bureaucrat who received or reviewed the grievance.

### State-Sanctioned Violence

The first form Anderson pulled out was an incident of state-sanctioned sexual violence toward a trans woman. A member of Las Amazonas recounted the story of what had happened to her to Norma, the president of the organization. Later, when Jefferson made a visit to the organization as part of the Tenth Round's System of Community Protection project, Norma recounted the details to him, and Jefferson filled out the form. Around 1:00 a.m., while the victim was standing at a street corner behind the city's sports coliseum, she was approached by a patrol from the auxiliary municipal police, or *el serenazgo*. The patrollers asked her for her identification card; when she did not furnish it, she was forced into the patrol vehicle. As the vehicle drove off, she realized that instead of traveling toward the municipal commissary, they were driving toward the hills to the northwest of the city. Inside the vehicle, the security officers began to harass her with suggestions that she perform oral sex on them. They also touched her inappropriately.

After she pleaded with them to let her go, the security officers threatened to drive her farther into the hills and leave her there. However, she was able to leave the vehicle at the very edge of town, where a heavily transited boulevard reaches a dead end atop a dramatic and deep precipice. Ten minutes into her walk back down the boulevard toward the center of town, a police patrol stopped her. They accused her of selling drugs, even insisting that she sell drugs to them. When she denied that she possessed or was selling drugs, the police officer threatened to plant drugs on her. Feeling threatened and intimidated by the police, she just kept walking and they eventually left.

### Discrimination at the Disco

The second case in the archive of the System of Community Protection was not a specific incident that had occurred but a composite case of discrimination that Norma and Jefferson co-authored during one of Jefferson's periodic visits to the Las Amazonas organization as an example to be used for pedagogical purposes (in fact, Norma had written "Example" at the top of the form), showing those gathered at the meeting what each element of the form was asking and the details that the description of the incident required. The composite case described an incident in which a trans woman was denied entry into a nightclub. The persistence of this story, even in the hypothetical version on this form, speaks more broadly to its endurance as a mode of exclusion that trans women across the community faced.

Norma described the incident in the first person, and while incidents like the one she described were frequent, she made clear that this was a hypothetical scenario. The security guards at the entrance to the nightclub refused to let her in, explaining that this been ordered by the nightclub administrators. After a discussion with the administrator, he said she was being denied entry because she was a transgender person. Upon hearing this, Norma opted to leave the nightclub.[8] The following morning, as she outlined in the form, she visited the INDECOPI office, and she included details such as what day and time she visited the office, the address of the office, and the names of those she talked to there. She indicated that she brought photographs of the incident as proof that she had been discriminated against at the nightclub.

## Even in Death They Are Discriminated Against

The third case described an episode of fraud committed by a municipal cemetery administrator, with the victim the sister of a young gay man who had recently passed away from an opportunistic infection associated with HIV/AIDS. Ramón brought the case to the attention of Jefferson, who introduced it into the System of Community Protection. The young man and Ramón had been neighbors, and Ramón heard about the incident through conversations with the deceased's sister.

As Ramón described in the written form, upon filling out the paperwork for the death certificate at the municipal civil registry office, the office administrator informed the deceased's sister that she would be required to pay an additional 600 soles (approximately $200) for the burial. But, the administrator added, if they conducted the transaction off the books, then the amount could be reduced. The reason she was given—and in the form, Ramón emphasized this as a direct quote from the administrator—was this: "These types of people cannot be buried with the rest. They have a special site, separated from the rest, and the plot has a thicker wall of concrete. This has a cost." The sister explained that they did not have this money, but the administrator insisted that the fee was obligatory and threatened to withhold the death certificate if it was not paid. The administrator continued, "When someone dies with that disease, they have to prepare the plot specially. I will call the man at the cemetery and see if he can lower the cost since you are my friend." A few moments later, the administrator reemerged and told the sister that she had been able to lower the price to 300 soles, but this was an obligatory fee required by the municipality. The sister then paid the administrator the money, but she was not given a receipt for the payment.

When I asked Ramón about the case, he explained that he had originally been approached by the sister of the young man who passed away to organize a *pollada* to help raise money for funeral expenses. It was in this process of organizing this *pollada* that Ramón found out what the municipal cemetery staff had been saying to the family. At the time, Ramón had a temporary contract as a community health promoter, so he was able to bring the incident to the attention of Jefferson. However, after some time, the family decided they did not want to follow through with the grievance:

they did not want to be identified, and they did not want to identify their brother as having been HIV positive.[9]

A few months later, when I was hanging out with Ramón at his family's corner store, he decided to take a walk and visit the cemetery. It was only a few blocks from his house; furthermore, he had heard that the cemetery's practice of extorting the families of people who had died with HIV/AIDS into paying additional costs was still happening. When we arrived at the cemetery, we found the row of thick, cement plots. When he recognized the name on a plot as that of a *compañero* or *compañera*, Ramón told me the nickname of the person: "This is La Cuchara . . . this is La Lluvia." It was an entire row of gay and transgender people, far apart from the rest of the deceased. He turned to me and said, "*Aun en la muerte están discriminados*"—even in death they are discriminated against.

The project specialists in Tarapoto understood the System of Community Protection as the centerpiece of their broader effort to cultivate a culture of denouncement, and, consequently, their pivotal contribution to mitigating the impact of discrimination and stigma across their communities. All of the cases collected through the project spoke to the lived and systematic realities of violence and exclusion experienced by those designated as key populations (and others) across Tarapoto. As chapter 3 indicated, trans women frequently circulated stories about encountering exclusion from the popular nightclubs in the city. The case of the cemetery fraud and the separation of the graves made visible the persistent stigma around HIV, a diagnosis that many gay and trans individuals and their families often kept highly guarded.

These three cases from the archive further highlight the new social tensions that project specialists encountered as they reoriented their efforts toward identifying emblematic cases of discrimination in their communities. The closure of the Tenth Round impacted the continuation of the project by pausing the long and time-intensive element of following up on discrimination cases and institutionalized practices of injustice. The cases were compiled in folders and sealed in boxes in the basement of CEDISA. But the story of the Tenth Round and its continuing impact on gay and trans social worlds did not end so neatly. Stories about the Tenth Round persisted even after it ended, and its consequences continued to affect the reputations of project specialists and their social relationships with their communities.

## Collaboration and Fragmentation

The freezing and subsequent termination of the Tenth Round was most palpably felt by the project specialists who ran community-based organizations. Rogerio, Olaf, and Arturo were project specialists outside of Tarapoto, in the cities of Chiclayo, Pucallpa, and Iquitos, respectively. They shared similar experiences of the serious crisis that transformed their position and social relations in their communities when the Tenth Round ended. This crisis obligated them to reconsider the long-term sustainability of the organizations that they now ran and the particular model of community health promotion that had been introduced through the Global Fund.

Project specialists often contended with allegations that they were mismanaging the projects or, more seriously, engaging in corruption or fraud. Capacity-building workshops connected with the System of Community Protection, for example, lacked the luster and spectacle of beauty contests and sports tournaments and, importantly, did not inspire others to engage in small forms of redistribution. Since they focused their efforts on identifying singular cases of discrimination, they were not perceived by others as contributing to or creating space for the system of collaboration. Some project specialists reported their sense of their shifting reputations to me in interviews and during informal conversations, but I also heard these ideas expressed by others in the everyday course of ethnographic fieldwork. For example, Rogerio, a project specialist who ran a gay community-based organization in the coastal city of Chiclayo, explained his awareness of what others said about him in an interview: "For me, before the Global Fund and before I became a project specialist, my activism was out in the street. But unfortunately, I had to go into the office more as a monitor. And because of this, there was more and more gossip about me, that I was profiting from the Tenth Round, that I lived off the Global Fund. But this was not the case. I was behind everything, helping plan and direct activities."

I suspect that these allegations were not rooted in actual moments of fraudulent or illegal practices at the level of community-based organizations. Rather, they reflected the changing roles of project specialists. While the new project specialists dutifully carried out the tasks associated with project monitoring and evaluation and meticulously archived the emblematic cases of discrimination that occurred in their communities, they spent less time planning the large spectacles that created opportunities for collective redistribution (i.e., *la colaboración*), the very spectacles through which they had earned their name in the community. Community members who were outside of the formal hierarchy of the projects experienced this shift with feelings of disillusion and disappointment and sometimes interpreted those feelings through the vocabulary of fraud, robbery, or corruption.[10] Thus, not only did the transformation from collaborator to project specialist predispose individuals to gossip, but these allegations intensified when the Tenth Round was terminated for reasons beyond their control.

When the Global Fund terminated the Tenth Round and many project specialists found themselves in a moment of crisis, they turned to redistributive activities like *polladas*, sports tournaments, and beauty contests to raise money to support the operating costs of their organizations. However, because in the recent past their efforts had been focused on the projects' new technical requirements, some found that they were not able to generate the same *convocatoria*, or turnout, for these redistributive activities that they might have been able to before becoming a project specialist. In our interview, Rogerio described his strategy for covering the expenses for the office space used by the community-based organization when the Tenth Round was terminated:

> On social media, everyone said I should do a *pollada*. "Okay, Rogerio, organize an activity," they said. And this put batteries in me to do a big, big, big activity, a *pollada*. So I did it, I organized a *pollada*. I sold tickets, but just to my personal friends; I did not get any help from the community. . . . It was not worth it, what we made from the *pollada* did not justify the work, selling tickets, and I grilled all the chicken. It was not a lot to ask, people could even just take the chicken to go. And so many people said they would come, but there was just no support.

Rogerio experienced the ending of the Tenth Round through the fragmentation of the social relationships that he had spent decades cultivating as an activist. He, too, felt disillusioned that the work he had done to formalize the community-based organization to bring the Global Fund's HIV prevention resources to his community went unrecognized. When he needed collaboration from others to help pay for the office space, he could no longer count on their support through traditional redistributive activities. The broader transformations that prompted opportunities for some individuals like Rogerio to become project specialists had significant social repercussions when the projects disappeared.

Olaf was a project specialist who operated a community-based organization in the city of Pucallpa. I conducted an interview with Olaf in 2015, several months after he received official word that the Tenth Round was terminated. Before he became a project specialist, Olaf was a popular seamster who created outfits for contestants in local beauty contests. He and a small group of friends eventually established a collective, where they would collaborate on the costuming, makeup, and hair for contestants in all kinds of beauty contests. Around 2008, he began to take on intermittent contracts as a community health promoter. By 2011, he formalized the collective into a community-based organization, and it was eventually selected alongside a few other gay, trans, and LGBT organizations to implement Tenth Round activities in Pucallpa.

As he recounted, a few months prior to the freezing of the Tenth Round, a team from Lima visited Pucallpa and required him to move his organization to a new site. He recalled that they told him the current site was too small to work as a "community center" and that moving to a larger site would enable more services and opportunities and meet the new requirements of the second phase of the Tenth Round. Olaf was hesitant to move the organization to a new site. He was proud of the reputation that he had established in the neighborhood and the broader community. Though small, the current site had been "won." He insisted that his organization had proven that they were good neighbors; even if they got a little too loud when they held activities, the neighbors did not get annoyed. They had put in a lot of work to "win" the community, and moving the organization to a new location would mean starting this process of "winning" the neighbors all over again. However, he eventually acquiesced and moved the community-based organization to a larger space.

A few months later, the Tenth Round was frozen and then ultimately terminated. During the period when the Tenth Round was frozen, before the CONAMUSA decided to terminate it entirely, Olaf recalled, he had been assured that the freeze was temporary. He insisted he had been told that the rent for the new space would be covered later, through a reimbursement. However, at the time of our interview, he found himself in a situation in which he was personally responsible for a backlog of several months of rent, and to a landlord with whom he had only recently established a relationship. He had been using the computers and office furniture acquired through the Tenth Round project as collateral and feared that the landlord would take everything because of the overdue rent. This, in fact, had happened to another community-based organization in a different district of Pucallpa: the land-lord locked the doors and kept all of the equipment, computers, and files until the rent was paid. Ultimately, Olaf lamented not just the move to a new space but, more importantly, what he perceived as the loss of his name in his neighborhood and community.

Arturo was a project specialist and the president of a community-based organization in Iquitos. He had several years of experience working on proj-ects, even prior to the start of the Global Fund's Tenth Round. When I con-ducted an interview with Arturo several years after the untimely ending of the Tenth Round, I asked him to reflect on his experience as a project spe-cialist at the time and for his organization. Arturo credited the introduction of a prior round, the Fifth Round, as his initial entry into HIV prevention efforts and the promotion of human rights. He specifically remembered a workshop that he had attended in Iquitos, run by activists associated with Movimiento Homosexual de Lima, as his starting point. However, over the course of the Tenth Round, he emphasized, the involvement of well-known LGBT activists associated with MHOL, especially Gio Infante, had helped him better understand the importance of human rights.[11] Even though the Tenth Round was specifically about HIV prevention, he recalled how conversations with these activists helped him and the *compañeros* and *compañeras* in his organization expand their focus beyond HIV prevention to include learning how to talk about and advocate for human rights more broadly.

Like Rogerio, Arturo was sensitive to the new pressures that came with the management of the Tenth Round project in his community. For example, the Tenth Round enabled community health organizations to increase the salary of *promotores*, or peer community health promoters. Before the Tenth Round, he explained, it was difficult to recruit *promotores* because the pay for the contracts was so little. He recalled that prior to the Tenth Round *promo-tores* were paid 300 soles per month (approximately $100). When the Tenth Round began, the budget for peer health promoters improved tremendously, and they were paid the same salary that "any other professional" would be paid. The drawback, though, was that this made the position of peer health promoter more desirable. Although Arturo selected peer health promot-ers based on their work history and their profile, he said, he was subject to allegations of favoritism by community members. Instead of project spe-cialists being perceived as engaging in "collaboration," which emphasized the creation of space for community members themselves to participate in collective redistribution, their selection of *promotores* appeared as a more personalized allocation of resources and opportunities to specific individuals, a role much closer to clientelism than collaboration. The result was that he was subjected to a new mode of social fragmentation he had not had to contend with in prior Global Fund rounds.

However, he insisted that the greatest fragmentation that occurred as a result of the Tenth Round took place when the round was frozen and in the aftermath. Arturo recalled that this caused *terremotos*, or earthquakes, all across Peru, but especially in the Amazonian region. The earthquakes, he explained, came from the fact that there was no plan for continuity. The Tenth Round offered community-based organizations across Peru resources, but it did not have a plan for how to sustain them: "I will give you a community center, I will give you computers and supplies, I will give you workshops and trainings. But what will happen next?"

The Tenth Round precipitated a restructuring of social relations among gay and trans communities across the country. For several of the gay and trans project specialists who implemented the Tenth Round at the level of community-based organizations, their former experiences organizing and staging collective redistributive activities as a means of responding to a crisis informed their strategies for responding to the new crisis they encountered with the freezing of the Tenth Round. However, for reasons outside of their control, they found that their hard-earned name as collaborators in the community had been diminished over the course of the project.

### The NGO Response

Directly above the community-based organizations in the hierarchy of the Tenth Round project was the nongovernmental organization selected as the regional sub-recipient. For the Amazonian region—which covered the community-based organizations in Tarapoto, Iquitos, and Pucallpa—the regional sub-recipient was CEDISA. Based in Tarapoto, CEDISA managed a wide range of sustainable development and human rights projects in the region. Mariana was the director of CEDISA, and Anderson was responsible for the administration of aspects of its portfolio related to the Global Fund. CEDISA, too, was impacted by the freeze of the Global Fund money and the later cancellation of the round, though to a different degree than the smaller community-based organizations. While many of the project specialists fell back on small redistributive activities like *polladas* in the aftermath of the Tenth Round's withdrawal in order to continue their work, Anderson and Mariana responded by drawing on their broader professional network. They emphasized the submission of new grant proposals, which resulted in new spaces for dialogue and reflection about the implementation and future of HIV prevention efforts.

As in other cities around the country, there were two main community-based organizations in Tarapoto involved in the Tenth Round: a transfeminine organization that served trans, transgender, and *travesti* communities and an organization that implemented programming that targeted gay men and MSM. Anderson and Mariana immediately mobilized to identify resources for the long-term operation and continuity of both community-based organizations in Tarapoto. Norma, the president of the transfeminine community-based organization Las Amazonas, had established its office in her house, so she did not have the issue with rent that many other organizations faced. The large patio in the center of Norma's multigenerational home always made sense as a meeting space for Las Amazonas, as well as her other enterprises of aerobics instruction and special-event hosting.

DISAM, on the other hand, confronted a problem that many community-based organizations encountered: how to pay for the months of past due rent incurred while the Tenth Round was frozen, and then how to sustain operations in the absence of direct Global Fund support. While for the purposes of the Tenth Round it was designated as the organization serving gay men and MSM, DISAM implemented a range of projects related to human rights promotion and broader LGBT advocacy. The Global Fund, though, supported a significant portion of the organization's rent. As a result, DISAM had recently moved to a new space on a bustling, centrally located road a few blocks from the city's main plaza. As soon as they received the news that the Tenth Round would be closed, the board of DISAM decided to vacate the new office space. They sold a television to pay for a moving truck and moved the computers, chairs, electronics, and office supplies to the house of the current president. Thus, DISAM modeled their response after Las Amazonas and moved the offices into an individual house.

To help ensure the continuity of the community-based organization DISAM, Anderson and Mariana quickly put together an emergency proposal to a European NGO that had previously funded smaller projects on LGBT and human rights in the region. Since he had studied in Iquitos and had worked closely with Arturo, Anderson prepared a proposal that also included temporary financial assistance for Arturo's community-based organization in Iquitos.

For Mariana and Anderson, the months following the closure of the Tenth Round felt like a swirl. They were constantly searching for and identifying new funding opportunities. As a nongovernmental organization with an existing record of project administration, as well as a large, modern office, CEDISA was better positioned than most of the community-based organizations to seek new streams of funding. Plus, this process unexpectedly became an opportunity to reassess the System of Community Protection, as well as a site to debate and reflect on some of the technical categories that HIV prevention had imposed in the local context.

Though it was developed and implemented as a strategy to mitigate HIV transmission by reducing discrimination and stigma, project specialists expressed a strong commitment to the goal of cultivating a culture of denouncement among gay and transgender communities. So even though the Tenth Round was no longer supporting the System of Community Protection, enthusiasm coalesced around finding new sources to fund its continuation. This was made evident when Mariana invited me to collaborate on a new grant proposal. She had recently found a request for proposals circulating from the Global Equity Fund, a US Department of State initiative composed "of like-minded governments and private sector entities dedicated to protecting and defending the freedoms of lesbian, gay, bisexual, transgender, and intersex (LGBTI) persons around the world."[12] She saw the short-term grant as an opportunity to maintain and continue the System of Community Protection.

She asked Anderson and me to come to the office one morning to begin putting together an outline of the proposal. Anderson was invited because of his extensive experience with the Global Fund in Peru, and I was invited because, she suggested, I might be able to offer insight from a North American perspective. The international cast of participants at the table was rounded out by a Dutch volunteer with extensive experience in international development and two Chilean contractors who specialized in environmental issues. With a copy of the request for proposals printed out in front of each of us gathered in the conference room, as well as a Google-translated version of the text projected on the wall, the group began discussing what might go into the two-page Statement of Interest that would need to be submitted to the Global Equity Fund before being able to submit the full proposal.

Mariana and Anderson settled on two initiatives to propose. The first would be sensitivity trainings conducted through a community theater group and presented at secondary schools throughout the department, which could be attended by students and their parents or other family members. CEDISA had implemented a similar program on human trafficking, and

Mariana suggested that the model could work for sensitizing students to and informing them about discrimination and stigma around HIV, sexual orientation, and gender identity.

The second initiative that would be proposed was a one-year continuation of the System of Community Protection. The group immediately set out to identify what might be the ideal strategies to undertake during the one-year continuation and what indicators might serve as markers of positive results, and settled on the support and success of one formal discrimination grievance. During this conversation, I asked why they were seeking to continue the System of Community Protection for only one year. Mariana, the director, responded, "It only lasts for one year because the point is to follow through with one case and set a precedent." Even though the objective was to cultivate a broader culture of denouncement throughout gay and transgender communities, the time-intensive realities of following through with a successful discrimination grievance obligated Mariana and Anderson to realistically imagine focusing on one incident and transforming it into an emblematic case.

The efforts to sustain community-based organizations in the aftermath of the closure of the Tenth Round foregrounded discussion about key differences between the experiences of gay men and trans women in Tarapoto and how to effectively distribute potential resources. The Global Equity Fund's call for proposals listed two objectives: one objective was geared toward the LGBTI population, and the other objective focused specifically on transgender women. NGOs had the option of submitting two separate statements of interest to correspond to the two distinct objectives or combining both objectives into one statement. The discussion over whether to craft two separate statements or just one turned into a frank and open conversation among those gathered.

With the precedent already established, as a result of Tenth Round requirements, to distinguish structurally between DISAM and Las Amazonas, there was now an opportunity to discuss whether this distinction would continue after the Tenth Round. Anderson posed the question to the group explicitly: Should they apply separately, with Norma submitting a statement on behalf of Las Amazonas and CEDISA submitting the statement for the LGBTI objective? Or should they combine the two objectives into one statement?

On the one hand, Anderson reasoned, there must have been a reason the call for proposals explicitly described the two separate objectives. Strategically, he continued, it would make sense to read between the lines and submit two separate statements. Mariana, however, disagreed. Neither Las Amazonas nor DISAM had the permanent infrastructure to be successful with this proposal. Las Amazonas was already located in Norma's own house, and as a result of the closure of the Tenth Round, DISAM had temporarily relocated to its president's house. As the conversation continued, it became apparent that this particular question touched on a recurring debate in Tarapoto regarding how and when it made sense for categories like "gay" and "transgender" to be combined and when it was more helpful to separate and distinguish the categories. Much like the debate over which division the lesbian soccer team would compete in during the soccer tournament (discussed in chapter 3), the meaning of sexual categories was constantly assessed and renegotiated.

They ultimately decided that it would make the most sense to submit one statement of interest that would combine both objectives; however, they would include letters of support for Las Amazonas and DISAM as annexes to the statement. Even though this statement of interest never came to fruition, as they later found that they did not meet the criteria to submit the application, the discussion itself illuminated the contours of debates that existed outside and beyond the proposal itself. Mariana and Anderson imagined that the continuation of antidiscrimination efforts in Tarapoto would require a combined effort between Las Amazonas and DISAM, while also acknowledging the structural differences between the experiences of the members of the two groups. Yet they still found it important to continue working in conjunction with both community-based organizations, suggesting how, in Tarapoto, categories were lived and experienced as permeable and emergent.

## Scandalous Stories of Unfinished Projects

The untimely end of the Tenth Round, a project that had brought tremendous promise and resources to efforts to improve the social conditions of gay and transgender communities in Peru, weighed heavily on Anderson. He was frustrated and disappointed with the decisions that were made in the CONAMUSA. His own professional trajectory was intertwined with the introduction of the Global Fund in the Amazonian region, and he valued the opportunities that it had given to him and to many of his gay and trans friends throughout the country. But this was not the first hardship he had encountered. His life was full of moments of crisis and adversity, many of which I learned about when he recounted those struggles in the form of stories of the scandals that punctured his life experiences. He was the youngest of twelve siblings, and his family was never fully supportive of his sexual orientation and desire to become a public-facing advocate for LGBT issues in Tarapoto. His stories ranged from the familial challenges he encountered as a young adult when he entered a Miss Gay beauty contest in Tarapoto to a contentious encounter with the dean of his law school in Iquitos, who tried to expel him for writing a thesis on violence and discrimination toward gay and trans people. His repertoire of stories was an experiment in living otherwise, an archive of his own journey in finding a place amid a social world that all too frequently limited his ambitions, his talents, and the change he aspired to make in the world.[13]

Many of his scandalous stories pivoted on an encounter with adversity and then, even when all seems lost, having a stroke of luck and coming out ahead. It is no surprise that the challenges of the Global Fund and the Tenth Round also became a subject of Anderson's storytelling. He often found moments during meetings to insert a moment of entertainment and captivate those gathered with these stories. For example, during the discussion about the application to the US Department of State's Global Equity Fund, Mariana observed that the proposal was an electronic application—no hard copies required at all. Mariana and Anderson gave a collective sigh of relief, much to the confusion of everyone else gathered. Shortly thereafter Anderson explained their relief with a scandalous story from years prior, back when CEDISA had first applied to be the coordinator of the Amazonian portion of the Tenth Round.

Years earlier, before CEDISA started coordinating the Tenth Round activities from Tarapoto, Anderson was living and working in Iquitos. When the call for proposals for sub-recipients for the Tenth Round was announced, CEDISA formed a coalition with a community-based organization in Iquitos (run by Arturo) and an LGBT activist group based in Lima to apply to coordinate the Amazonian portion of the intervention. From Iquitos, Anderson, Arturo, and others prepared the materials required for the application. However, the application had to be submitted in Lima, in person and in hard copy. "You could not submit any of the materials electronically," Anderson emphasized.

The night before the proposal was due, Anderson stayed up all night getting the documents, timelines, budget materials, and everything else in order. He was so focused on the task that he completely lost track of time, and before he knew it, the sun was already up and he had to leave to catch the first morning flight. (At this point in Anderson's telling of the story, he grabbed a stack of papers and used frenetic gestures and an exasperated tone.) He jumped into a *motocar* and rushed to the airport with the documents in hand. The driver went too fast, though, and as Anderson tried to transfer the papers from loose stacks into properly ordered and numbered binders, the wind blew all the papers out of order. He could barely keep the papers in his hand, but managed to hold on tight and did not lose anything to the wind.

He made it to the airport and ran to the gate, but, unfortunately, he was too late to board the plane, and so missed his flight to Lima. Now he would have to wait two more hours until the next flight to Lima, which was scheduled to leave at 10:00 a.m. This would be cutting it very close, as the deadline was 1:00 p.m. that day. He had no choice but to wait. If the flight left on time, he could be in Lima by 12:30, he told himself, and traffic from the airport in Lima at that time would not be as bad as during normal rush hour.

He got on the next flight to Lima, but while he was in the air, he remembered that he needed to make additional copies of the proposal, and each copy had to be in a binder. So he would need to stop at the partnering organization in Lima to make the copies and put them in binders. When he arrived at the office he found a group of queer *compañeros* and *compañeras* ready to get to work making the copies and putting the binders together. They "worked like ants" to get the binders together, but, alas, they missed the 1:00 p.m. deadline. Everyone was devasted because they had worked so hard to get the proposal together.

Anderson called the office of the principal recipient to inform them that they had been unable to get the proposal in on time. But he received good news: the other NGO applying to coordinate the Amazonian region also had missed the deadline. So both groups were granted extensions, and Anderson was able to turn in the appropriate number of binders. (Their proposal was eventually selected for funding, and that was how CEDISA became the sub-recipient to coordinate the Tenth Round in the Amazon.)

After turning in the proposal, Anderson went to his hotel in Lima and went immediately to sleep. He had built up so much anxiety and had become so tired after working all night that he proceeded to sleep for an entire twenty-four hours. When he woke up, he briefly did not even know where he was, and at first he didn't recall the episode with the proposals at all. (At this point Anderson concluded the story; his last wry observation, inserted to circle back to the topic at hand, was that they should definitely go ahead with the application because it was electronic and not a hard copy.)

The ethos of collaboration lay at the heart of the story's moral lesson. The story hinged on a moment in which Anderson believed there was absolutely no way of salvaging the situation. After a succession of missteps, misfortune, and bad luck, it was with the collective support of a team and a final stroke of good luck that things worked out. The scandalous scene of Anderson, who had tried to do it all alone, racing through the city of Iquitos with papers flying in the wind, contrasts with the collective support that he received when he finally made it to Lima, and which ultimately made the proposal come together. Through a coordinated effort—so coordinated that it was as if they were "working like ants"—they were able to overcome the unknown forces conspiring against them. To borrow a turn of phrase from Saidiya Hartman, Anderson's scandalous story was an "experiment in how-to-live" (2019, 228). That is, in narrativizing the episode as a scandal, reconfiguring it through the arts of exaggeration and embellishment, Anderson shared a broader lesson about navigating adversity even when all paths forward appeared closed. Despite the obstacles brought about by the "projectification" of the goal of ending AIDS, he storied a lesson about how to persist.

The richness of Anderson's story about what is normally a mundane process of applying for a grant is enhanced by the clear intertextual connections to the scandalous stories circulated among gay and trans communities. Scandalous stories about their romantic lives, about their experience with the internal armed conflict, and about what happened at social events were animated by the same twists, turns, and embellishments that Anderson used in the story about the application. Similarly, Martín's story, discussed in chapter 2, ended with a stroke of good luck resolving the problem after what felt like successive, and increasingly inescapable, moments of adversity and bad luck.

Anderson told this story in the middle of what felt like a real crisis for him and the other project specialists who had dedicated years to improving the social conditions of their communities. At a moment when it appeared as though all the efforts would come to an abrupt and unexpected end, Anderson insisted that the story of preventing HIV—in essence, the story of ending AIDS—was still unfolding and therefore still unfinished. And, as an unfinished project, the end of AIDS was a story best told in the subjunctive: "the grammatical mood that expresses doubts, wishes, and possibilities" (Hartman 2008, 11). Turning to the arts of embellishment and exaggeration, Anderson crafted a narrative in which, lingering in the background of the story, there was a horizon of an afterworld: what *could be* after the end of AIDS. The episode they were currently living, which had been brought about by the closure of one project targeting HIV prevention, was not yet over; there was, perhaps, still space for wishes and possibilities.

With just one moment of coordinated and collective effort—and, perhaps, a stroke of good luck—things might go their way.

## Anticipatory Imaginaries

Eventually, Peru elaborated a new "concept note" to implement renewed support for the national HIV/AIDS program for vulnerable populations in urban and Amazonian regions of the country.[14] A new principal recipient was selected, and HIV prevention programming among key populations resumed. Left fragmented and with much less infrastructure as a result of the closure of the Tenth Round, HIV prevention efforts became a more centralized project based primarily out of Lima. Community-based organizations selected to implement subsequent projects found themselves operating with new restrictions, like a prohibition on the purchase of new office or computer equipment. While capacity-building workshops and trainings appeared sporadically in the cities of Amazonian Peru, many individuals who had previously worked on the projects sought out new or different opportunities.

Arturo's community-based organization in Iquitos weathered the crisis of the freezing of the Tenth Round. Piecing together funding opportunities, he was able to keep his organization going not just through the decade but even through the unexpected crisis of the global coronavirus pandemic. In 2022, I visited Arturo at his office. It was the same space that he had used throughout the Tenth Round. Posters, pamphlets, and other ephemera from the Global Fund were still on the walls and neatly catalogued in boxes and shelves in the space. I also learned that, over time, he had been able to rebuild some of the communal and social relations fragmented by the Tenth Round. For example, in 2020, during one of the most intense waves of the coronavirus pandemic in Iquitos, Arturo co-organized a collection of basic, nonperishable food items that were distributed across the city to LGBT people in need of food.

I had come to visit Arturo, though, because he had asked me to help him translate documents related to a new funding opportunity that a colleague in Lima had mentioned to him. He wanted to learn more and see if his organization could be eligible to apply. As we went through the documents, we ultimately determined that Arturo and his organization were ineligible.

Although he decided he would not prepare an application, he still shared with me the projects that he would have proposed, continuing to imagine ways to support the rights and prospects of LGBT communities in Iquitos. I asked Arturo what he remembered about the Tenth Round and, more generally, the impacts of the Global Fund. Although so much had happened since the Tenth Round had been paused nearly seven years earlier, what he remembered revolved around how it could have been planned and implemented differently:

> For the Global Fund, it was just about meeting the numbers and spending the money, nothing else. I always had a much broader vision of the political transformations we could make in Iquitos, but it was limited by the format and requirements of the Global Fund. For example, say we had to do a workshop. What happened was that we would invite forty people to the workshop, as per the mandate, but only five would show up. Instead of going on with the day-long workshop at some meeting room in a hotel in Iquitos, I would have always wanted to plan a retreat for those five who would show up. Let's get out of Iquitos, maybe have some kind of exchange of new ideas and new practices.

As he looked back and recalled the Tenth Round, he landed on the example of workshops to summarize his assessment. Workshops had been essential to the Tenth Round and were one of the main programming elements for mitigating and reducing the social problems affecting HIV vulnerability. In his memory, they stood as one of his most difficult challenges as a project specialist back then: although organizers had the support and money to put on such workshops, they never had the *convocatoria* that they had anticipated or expected. For Arturo, this was one of the limits of the Tenth Round. He went on to describe what he imagined for a retreat activity:

> Imagine a retreat: We get out of the city, on a Sunday. Or we leave on a Saturday, and come back on a Sunday. We rent a small van, ask two people to bring food, a few others to bring materials, and we go, say, to a river, and we sit down and talk. You know, a place where people feel more relaxed. After working, we go to the river, we have breakfast and lunch together, and then go to the *maloca* and get to work. But the Global Fund wouldn't let us do this. We could not present this with the Global Fund. With the Global Fund, anything had to be in the city; it had to be at the Victoria Regia hotel. The capacity-building workshops had to have this schedule, at this hour, with these people, and it had to be like this or that. But we always wanted to do it differently. And we could have, even with half of the budget that went to the Tenth Round.

While Arturo's alternative proposal for a small retreat instead of, say, a workshop on the System of Community Protection might not have changed the ultimate outcome of the Tenth Round, his proposal was not necessarily about changing activities because one might have a "greater impact" or "better value" for improving "outcomes." Rather, it revealed his effort to reimagine HIV prevention through the ethos of collaboration. In this alternative vision, the role of the project specialist was not about collecting and archiving individual, emblematic cases of discrimination but about creating space for the reproduction of collective sociality within gay and trans communities. In Arturo's proposal, each participant brought a small but meaningful item to redistribute and, effectively, to make the retreat happen. This was, at its heart, the fundamental model of redistributive activities like *polladas*. Arturo's assessment of the Tenth Round was a reimagining of the unfinished project of ending AIDS refracted through the ethos of collaboration. And even though many social relationships were fractured as a result of the Tenth Round, Arturo projected a vision of the future that insisted on the significance of a social world held together through small acts of collaboration.

## Collaboration after Fragmentation

The HIV/AIDS component of the Tenth Round of the Global Fund coincided with the prominent circulation of a broader, global discourse about the status and possibility of an end to AIDS in the future.[15] In urban Amazonian Peru, the Tenth Round aimed at significant structural reconfiguration in gay and transgender communities, as a means of preventing HIV through social interventions among the communities already most vulnerable to and impacted by the epidemic. These transformations came in the form of new institutional arrangements, including the creation of formalized community-based organizations, as well as new individual opportunities, specifically the emergence of the novel "project specialist" subject position.

However, precisely at a time when, globally, enthusiasm for the prospect of ending AIDS was growing, gay and transgender communities in Peru paradoxically encountered a contraction of HIV prevention efforts through the abrupt and unexpected termination of the Tenth Round. The failure of the Tenth Round was no small matter; even if the project did not operate long enough for project specialists to go through the entire process of formalizing a discrimination grievance, its closure generated loss and precipitated social fragmentation. And it was the project specialists in cities such as Tarapoto, Iquitos, and Pucallpa who ultimately bore the brunt of the withdrawal of the Global Fund, despite having very little to do with the actions that ultimately brought about the end of the Tenth Round. Project specialists experienced the continued resonance of the Tenth Round's abrupt ending through a fragmentation of social relations and a loss of their hard-earned reputations as collaborators in their communities.

And yet, amid the crisis precipitated by the administrative closure of the Tenth Round, project specialists found ways to engage with the crisis through their practice of scandalous storytelling. There was an anticipatory lesson in their stories, a lesson that exceeded the insight generated through traditional techniques of project monitoring and evaluation. And while the scale of the Tenth Round might appear small within the grander scheme of the unfinished project to end AIDS, its sudden and unexpected closure anticipated some of the major setbacks that the global "end of AIDS" effort would encounter in the following years.[16] In Peru, project specialists subjected the story of the closure of the Tenth Round to stylized tropes and embellishments, thereby imagining how they could continue to promote the dignity and rights of gay and trans communities and, importantly, do so in a way that insisted on the centrality of the collaborative ethos.

5

## Stories That Count

The Pathways
of Discrimination Stories

In 2014, the Joint United Nations Programme on HIV/AIDS (UN-AIDS) announced the "fast track" toward ending AIDS by 2030. The strategy entailed three numerical targets, known as the 90-90-90 targets. In order to stay on track to end AIDS by 2030, by the year 2020, 90 percent of all people living with HIV/AIDS would know their status, 90 percent of those living with HIV would be on anti-retroviral therapy, and 90 percent of those on antiretroviral therapy would reach undetectable viral loads. These targets were intended to synchronize efforts across multiple settings and scales, as well as to create a set of standardized disciplinary metrics to incentivize accountability (Kenworthy, Thomann, and Parker 2018; Sandset 2021). Amid the curtailment of HIV/AIDS funding that characterized the period, it became more and more incumbent on countries and communities to evidence progress toward these standardized, universal numerical targets. However, despite the universalizing ambitions of the 90-90-90 targets, access to robust and up-to-date data was not always universal. In Peru, as Cáceres et al. (2013) observe, data essential for HIV prevention and ending AIDS—such as estimates of key populations, cumulative case reports, and total numbers of people living with HIV/AIDS—was frequently inconsistent across the country. This meant that in the country's Amazonian region, far outside of the capital city, project specialists engaged in HIV prevention advocacy within a context of what Adams (2016) refers to as the problem of "data deprivation," or the lack of data.[1] As efforts to control HIV/AIDS increasingly turned toward the numerical and quantitative, this chapter poses an alternative question: What knowledge practices develop when data is inaccessible or unreliable?

Project specialists navigated complex and dynamic fields of knowledge in their effort to advocate for their communities. On the one hand, they were closely involved in HIV prevention. Because of the concentration of the epidemic among gay men, trans women, and men who have sex with men, this meant that their activities and advocacy primarily focused on gay men and trans women. More specifically, in Peru they focused on alleviating the impacts of discrimination as a means of reducing the transmission of HIV. However, they were also part of broader LGBTQ social movements. These movements developed specialized knowledge practices that often paralleled the quantitative methods dominant in the global health sciences. Through a process of conversion—that is, the effort to make stories of discrimination quantifiable—project specialists collected cases of discrimination on the ground in diverse regions of the country, then sent these stories to NGOs and activist collectives in Lima, which coordinated efforts to quantify and analyze the cases. Through reports, diagnostics, and surveys, nongovernmental organizations and LGBTQ activist collectives codified and concretized discrimination by turning individual episodes into objective and authoritative knowledge, and creating what I call "stories that count." These reports made their way back to project specialists, who then used the data as a "credibility tactic" to engage in HIV prevention advocacy *and* the promotion of LGBTQ human rights (Epstein 1996). Along the way, project specialists navigated shifting and murky categorical waters. Sometimes they focused broadly on the human rights of lesbian, gay, bisexual, transgender, and queer communities, while at other times they focused narrowly on HIV prevention among gay men and transgender women. Still, they brought these adjacent, though autonomous, fields of knowledge together as a strategy for circumventing the limits of data deprivation.

In tracking the conversion of experiences of discrimination from first-person stories to quantifiable evidence about discrimination toward LGBTQ people across the country, I show how the process of conversion—the effort to make stories of discrimination quantifiable—in turn transformed social relationships and created the space for novel queer subjectivities to emerge along the way. In this chapter, I focus specifically on moments of data collection that I observed in the popular, communal space of volleyball games. By making use of the capacity of volleyball games to bring together large numbers of gay and trans people, I further show how the ethos of *colaboración* sustained ongoing efforts to document discrimination. And while the process of storying one's own experience of discrimination can be cathartic, ethnographic attention to the everyday experience of doing so makes visible the diverse ambivalences and hesitations that some individuals felt toward the effort to assume authorship of their own experience of discrimination. Likewise, an examination of the intersubjective moments that emerged when multiple research projects converged—moments when interlocutors reversed the ethnographic gaze and conscripted me into the position of a "research subject"—can open new vantage points for examining emergent cultural processes and transforming social relations.

### Diagnostics and Reports of LGBT Rights in Peru, 2005–2016

In the early to mid-2000s across Latin America, researchers associated with human rights and LGBT social movements, activist collectives, and non-governmental organizations began to engage in efforts to survey and assess the status of LGBT and trans rights across their respective national contexts using quantitative methods and techniques. In Argentina, Lohana Berkins and Josephina Fernandez published the seminal and groundbreaking study *La gesta del nombre propio* (2005), which was followed up by Lohana Berkins's (2007) *Cumbia, copeteo y lágrimas: Informe nacional sobre la situación de las travestis, transexuales y transgéneros*. Hanssmann (2020) considers these studies to be exemplary of the genre he terms "epidemiological biographies," studies undertaken by social-movement-affiliated community-based researchers and activists that combine biographical narrative with statistical data and exhibit an explicitly political tone and orientation. As Sosa (2023) documents in the case of Brazil, a range of efforts to monitor and quantify homo- and transphobic violence persisted over the same period, including activist manuals for collecting journalistic accounts of violence, the collection of statistics by official government agencies, and policy plans for combatting LGBTQ violence and discrimination.

These efforts paralleled an increasing and broader global turn toward the hegemony of quantitative metrics in global health that emerged alongside efforts to scale up access to HIV treatment around the world. Yet despite claims regarding the comprehensiveness, universality, authority, and neutrality of quantitative metrics, critical medical anthropologists have shown how the use of quantitative metrics in health contexts can be limited, contested, and context-specific (Adams, Burke, and Whitmarsh 2013; Biruk 2018; Briggs and Mantini-Briggs 2003; Fan 2017; Guerra-Reyes 2019; Sangaramoorthy 2012; Sangaramoorthy and Benton 2012; Storeng and Béhague 2014). One of the more novel transformations in global health, as scholars have pointed out, has been the ways in which global health interventions require not just evidence of health outcomes but also data that can be scaled up and applied at other sites across the world.[2] As a result of the increasing use of public-private partnerships in global health, emphasis has shifted toward demonstrating that an intervention can produce robust, generalizable data through accepted scientific methods. The way to entice private investment was no longer just to show that a strategy was effective but also to demonstrate that it could be co-branded and sold for profit elsewhere (Adams 2016). Because of the shifting dynamics of legibility in global health, data deprivation could be considered by some as "even more tragic than lacking health" (Adams 2016, 44).

To my knowledge, efforts to produce technical diagnostics in the form of annual reports regarding the status of sexual rights among and discrimination toward LGBT people first emerged in the early 2000s in Peru within social movement and activist spaces, and in response to a paucity of systematic data about LGBT communities across the country. As activists and scholars associated with the organization Movimiento Homosexual de Lima, Jorge Bracamonte Allaín and Roland Alvarez Chávez (2006) authored a groundbreaking *informe anual*, or annual report, assessing the situation of LGBT human rights in Peru. The organization and layout of the report suggest an important connection to the final report of Peru's Truth and Reconciliation Commission, which had been published only a few years earlier. Importantly, Bracamonte Allaín and Alvarez Chávez collected and catalogued the testimonies of LGBT victims of violence from both during and after the internal armed conflict. The authors not only cited testimonies collected and published previously in the Truth and Reconciliation Commission's final report but also included testimonies that their organization had collected that did not appear in the final report. The anecdotes were woven together to elaborate a broader narrative about the forms of discrimination LGBT Peruvians have experienced, to describe who the primary perpetrators of violence and discrimination toward LGBT people have been, and, finally, to provide recommendations in the form of legal reforms that the state ought to implement. The authors explicitly describe the adverse impact that the discrimination and violence experienced by LGBT people have on the transmission of HIV, and use the collected cases to evidence the persistence and breadth of discrimination. The activist orientation of the authors of this first study set a crucial tone that persisted in subsequent efforts to diagnose and assess the status of LGBT communities in Lima and throughout the country.

The feminist nongovernmental organization Centro de Promoción y Defensa de los Derechos Sexuales y Reproductivos (PROMSEX) and the Red Peruana de Trans, Lesbianas, Gays y Bisexuales (Red Peruana TLGB), both based in Lima, continued the effort to collect and analyze the status of LGBT human rights in the country through the publication of annual reports and diagnostics. Over the period under consideration, PROMSEX published eight comprehensive annual reports on the human rights of LGBT people in Peru, covering the years 2008, 2009, 2010, 2011, 2012, 2013–14, 2014–15, and 2015–16.[3] Overall, the cases of discrimination, violence, and human rights violations that are documented in these reports tend to skew toward Lima, though the reports do include cases from around the country. There are a few notable shifts that can be observed in the comparison between the initial MHOL report and the subsequent PROMSEX/Red Peruana TLGB annual reports. While the focus on experiences of discrimination persisted, issues of health, including HIV/AIDS, were not emphasized or foregrounded. The themes of the rights to education, political participation, and forming a family, for example, were used to structure the reports. The various authors and coordinators of the series of PROMSEX/Red Peruana TLGB reports specifically note the use of the 2006 Yogyakarta Principles as a reference point, suggesting that some of these transformations were influenced by the introduction and global dissemination of the Yogyakarta Principles.[4] Another significant difference between this set of annual reports and the MHOL report was the sheer number of cases arranged and collected. Whereas the MHOL report emphasized the solicitation of detailed testimonies from victims, the PROMSEX/Red Peruana TLGB reports tended to focus on enumerating and archiving cases. This meant that while more cases and examples were included in the PROMSEX/Red Peruana TLGB reports, there was less emphasis on first-person narrative or detail. Instead of focusing on longer testimonies or descriptions, these reports arrange data about episodes of violence and discrimination in rows and columns with the name of the victim, the terms regarding sexual orientation and gender that the victim may have been known to identify with, who the aggressor was, the location where the discrimination or violence occurred, and a description of how the authors discovered or otherwise found out about the case.

A third set of technical reports for the period under consideration came from the activist collective No Tengo Miedo. This collective published two comprehensive studies in the period under consideration: *Estado de Violencia* (Machuca and Cocchella 2014) and *Nuestra Voz Persiste* (Machuca Rose, Cocchella Loli, and Gallegos Dextre 2016). The first focused on metropolitan Lima, while the second report expanded the scale to include Lima, Callao, and four other departments in Peru. Together, the No Tengo Miedo reports marked a third transformation in the existing tradition of LGBT human rights activist research. Like the MHOL and PROMSEX/Red Peruana TLGB reports, the No Tengo Miedo reports outlined different forms of violence and discrimination, different spaces where these might occur, who might be involved, and what steps were taken for each of the cases. In addition to the introduction of new categories of selfhood, such as "gender non-binary" and "queer," a characteristic that distinguishes the No Tengo Miedo publications from the other two sets of reports was the incorporation of statistical analysis.

The output of the No Tengo Miedo reports most closely coincided in time with the antidiscrimination efforts that were implemented as part of the Global Fund's HIV prevention activities, such as the System of Community Protection. However, they take a more expansive view of health, well-being, and discrimination than traditional health science literature by describing diverse forms of violence and casting a much broader net in terms of subject population. The reports catalogue and analyze discrimination not just through the collection of individual, first-person testimonies but also through elaborate quantitative techniques including distributions, frequencies, and percentages. They consider the data in relation to the LGBTQ population as a whole, as well as broken down by each constitutive category of the acronym. Through their technical combination of biographical and quantitative data, these two studies thus appear closest to the genre of activist research that Hanssmann (2020) termed "epidemiological biographies." There is a seamless intertwining of statistical data and biographical narrative, artfully arranged alongside photographs and figures.

## Responding to Data Deprivation

The trajectory of activist and community-driven studies regarding the human rights of LGBT communities in Lima and across Peru represents an effort that is adjacent to, though autonomous of, the HIV prevention projects profiled throughout the book. Most significantly, in terms of the population under examination, the two efforts cast nets of drastically different sizes. HIV prevention focused on "key" or "vulnerable" populations in Peru, with an emphasis on communities of gay men and transgender women in urban Amazonian Peru, as explored throughout the book, and in the major cities of the country's coast. Thus, since discrimination and stigma were social forces that could determine or impact the transmission of HIV, antidiscrimination efforts sought to mitigate the effects of discrimination on key populations. On the other hand, the activist and community-based diagnostics that sought to document and analyze discrimination and violence toward LGBT communities took a broader and more expansive approach in order to assess and promote the human rights of those communities. Studies not only included gay, lesbian, bisexual, and transgender groups but also, over time, expanded to include other categories of sexual and gender diversity, including "queer," "intersex," and "nonbinary." Although they represented a separate project from HIV prevention, the efforts to compile and collect cases of violence and discrimination for the purpose of assessing the status of LGBT human rights in Peru came together with the efforts to collect cases of discrimination for the purpose of HIV prevention on the ground. Project specialists who had been contracted to perform diverse HIV prevention projects through the Global Fund adapted their training and drew on their existing social relationships and reputations to support adjacent efforts to document LGBT human rights. In the process, project specialists encountered a range of categorical slippages, maneuvering around shifting terms of sexual orientation and gender identity, as well as fields of knowledge (e.g., health sciences, epidemiology, public policy, and human rights). Yet the focus on discrimination—on making it knowable and quantifiable— enabled on-the-ground project specialists to work within the limits of categorical slippages.

As part of the System of Community Protection, some project specialists in Iquitos, Pucallpa, and Tarapoto spent time reviewing local periodicals for cases of discrimination relating to sexual orientation and gender identity. Arturo, a project specialist in Iquitos, explained that when he identified cases in local periodicals, he would collect them for the archival purposes of the

System of Community Protection (even in periods when funding for the program was frozen), but he also sent the same cases to his collaborators and contacts at NGOs based in Lima:

> They have asked me for the data and I only have told them what has happened, that is all. In Iquitos, we collected newspaper articles. But we also send them to the organizations that collect the discrimination data. PROMSEX creates an annual report about human rights and discrimination toward the LGBT community. Sometimes I look in the newspapers for cases, and send them so that I do not have to go all the way to Lima, but that is what the cases are for, for these reports, to show what rights were violated and the year that it happened.

The journalistic accounts of discrimination that were collected and archived throughout the Amazonian region while carrying out HIV prevention efforts were also sent to other NGOs in Lima to support their efforts to document violence and human rights violations against LGBTQ people. When NGOs or other researchers reached out to him for data or information, Arturo forwarded the research that he had conducted. This two-pronged approach of collecting discrimination cases for both HIV prevention efforts and LGBT human rights research, he further explained, was motivated by his own sense of data deprivation about LGBT people in Peru:

> There is simply no data about how many LGBT there are in Peru. From the census, we do not have this kind of information, and the state does not care to collect it. Because of this, the state does not include in its plans support for cases of hate crimes, support for people living with HIV/AIDS, support for young people who are excluded from education because of homophobia and bullying, and so as activists we have to create the data about LGBT in Peru, but from the Global Fund and from international cooperation.

Arturo recognized the significance of data. He and others in the Amazonian region navigated a complex and far-reaching ecosystem that extended beyond the cities of the Amazon, to Lima and to the international entities that supported the promotion of LGBT human rights in Peru. While the primary source of funding for his organization and his own efforts in Iquitos was the Global Fund under the rubric of HIV prevention, he also positioned himself to connect and collaborate with organizations and researchers who worked outside of HIV/AIDS and the health sciences. However, the training and support that he received through the various workshops and programs that arose because of the Global Fund's Tenth Round proved to meaningfully support his work and his ability to adapt and be nimble even after the round ended.

## Collecting Cases of Discrimination in Tarapoto

Like Arturo, Anderson's experience with the Global Fund's projects helped him collaborate with a range of entities promoting LGBT rights beyond HIV prevention. As a project specialist responsible for activities throughout the Amazonian region for the Tenth Round and other Global Fund programs, Anderson frequently traveled between the cities of Tarapoto, Iquitos, and Pucallpa. He "won his name" not just in his own community but across many other cities as well. For nearly a decade, he was involved in various capacities in the Global Fund's projects in Peru. Having grown up in Tarapoto, studied law in Iquitos, and amassed tremendous experience and technical acumen in project management, program monitoring, and evaluation, he possessed a unique combination of "local" expertise, specialized skills, and a reputation as a collaborator in communities across the region. He was a workaholic who put in long hours, frequently working late at night to finish a project, compose a grant proposal, or prepare for an upcoming meeting or workshop. While he was a founding member of the DISAM community-based organization in Tarapoto, he collaborated with other organizations in Iquitos and Pucallpa to develop grant proposals, often identifying opportunities and submitting them on behalf of several organizations at once. However, despite his unique expertise and years spent accumulating social capital across the cities in the Amazonian region, Anderson struggled to find long-term employment opportunities. Many of the contracts that he received through Global Fund projects were short-term or based on the completion of a specific project. He was often managing multiple projects at once from different funding sources, and he also would experience periods with no projects or work opportunities at all. The closure of the Tenth Round was a particularly challenging time for him professionally.

He was a pivotal contact person for nongovernmental organizations based in Lima when the organizations required assistance with, information about, or support for activities in the Amazonian region. While HIV prevention had dominated his professional activities, he considered himself a human rights activist and could provide support for a range of projects related to sexual and gender diversity. While I accompanied him to the offices of CEDISA to observe activities related to HIV prevention, one afternoon he surprised me by asking where we should go to watch volleyball. "*Gringa*," he said to me one afternoon while I was hanging out in the CEDISA office, "where are they playing volleyball right now? Let's go! Come with me!"[5] Though he was a fan of volleyball and had played a lot when he was younger, he was typically so occupied with project coordination that he rarely went to the spaces that gay and trans people took over each afternoon to play volleyball. At first I was surprised that Anderson wanted to watch volleyball, but he then explained that the purpose was to connect with community members and to see if there were any cases of discrimination to collect. Though the System of Community Protection was dormant at the time because of the freezing of the Tenth Round, he had recently been asked by a nongovernmental organization in Lima to provide information on any cases of discrimination that could be added to the organization's efforts to assess the status of LGBT rights in Peru.

At my suggestion, we went to a park at the edge of the Banda de Shilcayo district of Tarapoto. The park was packed by the time we arrived. *Motocars* and motorcycles were lined up in neat rows around the field, and people were sitting either in the *motocars*, on them, or next to them on the ground. Further back, there were rows of barbeque grills, operated primarily by women from the neighborhood selling typical afternoon snacks such as grilled plantain accompanied by peanuts or cheese, *tacacho*, and *juane*. And a thrilling volleyball game was happening in the center of it all: the game pitted the teams of Paula and Angel against each other, two volleyball rivals who both owned salons and likely had spent a good part of the day recruiting other players for their teams that afternoon. Judging by the enthusiasm of the crowd, a significant amount of money had been bet on the game.[6] I wandered around chatting with various interlocutors who also happened to be there, while Anderson immediately started looking for individuals who would fill out a form to document an experience of discrimination.

While I sat beside Axel to watch the game, Anderson quickly recruited Jorge to fill out one of the forms. Jorge was openly living with HIV and had been contracted as a health promoter for various Global Fund–related projects in Tarapoto. He was well known as an outstanding and entertaining volleyball player, though that evening it appeared that he was there to watch and hang out, not to play. Though he was not at the time working on a contract for the Tenth Round, he had attended many capacity-building workshops

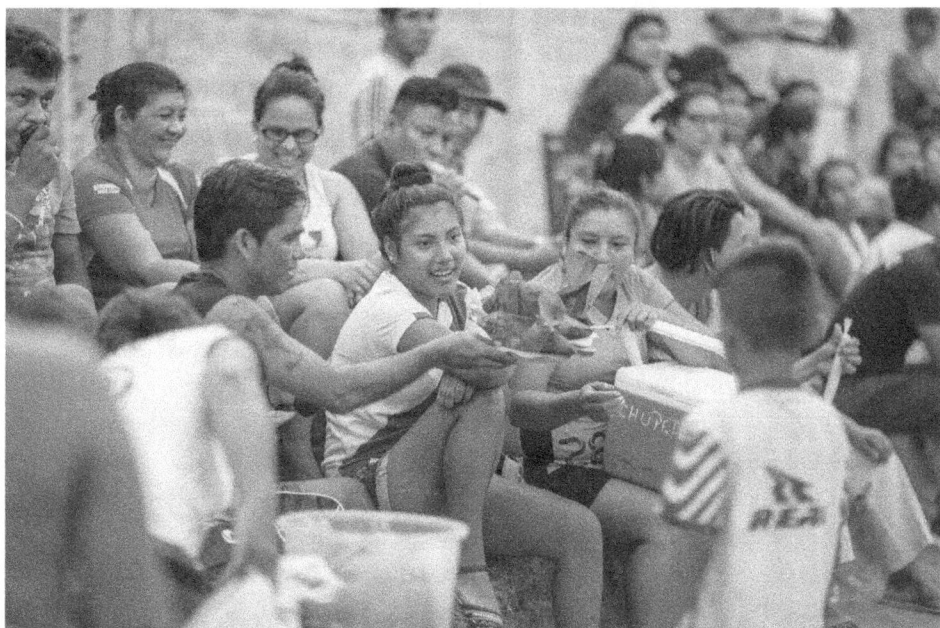

**Figure 5.1.** A vendor sells *juane*, a boiled mixture of rice, egg, and meat, to spectators at a volleyball game in Tarapoto, Peru. (Photograph by Marlon del Aguila Guerrero)

and was familiar with the form that was used to document discrimination as part of the System of Community Protection.

Anderson was seated on a large rock close to the volleyball court, and the act of someone walking up to him and filling out a form might have been a peculiar rupture in the flow of what was otherwise a typical social scene in Tarapoto. It was awkward to fill out surveys there, because the craggy, uneven rock provided a poor surface for pen and paper. Also, everyone gathered was watching because Anderson had chosen a spot so close to the volleyball game itself. Axel and I made our way over to Anderson, who quickly convinced Axel to fill out a form. A few weeks earlier, I had accompanied Axel to the medical post in Morales during the time set aside for "vulnerable populations" to take HIV and STI tests and receive treatment. When we arrived, though, we were told that the staff that attended to "vulnerable populations" were not available. If we wanted a test, we would have to use the regular paid services or go to a private clinic down the street. Anderson explained to Axel that because the medical post received funding from the provincial government to provide this service, this was a clear episode of discrimination.[7] He convinced Axel to fill out a form about this incident.

Once Axel completed the survey, Anderson requested that he bring over anyone else he knew who might be willing to fill out a survey. He told Axel to emphasize that anyone who filled one out would receive 10 soles.[8] Anabella, a trans woman who often played volleyball in the afternoons but was not playing this particular day, eventually joined us at the rock. After a stylized performance of cheek kissing and pleasantries among the four of us, Anderson asked Anabella if she had experienced discrimination in the past year. Anabella had not, and went on to explain why: "I don't experience discrimination because I know how to defend myself now. Maybe a couple of years ago, yes, but not anymore. Maybe the girls who do sex work might be able to fill this out." While Anderson lamented that by not filling out the survey Anabella was missing out on a chance to earn a little money, Anabella felt confident that she had nothing to write about.

At first Annabella's ambivalence toward the exercise might appear to confirm the hypothesis that was sometimes circulated among HIV prevention project specialists and community promoters about gay and trans communities in Tarapoto: that they lacked a "culture of denouncement." Indeed, after we left the volleyball game that evening Anderson mentioned the continued importance of cultivating a culture of denouncement. However, her hesitation might also be read as her intrinsic sense of some of the methodological limits of the form she was handed. In his analysis of similar efforts to count LGBT violence and discrimination in Brazil, Joseph Jay Sosa develops the framework of epistemic doubt and affective certainty to describe how some LGBTQ social movement activists at once critiqued the limits of statistical measurements of homo- and transphobia while also maintaining "affective certainty that they are documenting something real" (2023, 113). Annabella did not *deny* that the experience of discrimination was real and vividly felt among her friends and throughout her community.[9] Yet she also acknowledged some of the limits of the effort to put forward and share individuals' traumatic experiences. I extend the benefit of the epistemic doubt (the concept used to describe the orientation of some activists, like Anderson) to also include some of the subjects who encountered the request to write about their experiences of discrimination. Perhaps Annabella's hesitation came from the fact that she did not know where or how the story would circulate. She did not know who would see it and what, if anything, would be done with the story. Not to mention that the request came at an inopportune time—we were interrupting what was otherwise an entertaining afternoon and evening of volleyball.

## Collecting Cases with Las Amazonas

Anderson's enthusiasm for collecting more cases continued later that very same evening. He asked Norma to call a meeting of the Las Amazonas organization in order to have members fill out a survey and, in return, receive the payment of 10 soles. Anderson again invited me to come along, and we agreed to reconvene at Norma's house, where the organization was based. I knew that the event would start a little after 9:00 p.m., but by the time I arrived, about fifteen minutes later, there were only three people in the meeting space: Norma, the president of Las Amazonas; Maritza, a young trans woman and a member of the organization; and Anderson. After waiting another twenty minutes to see if more community members might arrive, Anderson determined it was time to start. He pulled out copies of the survey and explained that they were for a report about discrimination among LGBT people in Peru compiled every year. He even brought a copy of a prior year's annual report to show those who were at the meeting. He explained that filling out the surveys was a way of representing the Amazonian region in this report.

"Does anyone have an example of discrimination?" Anderson asked the three of us, to which Norma replied that she had several examples. A couple of weeks earlier, she explained, she had accompanied members of Las Amazonas to the two street corners in the Huayco neighborhood of Tarapoto where they typically congregate for sex work. A police patrol drove by and told them all to continue walking, and harassed them with demeaning names and slurs. When someone yelled back at the policeman, he got out of his truck, asked her for her identification card, grabbed her purse, and dumped all of the contents out onto the street. Before explaining how this story ended, though, Norma quickly moved to her second example. This one had happened that past weekend. She and her boyfriend had gone out to the La Mega disco with a group of transgender women and their boyfriends. As they were drinking, a group of men started yelling names at the group in front of the entrance of La Mega. Norma was so upset, she explained, that she turned around and punched one of the men in the other group. A tussle broke out and a security guard grabbed her boyfriend. However, she convinced the security guard to let him go, promising that they would leave and not cause a scandal. After Norma gave these two examples, Anderson commented that they were both instances of stories that could be written on the form. He also said that if anything like that had happened to either Maritza or myself, we too could write it on the form.

Anderson then reminded me that I had been with Axel when he was denied services at the medical post, and suggested that I fill out a form. Perhaps in his effort to normalize a "culture of denouncement," Anderson took the opportunity to include me alongside Norma and Maritza. Discrimination could happen to any LGBT person, and, he likely reasoned, we were all doing our part by codifying and submitting examples on this form. To be conscripted as an informant for Anderson's research project—in the middle of what I thought was my effort to conduct research about Anderson—was disorienting. As an outsider, I was at first hesitant to go along with his request. But I realized that it was an important moment of reciprocity. Anderson had been a key interlocutor for my research, and this was a request to reciprocate, to be an informant for his research. In reversing the roles of researcher and subject, Anderson instrumentalized my presence as an informant and a potential source of data for the knowledge-making project with which he was engaged, further illuminating the intersubjective possibilities of long-term ethnographic research.

Thus I wrote my version of the incident on the survey, which was compiled into a larger document alongside the other surveys collected by Anderson, and then sent along to Lima. I found it was not an easy task to fill out the form: How would I arrange the sequence of events? How would I explain my presence? What other information about the situation did I need to include so that someone analyzing the survey form would be able to situate this specific incident appropriately alongside other stories? How different would my account be from Axel's account? I thus started my narrative with an explanation of the context of the medical post. I explained how in Tarapoto there was a medical post funded through a tripartite agreement between the provincial government, the social security health system (EsSalud), and the LGBT organization DISAM to provide HIV/AIDS and STI services and call attention to those diseases. The provincial government agreed to cover the rent for the space, EsSalud would staff it with the necessary medical professionals through PROCETSS (the Program for STI and AIDS Control), and DISAM would ensure that the services were sensitive to and culturally appropriate for the diverse members of these vulnerable populations and would use its links to local communities to conduct necessary outreach. I figured that some of those who might eventually encounter my account (or Axel's version) on the form might not be familiar with this context, and also that it was important to remind those in Lima of the advancements and efforts that localized social movements have made outside of the capital city. Though I never saw the form Axel filled out, I also thought that a separate form written from my perspective might corroborate his experience.

As I recalled the episode and narrativized it for the form in that moment, I noted how Axel and I had arrived at the medical post on a Thursday afternoon.[10] We entered and asked the receptionist where one would go for an HIV test. He indicated where in the complex we would go, but also explained that the staff specifically assigned to the "vulnerable populations" office were not there presently. If we wanted the HIV test, we would have to use the regular medical services, and that would cost 25 soles for each person. But if we went to the private clinic three blocks down—which, as Axel later explained to me, and to which I then added to the narrative, happened to be owned by a high-ranking doctor in the regional offices of EsSalud— then it would cost only 15 soles. Axel was convinced that this was *una estafa* (or, a scam), and wanted to leave. But I suggested that before we left we should walk over to the "vulnerable populations" office anyway. The staff were there, it turned out, but asserted that they were not supposed to work with "vulnerable populations" outside of the designated days of the month. On the form I pointed out that the testing should be covered for Axel at the medical post, and he should not have to go to a private clinic down the street in order to access the services to which he was already entitled. Even though the municipal government was paying for the staff at the medical post to provide specific care, the staff had not fulfilled their obligations, which was discriminatory.

As we finished up at Las Amazonas, Anderson gave Norma and Maritza 10 soles for each of the forms they filled out. He expressed his appreciation for each of us because collectively we were able to show the LGBT activists in Lima that there was a culture of denouncement in Tarapoto. He returned to the office to compile the forms he had collected that day and to send them out to Lima.

For me, filling out the form provided a perspective on the effort to "cultivate a culture of denouncement" and the act of narrating an experience of discrimination. It was a challenging experience: not just sequencing the elements of an experience of trauma or vulnerability in a meaningful way, but also making that experience legible to an unknown reader. I do not know what eventually happened to the form I filled out, nor to the one Axel filled out. Though cases from throughout the Amazonian region found their way into the diagnostics and reports discussed previously, I have not been able to identify a report or diagnostic that included Axel's story. I also see the wisdom and reasoning on the part of those who decided not to come to the meeting that evening or who, like Annabella, decided not to disclose a story or experience of discrimination. Through their absence, the other members of Las Amazonas likewise challenged the transformation of their stories into a report. Perhaps somewhere else—in a social situation that included neither Anderson, Norma, nor myself—someone was recounting an exaggerated, embellished, or otherwise scandalous version of an experience of discrimination to an even larger group of people and, in their own way, narrativizing and circulating the story to a wider community.

## Collecting Discrimination Cases in Callao

The December 2014 holiday season was stressful for many of the gay and trans leaders of community-based organizations throughout the country involved in the Global Fund's Tenth Round. While a vibrant discussion had been occurring over the past few months on the popular "Vulnerable Populations" email listserv regarding the status of the Tenth Round, stories of the impending termination of the Tenth Round circulated offline between many of the leaders of the community-based organizations. The listserv included leaders and project specialists of all of the community-based organizations involved in the Tenth Round, as well as other individuals involved in HIV prevention programs throughout the country, and it fostered connections and social relationships between community leaders around the country.[11] In the weeks before the country coordinating mechanism ultimately decided to terminate the Tenth Round, many project specialists and community leaders were in the midst of strategizing how to prepare for the withdrawal of Global Fund support, as well as beginning to address the issue of the rent payment backlogs that many had amassed over the months in which payments had been paused (see chapter 4). For many, the obvious strategy was to organize a *pollada* or another type of spectacle to raise funds to support their organization.

For a few days in late December, I found myself in Lima. Late on Friday night, perhaps already into Saturday morning, I was at the La Jarrita bar with a friend when I heard, "*¡Justina! ¡Ingrata! ¿Que haces aqui?*" (Justin! Ungrateful! What are you doing here?). To my surprise, it was Juan Manuel. Juan Manuel was a project specialist at a community-based organization in Callao.[12] I had known Juan Manuel for several years, as he was a key interlocutor from a prior research project.[13] Juan Manuel knew that I was based in Tarapoto, and his comment expressed his own surprise at seeing me at the bar—as well as a joking comment that I had not told him ahead of time that I would be in Lima.

He invited my friend and me over to his corner of the bar, where he was gathered with a group of gay and trans *chalacos* and *chalacas*.[14] Circulating a plastic cup and an entire bottle of whiskey brought into the bar from outside, the group was chatting and dancing in a circle to the Peruvian cumbia music playing inside. Out of curiosity, I asked Juan Manuel how his community-based organization was handling the current crisis involving the Tenth Round. He replied by inviting me to a volleyball tournament and *pollada* that they were organizing that very Sunday as a joint fundraiser for the two community-based organizations that worked on the Tenth Round project in Callao. The objective was to raise enough money to pay for the rent for both of the organizations while they waited for a resolution to the situation. The tournament and *pollada* would start the next day at 11:00 a.m. in the Ciudad de Pescador neighborhood.

By the time I arrived the next day, preparations for the activities were in full swing. Some organizers were tasked with painting the lines of the volleyball court, while others were setting up the awning and organizing chairs for spectators. Juan Manuel and I were coordinating the food that would be sold to the spectators who gathered to watch the day's entertainment. There was *causa*, an appetizer of layered mashed yellow potatoes and a filling such as chicken salad or tuna salad molded into a square, as well as *chanfainita*, a spicy stew of diced potato and cow lung. Eager to help, I offered to arrange the food on the table and prepare it to be sold. The *causa*, though, made in a large sheet, had been covered only by a plastic bag, and as I reached down to grab it, I planted my entire hand onto the bag, leaving my handprint on the *causa*. "The *gringa* destroyed the *causa!*" I heard immediately from behind me, and everyone else who was gathered around immediately erupted in laughter. As the story spread like wildfire across the whole group, Juan Manuel came to the rescue, fluffed the *causa* back up, and cut it into squares to serve. I would never live down leaving my handprint in the *causa*—even after I left Peru, I received messages on social media telling me that Juan Manuel and others had recounted the story at workshops and meetings related to the Global Fund. Even people in Tarapoto, Iquitos, and Pucallpa would come to know this story, and in turn might tell of my "fly in the *chicha*" incident.

As preparations were underway, two members of the No Tengo Miedo collective arrived at the tournament. No Tengo Miedo (the name translates as "I am not afraid") is an activist collective that has as its mission "the promotion of social justice, liberation, and equitable access to resources for the LGBTIQ population, from a transfeminist and intersectional perspective" (Machuca Rose, Cocchella Loli, and Gallegos Dextre 2016; author's translation). Like me, they were fortunate to be able to connect with the organizers of the event in order to take advantage of the sizable crowd that the day's activities and spectacles promised, in order to advance their research. As soon as they arrived, they went to work setting up a photo opportunity for individuals to share on social media. With a giant purple cardboard cutout of a *carnet*, or identification card, they sought out individuals to pose for pictures with their face peeking through a hole in the mock ID card. The bright, colorful *carnet* read "I am [blank] and I am not afraid." Anyone who had a picture taken would be able to fill in the blank however they pleased. They could, for example, write their name, like on a national identity card. Alternatively, they could write their sexual orientation or gender identity— that they were gay, lesbian, bisexual, transgender, queer, or any other term relating to non-normative sexual orientations or gender identities. Or, as the members of the collective explained to me, they could write any adjective describing a feeling they might have been having that day, such as *alegre* (happy) or *libre* (free). Since the day's main activities had not yet started, the giant ID card really was the center of attention for those who were beginning to gather. Juan Manuel, who knew that the members of the collective would also be coming to the event, decided to go up and have his picture taken, hoping he might inspire others to participate.

At the encouragement of Juan Manuel, I followed him over. I was greeted with enthusiasm and smiles, and with a protocol I was familiar with as a social scientist conducting research with human subjects: a form detailing the project, including a description of how the photograph might be used on social media or in publications and a field for the date and my signature to document my consent. Like the moment when Anderson reversed roles and conscripted me into his effort to collect cases of discrimination in Tarapoto, to be on a different side of a research relationship was, at first, disorienting. As I explained to the activists, I was not actually from Callao, or even from Peru, but rather here conducting my own research on the Global Fund's Tenth Round. Perhaps because Juan Manuel and I were the only ones who had gone up, they still encouraged me to have a photo taken. I asked Juan Manuel for a suggestion of what I should write in the blank, to which he replied that I should write *loca*. One of the members of the activist collective suggested instead that, since I spoke Spanish with an accent and I was not from Peru, I should write *extranjero*, or "foreigner." After Juan Manuel

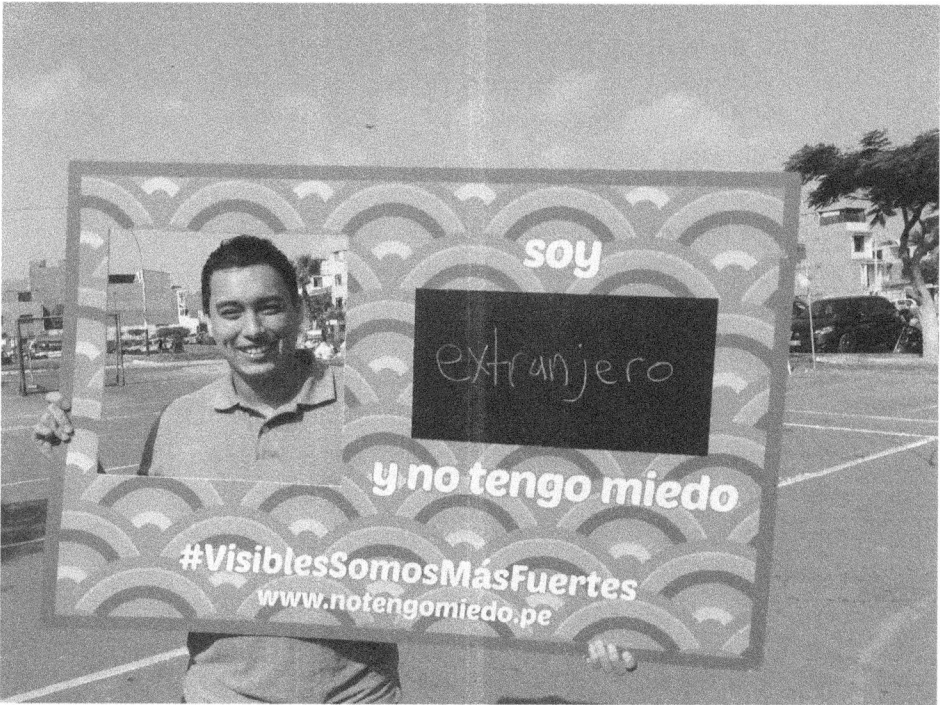

**Figure 5.2.** The author posing with the No Tengo Miedo *carnet*.

and I had our pictures taken, three other people from the event came up and had theirs taken.

In a moment when many of the efforts to support LGBT communities were primarily focused on gay men and trans women because of their vulnerability to HIV/AIDS, as I looked at the picture I began to imagine how powerful participating in the project could be for someone of a non-normative sexual orientation or gender identity. Even if an individual did not explicitly fill in the blank with a category from the LGBTQ spectrum, the very logic of the disclosure signaled by the phrase "I am [blank] and I am not afraid" had the effect of implying that anyone pictured with this identification card might imagine themselves as part of an "us" of sexual diversity. The project of collecting and compiling these photographs empirically illustrated that there was indeed a community of Peruvians who identified with a range of sexual orientations or gender identities. The use of the hashtag "#VisibleWeAreStronger" at the bottom of the *carnet* signaled to the individual who had their picture taken and who might later reexamine it that, no matter what they had written on the card, they were part of a larger collective that was only getting stronger as more people joined the ranks. On the part of the collective that took the picture, the hashtag might indicate their work of compilation and curation. A picture might circulate in unintended directions, whether on social media or in real life, but the hashtag symbolizes trackability. If one searches, one might be able to find and compile all of the instances in which that particular hashtag appears.

Eventually, once the freshly painted lines on the concrete had dried, the first athletic event began. It was a soccer game, and both teams were composed entirely of lesbian soccer players from different neighborhoods of Callao. This was one of the rare moments from my fieldwork when an activity that was centered on HIV prevention issues (in this case, to mitigate the pending impacts of the freezing of the Tenth Round) included lesbian participation. After the soccer game replaced the No Tengo Miedo photograph project as the center of attention, the No Tengo Miedo team put away the cardboard cutout and brought out a stack of forms. Titled "*Cuéntanos tu historia*," or "Tell us your story," the form was three pages and primarily asked the individual to write a paragraph or two about a time they experienced violence or discrimination for being LGBTQ as well as a paragraph about a time they were supported or celebrated for being LGBTQ.

There were some apparent similarities between the form distributed by the No Tengo Miedo collective and the forms that had been developed and distributed through the System of Community Protection and the Tenth Round–related efforts. For one, both types of form asked the individual to narrate their experience of discrimination in an open-ended format. However, the No Tengo Miedo forms took a much more expansive perspective regarding the possible units of analysis. In addition to the space for writing these longer stories about instances of discrimination or instances of celebration, there were additional demographic questions. These ranged from name, email, and age to sexual orientation, gender identity, and HIV status. One question asked if the person identified with any in a list of additional categories besides those represented by the LGBTIQ acronym, including "*pasivx*," "*activx*," "*modernx*," "*fluidx*," "*maricón*," or "*machona*." The form asked the person to select any of a range of racial and ethnic categories (e.g., "Quechua," "Aymara," "mestizo") and, following the space set aside for the description of the instance of discrimination, asked if the person felt that any other categories applied as a cause for discrimination (e.g., race, class, gender, age, disability, or religion, among others). The form was visually engaging, easy to read, and easy to fill out, yet captured extensive details about an individual and their life experiences.[15]

The form further lent itself to rich possibilities of qualitative and quantitative analysis. On the one hand, it collected discrete instances of discrimination on the basis of sexual orientation and gender identity. Each form that was fully filled out would contain individual narratives of an experience of discrimination and an experience of celebration. And even if these narratives were not particularly detailed, the additional questions, such as indicating who the perpetrator of the discrimination or violence was, or with which entities a grievance or complaint might have been filed, enabled a detailed and comprehensive analysis. The stories and anecdotes associated with qualitative methods like ethnography could be collected, compiled, and interpreted via this form. But the form also enabled a detailed and sophisticated statistical analysis. Correlations and interconnections between, say, HIV status, sexual role, and discrimination could be statistically represented through the collection of these forms.

Despite the form's ease of use and the enthusiasm of the No Tengo Miedo team, only a handful of people filled them out. Juan Manuel recruited the members of his organization to complete one each. He also encouraged me to fill out a form. Having recently filled out a similar form in Tarapoto at the encouragement of Anderson, I obliged Juan Manuel's request and wrote the same story that I had written previously, recounting again the time Axel and I were unable to access services at the medical post in Tarapoto during the time set aside for "vulnerable populations." Having written the story one time already, I found that I was able to craft the narrative of the incident more confidently this time around. I had the details and sequence down and, with the help of Anderson's initial encouragement and support the first time I wrote about the incident, I felt that I could better explain why it was an instance of discrimination. The iteration improved my own storytelling. And it felt cathartic to contribute the story to the project and make it "count" in a new way. As a young professional from a *provincia*, Axel struggled to make his way into a professional career several times in Lima over the years of my fieldwork, often moving from Tarapoto to take on promising professional opportunities that turned out to be far less than promised or did not materialize into more long-term opportunities. To document just one of the *estafas* (scams) that he encountered felt like a meaningful way to contest injustice in the moment at hand. And although in this case the collection of the story was motivated by different research objectives and with the aim of representing differing constituencies, recounting a story that revolved around the challenges of HIV prevention effectively prepared me to narrate an episode of discrimination for an adjacent but autonomous project. I can imagine that those who also filled out the survey that day might have had a similar experience, considering their prior involvement in Global Fund projects. Through their participation in workshops and trainings related to HIV prevention, they were prepared to narrate a story of discrimination for the purposes of broader LGBTQ human rights promotion. In that sense, the lessons and effects of the Tenth Round projects persisted even after the project was frozen.

Multiple community-based and activist research projects intertwined at the soccer and volleyball fundraiser that Juan Manuel and his collaborators organized. This included my own investigation of the consequences of HIV prevention, but also the projects of others who were studying and surveying the status of discrimination, human rights, and violence among broader LGBTQ communities across the country. Even amid the breakdown of the Tenth Round, and the resulting jeopardy in which community-based organizations around the country found themselves, Juan Manuel insisted on the continuation of the social practice of collaboration. By organizing the spectacle of the soccer and volleyball tournaments, he was able to convoke a large crowd to come out for the day. By selling *causa* and other food items, he raised money to support the two community-based organizations in Callao while they weathered the crisis brought on by the Tenth Round. He then encouraged and connected individuals to the two research projects undertaken that day, both of which were able to make use of the established reputation of Juan Manuel as a collaborator who had "won his name" in the community. Even in the moment of crisis generated by the Global Fund's decisions, the practice of collaboration continued to be a mode for generating social relations and opening new possibilities for representing, talking about, and quantifying discrimination.

**Stories That Count**

Although they had the support of project specialists and community leaders, the gay and transgender individuals who denounced discrimination in Tarapoto found redress elusive. The deeply entrenched structures of race, class, and gender often intersected with ideas about respectability and scandal, which, as explored in chapter 3, made the administrative process of pursuing a discrimination grievance challenging and time-consuming. And though the archiving of an incident of discrimination for the purposes of the System of Community Protection and the submission of a case to NGOs based in Lima did not necessarily lead to redress, the stories sometimes made their way back to Tarapoto in new forms. Specifically, the conversion of narratives about discrimination into quantifiable reports enabled community leaders like Anderson to advocate on behalf of vulnerable communities with experts and public officials in a range of settings. In short, the quantification of discrimination offered what Epstein (1996) terms a "credibility tactic." As Anderson traversed dialogues with doctors, public health officials, police, security personnel, elected officials, and others, he drew on the data produced about discrimination to establish and legitimize his authority.

Though the Tenth Round was no longer supporting prevention activities, Anderson and his team at DISAM still sought to plan an activity for World AIDS Day. Taking advantage of the legibility of the internationally recognized day, they decided to plan a workshop and sensitivity training for various employees of the municipal government. In coordination with Norma and Las Amazonas, they extended the invitation to the auxiliary municipal security, or *serenazgo*; this was in response to the persistent harassment and discrimination perpetrated by *serenazgo* patrols toward the members of Las Amazonas.

The workshop was intended to be brief, taking up only a portion of the morning. There would be three presentations of thirty minutes each, given by representatives of different stakeholders from the regional HIV prevention coordinating mechanism. Melissa, the *obstetra* (obstetrician) who conducted HIV testing at the medical post funded through the tripartite agreement, would give a presentation titled "Epidemiological Situation of HIV in Peru and San Martín." Anderson was to give a presentation titled "The Social Situation of Vulnerable Populations and the Response of the Global Fund." And finally, Dr. Enriquez, a consultant for the Ministry of Health and a professor at the local university, would complete the series with a presentation titled "Multi-Sectorial Articulation of HIV Prevention."[16] Unfortunately, these presentations never happened for the intended audience: the municipal security guards never showed up to the training, nor did the various other health professionals who were invited.

Taking advantage of the opportunity to have a discussion with the small group gathered, Anderson suggested that the presentations originally intended for the workshop participants simply be shared with each other. When Melissa and Dr. Enriquez shared their statistics about HIV incidence in 2014, Anderson realized that their numbers were different from his and from each other's. Furthermore, Anderson observed, all three presenters had different data on prevalence among gay and transgender populations. "*Obstetra* Melissa," he said, "your numbers must be from the beginning of 2014, because they are not up to date at all." He showed a copy of his slides to the group and went on, "If we are to talk about projections, the rate of new HIV infections among gay and transgender people will increase by 400 percent compared to the last ten years." Dr. Enriquez and Melissa responded with alarm, agreeing that they, as a group, needed to talk about this more with the government because, as Dr. Enriquez fittingly observed, "*la gente se mueva por numeros*" (that is, "people are compelled by numbers"). Then Anderson added another figure, this time bringing in the social context: "Thirty percent of transgender and gay Peruvians are HIV positive, and this is because of discrimination." Although they seemed convinced by Anderson's assertions about the socio-epidemiological landscape, Melissa and Dr. Enriquez still had one more question. Commenting that Anderson was a lawyer, and not trained in any medical profession, they asked how and why he knew these figures.[17] He replied that while, yes, he was a lawyer, he had had a decade of experience with the Global Fund in Peru. But, more importantly, he was an activist, and as an activist, he needed to understand how HIV/AIDS-related discrimination affected his community. He then pulled out a copy of a PROMSEX report from a prior year. Though he had not been involved in the compilation and analysis of the report, presumably he had contributed in small ways to it by sending along cases of discrimination to the coordinators. Anderson often carried copies of the PROMSEX reports to meetings, even though they were about the status of human rights among LGBTQ communities across Peru. Anderson handed the report to Dr. Enriquez as an opportunity to make a claim about discrimination and HIV among gay men and trans women, and also as a statement about his authority to make that claim.[18] However, ultimately they were dealing with two different units of analyses: Dr. Enriquez and Melissa had been talking about *HIV incidence*, whereas Anderson had come to talk about *discrimination*. Yet Anderson was able to work within the limits of these two fields of knowledge and within categorical slippages to establish a moment of commensurability. Drawing on his knowledge of discrimination enabled Anderson to credibly establish a claim about the status of HIV/AIDS in his community within the limits imposed by the hierarchy of medical practice.

Numerical data can travel in unexpected and unanticipated ways. In their ethnography of a cholera outbreak in Venezuela, Briggs and Mantini-Briggs (2003) found that statistical data about cholera both worked to create the category of a modern, sanitary citizen and, paradoxically, stigmatized those most affected by the cholera outbreak and intensified existing inequalities. They remind us: "Numbers travel longer and farther than their producers anticipate or desire; clearly, they can be used for purposes that are deemed inflammatory or illegitimate" (Briggs and Mantini-Briggs 2003, 267). Numbers can still find their way to distant places, far from the location in which they were produced. In a context characterized by data deprivation, project specialists reintegrated new data about discrimination in order to challenge the stigmatization of gay and trans communities. In a sense, they became a new type of numerical subject.[19] The demands of this context obligated the emergence of a queer subject who could effectively manage and translate numerical data into multiple contexts and fields. And this required curation and quantification of discrimination—in effect, a subject who could find ways to make stories of discrimination count.

## Countering Data Deprivation

Project specialists encountered a complicated problem in the form of data deprivation—and this problem emerged at an inopportune time. Precisely at a moment when the prospect of the "end of AIDS" and the justification of continued investment in HIV prevention efforts in the country came to hinge more and more on the production of specific numerical metrics tied to testing and treatment, project specialists involved in HIV prevention encountered inconsistent and out-of-date data about their communities. For project specialists outside of Lima, like Anderson and Arturo, this problem was intensified. Not only was data about the status of the HIV/AIDS epidemic often out of date, but also the project specialists were involved in advocacy for HIV prevention in spaces that were culturally and geographically distant from where the majority of accessible data was produced. In other words, their challenges bring to light how inequitable access to data between the Global North and the Global South can also be reproduced within different contexts of the Global South.

Project specialists traversed scenarios that required them to establish credibility and authority to convince regional medical experts and public officials about the vulnerabilities of gay and trans communities. However, because they often did not have at their disposal up-to-date health and demographic data, they invoked and drew from data that nongovernmental organizations and activist collectives produced about the human rights of LGBT Peruvians—the collection of which was itself supported by the practice and ethos of *colaboración* that many project specialists developed even before they became involved in the administrative or technical aspects of HIV prevention. Project specialists contributed to a broader process of conversion, whereby they collected stories of discrimination on the ground and, in return, received a powerful and important body of human rights knowledge authored by LGBT activist collectives, community-based organizations, and nongovernmental organizations that emphasized the quantification of discrimination. In spaces of everyday advocacy, this became a crucial source for establishing credibility and making authoritative claims about HIV/AIDS, discrimination, and the vulnerabilities encountered by gay and trans communities.

In creating stories that counted, the quantification of discrimination stories made discrimination—and therefore vulnerability to HIV—a knowable, empirical social force in situations characterized by data deprivation. Project specialists navigated categorical slippages and community members' varying ambivalences toward the codification of discrimination. Anderson, Arturo, and Juan Manuel found ways to work through the limits of categories and bring together distinct fields of knowledge. The context of data deprivation required flexibility and nimbleness on their part—and, paradoxically, created a space for the emergence of new social relations. They encountered and navigated multiple fields of knowledge, each with different methodological priorities and theoretical horizons, different modes of categorizing sexual orientations and gender identities, and different sensibilities about social exclusion and marginalization. The stories that they collected on the ground—in parks, at volleyball games, and at a range of social settings—made their way back to their communities. Though not always in a form that allowed redress for discrimination, the stories they collected came to be part of a broader process of conversion and supported moments of advocacy when data was sparse. Emergent, too, from this shifting and changing social field was a new queer subject—a calculating one.

The System of Community Protection—a brief experiment in collecting and archiving incidents of discrimination for the purposes of mitigating its impacts on the transmission of HIV—continued to resonate in unanticipated yet significant ways. Though funded through the short-lived Tenth Round of the Global Fund's HIV/AIDS interventions in Peru, the program created the infrastructure, relations, skills, and opportunities for some to practice denouncing discrimination. This did not end with the closure of the Tenth Round. The effort to catalogue and quantify discrimination and the will to denounce it persisted, fortifying other modes of representing and studying the status of diverse LGBTQ communities around the country.

It has been my intention throughout *Queer Emergent* to convey just how deeply transformative the HIV prevention component of the Tenth Round of the Global Fund was for the gay and transgender communities in urban Amazonian Peru conceived as its subjects. After the Peruvian state assumed responsibility for the universal provision of antiviral therapies for people living with HIV/AIDS, opportunities for international financing pivoted exclusively on the prevention of HIV in vulnerable populations through social interventions. Though a (relatively) small and brief experiment of HIV prevention, the Tenth Round was an experiment that subsumed social problems—like discrimination and stigma—into a novel project of health and sexual governance. Throughout the on-the-ground implementation of the program, gay and transgender individuals in urban Amazonian Peru attended capacity-building workshops, participated in meetings and events at gay and transgender community-based organizations, and encountered a new vocabulary for making sense of and challenging discrimination and injustice. But they also inhabited a wide and vibrant social world that extended beyond the parameters of HIV prevention projects. They organized, participated in, and attended beauty contests; they played soccer and volleyball games in parks and on streets; and they hung out in beauty salons to catch up on news and gossip. They made sense of the new obligations that arose from ongoing HIV prevention efforts—obligations that ranged from the imperative to denounce discrimination through formal grievances to the obligation to reform their transactional sexualities and assume egalitarian romantic and sexual relationships—through the scandalous stories they circulated in the spaces of quotidian social life. Through the arts of embellishment, exaggeration, and an exactness, gay and transgender Peruvians authored moral stories as the "end of AIDS" project unfurled in their social world. Their stories capture not just how they lived and experienced these transformations but also, and more importantly, how they responded to them on their own terms. It mattered what stories they told—even if those stories were not strictly "factual"—because they were true to the relationships they formed and to the social worlds they shared. Close attention to these stories not only makes clear how the technical conceptualization of the effort to end AIDS both transformed sexual cultures over the 2010s, but also makes visible the deeply entrenched ethno-racial, gender, and class hierarchies that have inevitably confounded the ambition to "end AIDS."

The introduction of the Global Fund's HIV/AIDS projects into the cities of Peru's Amazonian region transformed the infrastructure of gay and transgender community advocacy and brought new professional opportunities. The gay and transgender individuals who became project specialists in their communities faced new obligations and shifting priorities, alongside new challenges of establishing credibility as HIV prevention advocates within entrenched hierarchies. Importantly, the kinds of obligations that community health promoters encountered around the world so vividly described by anthropologists studying the scale-up of HIV treatments (e.g., modeling "positive living," encouraging adherence to treatment, etc.) were different in urban Amazonian Peru as the effort to end AIDS began to unfold during the 2010s. Project specialists encountered imperatives to encourage others to denounce homo- and transphobic discrimination, to collect cases of discrimination and accompany individuals through the administrative grievance process, and to organize workshops and trainings. This meant that many of the project specialists momentarily left behind the kinds of redistributive activities that they formerly organized. Members of wider gay and transgender communities—in a sense, the constituents of the project specialists—refracted these transformations through a social ethos and relational mode they termed *la colaboración*, or collaboration. As opposed to clientelism, which pivots on the capacity of certain individuals to mediate redistribution, collaboration hinged on the creation of conditions that would inspire others to themselves redistribute resources, however small, to those in need. And as opposed to the ongoing social obligations typically associated with systems of reciprocity, the redistributed relations generated through collaboration were ephemeral. Rather, those who garnered a reputation and "won their name" as collaborators were constantly organizing activities, thereby multiplying opportunities for new and more moments of collaboration.

It was the project specialists who ultimately bore the brunt of the overall dissatisfaction with the freezing of the Tenth Found and the contraction of the Global Fund's investment in HIV prevention in Peru. No longer creating the moments of collaboration that others had expected of them, they were subjected to allegations of fraud and experienced great loss to their names— names they had won over years of organizing collaborative spectacles and animating the social world. They most acutely and palpably experienced the administrative freezing of the Tenth Round through fragmentation of social relationships. And yet in the aftermath of the untimely termination of the Tenth Round, a moment when the experiment in ending AIDS also appeared to unexpectedly and momentarily end, project specialists returned to the practices that had made them known in the first place, organizing *polladas* and putting on sports tournaments. Albeit only temporarily putting off inevitable loss, doing so perhaps opened a seam for a rearticulation of social relations through collaboration. And they made sense of and contested these changes through their scandalous stories. In recirculating old stories and crafting new ones amid the crisis of the Tenth Round's closure, they made visible how queer social life endured despite the new obstacles and challenges brought about by the ending of AIDS.

### Emergent Horizons from "Failed" Ends

In 2018, I returned to Tarapoto. The palpable sense of crisis that had overtaken DISAM and CEDISA as part of the fallout of the Tenth Round closure no longer lingered, though certainly stories of the crisis persisted. In the meantime, the Global Fund resumed its investment in HIV/AIDS for Peru and finished out the Tenth Round in 2018. The Ministry of Health and a Lima-based NGO were working on a proposal for an extension of funding from the Global Fund to continue expanding the national response to HIV among vulnerable populations. The vulnerable population category was now broadened to encompass not just gay men, transgender women, and men who have sex with men but also indigenous Amazonians.[1]

Part of the process of submitting the proposal included public meetings with members of the vulnerable populations. Two days before one of these meetings was to take place in Lima, an invitation to participate was extended to "members of community-based organizations and unaffiliated activists in Lima, Callao, and the regions" though an email listserv. The meeting was scheduled for 3:00 p.m. at a hotel in the Lince neighborhood of Lima, a mere stone's throw away from the main offices of the Ministry of Health. While the venue might have been close to the Ministry of Health, it was very far away from "the regions." Back at the CEDISA office in Tarapoto, where Leyla and Mariana were finalizing Global Fund activities for 2018, Leyla wondered out loud how anyone from the regions could possibly make it to this meeting given such short notice.[2] And Tarapoto was considerably well connected to the country's transportation network, with an airport and a highway. For some of the remote, small-scale indigenous communities of the Amazonian region, travel time to Lima would be significantly greater.

Mariana, the director of CEDISA, wanted Leyla to attend the meeting. Her reasoning was strategic: if they were proposing a model in which a regional NGO would be subcontracted to oversee the regional implementation, it would be important to know ahead of time so that CEDISA could begin preparing its proposal. Although Leyla at first expressed hesitation about taking the trip to Lima, I volunteered to accompany her on the short trip. Furthermore, I asked, "Who else from the *selva* will be there? If not you, then who?" This must have been enough to convince her, because that afternoon we reserved our tickets for the first flight out of Tarapoto the morning of the meeting and a return later that evening.

After a quick flight and an arduous taxi ride from the airport in Lima to the hotel where the meeting took place, Leyla and I arrived at the meeting and sat alongside the other representatives from the gay and transgender community-based organizations from Lima and Callao. Our entrance into the room caused quite a stir among the participants. Many of Leyla's longtime acquaintances and colleagues from Lima were unaware of her transition; other participants were unaware that I was back in Tarapoto. I spotted and chatted with Juan Manuel and the contingent of representatives from Callao, while Leyla talked to a group of Limeña transgender activists. It appeared as though there were going to be separate sessions for, on the one hand, the "gay, transgender, and MSM" groups and sex worker organizations and, on the other hand, the groups representing indigenous Amazonians.[3] As we had predicted, Leyla was not just the only person from the *selva* there but also the only person from outside of Lima or Callao.

During the meeting, a representative of the Ministry of Health went over a PowerPoint presentation describing each of the proposed program's objectives, activities, and indicators for monitoring and evaluation. The vision of the proposal was to outline the steps that Peru would take in order to approach the 90-90-90 targets set out by UNAIDS. "We all know," began the presenter, "that Peru is probably not going to meet the targets by 2020. This proposal may help us get there, or at least close, by 2022."

In some ways, the proposal and the meeting itself felt very familiar, much like what I heard about and observed during my primary fieldwork in 2014–15. I saw individuals with whom I had attended countless activities, capacity-building workshops, and meetings. Yet there were also some notable differences. For one thing, the inclusion of indigenous Amazonians was a new development. But also I heard about strategies and concepts that I had not encountered four years earlier, such as an explicit foregrounding and a realistic assessment of the 90-90-90 targets. Likewise, instead of intervening in transactional sex, engaging in capacity-building workshops, or cultivating cultures of denouncement, it appeared as though the emphasis was reoriented toward biomedical interventions. Specifically, the proposal emphasized plans to prepare communities for a future rollout of pre-exposure prophylaxis. Proposals to implement pilot PrEP programs and cost-benefit analyses across the country now replaced the initiatives to encourage the denouncement of discrimination, develop a System of Community Protection, and train community health promoters in the administrative process of filing discrimination grievances, as well as the other activities that had characterized the vision of HIV prevention during the implementation of the Tenth Round.

On our trip back to Tarapoto, Leyla and I had the opportunity to exchange observations about the presentation and update each other on the gossip we had collected in our informal conversations with the other participants. Leyla wondered what everyone must have thought about her now, since hormone treatment over the past two years had visibly feminized her features. "*Que tú eres más regia, guapa y divina que nunca*," I reassured her—that she was more regal, pretty, and divine than ever before. After we gossiped a little more, I shifted the topic to the presentation itself. I asked Leyla for her perspective: "What did you think about the presentation? Do you think Peru can meet the 90-90-90 targets?" Leyla was ambivalent, particularly when it came to the very nature of the statistics that had been presented. "The baselines that they were using were from the spectrum estimations from 2014 and the sentinel surveillance from 2011. There is no way these are accurate baselines," she explained. It appeared that the challenge of data deprivation continued to impact Leyla's advocacy. There was too much that was unknown, and she was frustrated that, despite all of her efforts over the past decade to assist in the implementation of the Tenth Round in the Amazonian region, the Ministry of Health had no sense of what its effect had been in terms of how many gay and transgender people were aware of their HIV status, how many of them were receiving ARV, and how many had achieved viral suppression. While the tables, statistics, and estimates presented that afternoon might have been helpful baselines years ago, for Leyla they were now simply distractions from the fact that the Ministry of Health did not have accurate data on HIV at the present time or, importantly, on what the impacts of the Tenth Round were among gay and transgender communities in terms of preventing new cases of HIV. Furthermore, she added, transgender women and gay men continued to be discriminated against; she cited examples from the past year with which I had been unfamiliar. Ultimately, whether Leyla was right or wrong in her questioning of the statistics presented that afternoon is not the issue here.[4] Rather, in questioning the Ministry of Health's authority as well as the validity of the statistics they presented, Leyla insisted on the significance of the antidiscrimination efforts that she had been so involved with over the past years, and on their ability to offer a more knowable body of evidence.

We encountered another drama on our way back. Leyla was to attend a LGBT human rights training institute in Barcelona, Spain, in a few weeks. However, she did not have a suitcase large enough for the month that she would be traveling. So on our way to the airport I suggested we swing by Polvos Azules, a large market in the center of the city that sold shoes, clothing, electronics, and a range of other items like backpacks and suitcases. However, we did not consider the traffic that we would encounter on the way to the airport. By the time we arrived at the airport, we were told it was too late to check baggage for the flight to Tarapoto. Either we would have to miss the flight and wait until the next day, or we would have to ditch the large suitcase Leyla had just bought. In a split-second decision, we left the suitcase behind and sprinted across the airport to board the last flight to Tarapoto. Leyla lost the new suitcase but did get a new story about another misadventure with the "*gringa* anthropologist."

Soon after I left Peru again, Leyla moved to Spain. In fact, she was able to successfully petition for asylum and has since made a new life for herself in Barcelona. Leyla confronted many "ends" over the course of the 2010s: the promise of the "end of AIDS," the unexpected end of the Global Fund, the end of her former identity, the end of her time in Peru. Ends sometimes occlude moments of transformation, unfinishedness, and emergence. In confronting these ends, Leyla imagined new horizons.

## A New Stage of HIV Prevention in Peru

In June 2023, Peru's Ministry of Health announced the free and universal provision of PrEP as part of a new "combination" strategy for HIV prevention among vulnerable and high-risk populations.[5] The announcement describes the criteria for each of the eligible population categories (MSM, trans women, sex workers, and serodiscordant couples) as well as the steps regarding consultation and follow-up to be taken with those receiving treatment.[6] The plan was to roll out the program over a period of years, beginning in late 2023 in Lima and Callao.

Clearly, the COVID-19 pandemic had played a significant role in derailing the plans to provide PrEP that I heard discussed during my final months of fieldwork in 2018. However, I was also struck by how vastly different the experiences of HIV prevention in Peru had been over the course of a decade compared with other contexts in the Global North. Consider, for example, that PrEP was approved in the United States in August 2012. This approval was in part based on the results of the iPrEx clinical trial, conducted from 2007 to 2011. Though the trial took place in sites across the world, many of the participants were enrolled in study sites in Peru. So even though gay and transgender Peruvians had contributed tremendously to making new forms of HIV prevention possible by participating in the trial, it took more than a decade for these very same technologies to be made available to them. Over the 2010s, their experience of HIV prevention was in the realm of antidiscrimination advocacy and the other social transformations catalogued throughout *Queer Emergent*. It was not until the 2020s that PrEP became a real part of the "end of AIDS" project for gay and transgender Peruvians.

The announcement about PrEP marked a new stage of HIV prevention efforts in Peru and, by extension, how the end of AIDS would continue to unfurl for gay and transgender communities in urban Amazonian Peru. Researchers broadly interested in the enduring inequalities that continue to shape the efforts to bring about an end to AIDS may want to consider the continued gap between the abstract, idealized imaginary about this future and the realities of who has been excluded. I hope the scandalous stories of gay and transgender Peruvians not only expose this gap but also illustrate how communities collectively make social life possible amid exclusion and discrimination. And as critical scholars continue to analyze the ongoing experience of the "end of AIDS" in Peru, I hope the insights in *Queer Emergent* can provide a conceptual and methodological springboard from which to embark, as well as a set of new questions to consider: Will a "culture of adherence" supplant the idea of a "culture of denouncement"? And how might the same entrenched hierarchies that impacted the capacity to denounce shape the capacity to adhere? Which new social roles and professional opportunities will the distribution of PrEP entail for project specialists and community health promoters? And how will this transform social relations and sexual cultures? No matter the outcome of Peru's effort to integrate PrEP into the national response, I write with certainty that success—however it is determined—will depend not just on an appreciation for the collaborative, redistributive relationality central to queer world-making and social life in Peru but also on the willingness to listen to the extraordinary, and even scandalous, stories that emerge along the way.

### Introduction

1    This element of Paula's story was no exaggeration. Whenever I saw her at the La Anaconda disco, she was always at the same corner of the bar right next to the main, elevated stage where the DJ was located. Part of the story is that the listener typically knew that Paula was a regular at La Anaconda and even had a signature spot.

2    That Paula played with gender presentations in her everyday life was clear to anyone who might see her. Her height (she was nearly six feet tall) and her broad shoulders, which were a constant source of playful banter among her friends, juxtaposed starkly with the jet-black eyeliner, applied with a thick wing tip extending to her temple, which she wore every day. Her long black hair was always put into a ponytail and always covered with a floral-printed bandana. I never heard her assume the identity terms *travesti*, *trans*, *transfeminine*, or *transgender*. These were the more common terms used in the region among those who assume a gender identity, style, or social role that differed from the sex they were assigned at birth (Pierce 2020). These were also the terms typically used in global HIV prevention initiatives, which had been increasingly present in cities throughout Peru's Amazonian region. Paula always referred to herself by feminine pronouns, though, and although she referred to sexual orientation in her story, in the formalized version her complaint became one of discrimination on the basis of gender identity. Paula also played with grammatical gender in her

story. She often interpellated a listener as *amiga*, using the grammatical feminine, regardless of how the listener might identify.

3     People choose to identify with the term *travesti* in contexts throughout Latin America and, through circuits of transnational migration, in countries around the world as well (Silva and Ornat 2015). Across these diverse contexts, *travesti* generally "refers most frequently to people assigned male sex at birth who feminize their bodies, dress, and behavior; prefer feminine pronouns and forms of address; and often make significant bodily transformations by injecting silicon or taking hormonal treatments but do not necessarily seek sex-reassignment surgery" (Pierce 2020, 306).

4     In total, my fieldwork in urban Amazonian Peru lasted from 2012 to 2018. I conducted brief periods (two to three months at a time) of fieldwork in 2012, 2013, 2017, and 2018 in addition to fifteen months of sustained fieldwork in 2014–15.

5     This is queer anthropology's legacy of what Weston (1993) termed ethnocartography—the impulse to salvage traditional, non-normative sexual categories in the non-West before they seemingly disappear.

6     The Global Fund's Tenth Round in Peru specifically sought to target three categories: "gay men," "transgender women," and "MSM." Though some parts of the study reference broader LGBT social movements, in order to direct critical attention to the effects of HIV prevention, and because the Global Fund specifically directed prevention efforts toward gay men, transgender women, and MSM, I do not include equal amounts of ethnographic data on how people in urban Amazonian Peru encountered and experienced other categories of the expansive LGBT+ acronym, including "lesbian," "bisexual," "nonbinary," "transmasculine," or "intersex." Readers of *Queer Emergent* may also note that I make little mention of "MSM." This is for several reasons. The first reason is purely a response to the ethnographic realities of field sites. In practice, throughout Tarapoto and other cities of urban Amazonian Peru, those who might have been considered "MSM" (and not "gay") simply did not actively participate in HIV prevention programming, nor did they become involved in LGBT community-based organizations. This does not mean there were not men who had sex with men but who did not identify as gay. They were typically called *maperos*, and in chapter 1 I analyze at length the stories that gay and transgender interlocutors told about *maperos*. The second reason is methodological and related to some of the limits of ethnographic methods. I was out playing volleyball, hanging out in beauty salons and discos, and being visibly connected to the public social milieu of gay and transgender collaborators. Even if there were individuals who considered themselves "MSM" (and not "gay"), they would have valued discretion. My presence was not discreet in a way that could have accommodated rapport with

them. This is a personal limitation of this particular researcher; perhaps a future study could shed more light on this and fill in gaps.

7    Drawing on the work of Portocarrero (2007a), further discussion of the "individualization" of ethno-racial hierarchy in Peru is in chapter 3.

8    As Garro and Mattingly (2001) observe, anthropological theorizations of "story" and "narrative" do not necessarily align with how the terms operate within literary theory. Literary scholars maintain key distinctions between narrative and story, the former referring to a specific "discursive rendering," and the latter to the "underlying events that the narrative recounts" (Garro and Mattingly 2001, 12). Following Garro and Mattingly—and the general conventions of anthropology—*Queer Emergent* does not maintain as rigid a distinction between these terms. First, scandalous storytelling emphasizes embellishment and exaggeration, to the extent that any underlying sequence of events, if such a thing exists, is not actually what is most socially significant. And, second, my fundamental interest is to understand emergent and unfinished social phenomena. I thus use the terms *narrative* (and *narrative practice*) and *story* (and *storytelling*) interchangeably.

9    Ochs and Capps (2001) term conversational narrative an approach to storytelling that both emphasizes the everydayness of stories in social interactions and shows that stories have social roles and animate social life.

10   Other social scientific scholars working in Peru have observed how the concept of "scandal" was used by gay men to differentiate themselves from others. For example, Alcalde (2018) documented an upper-middle-class gay interlocutor from Lima who expressed ambivalence toward public demands for LGBT rights through protests and marches because he saw them as scandalous. To be scandalous, Alcalde's interlocutor explained, was "to participate in public protests and to yell in public to make demands" (2018, 138). Studying gay Peruvian immigrants, Vasquez del Aguila (2012) observed that the popular saying "*Dios perdona el pecado pero no el escándalo*," meaning "God forgives the sin but not the scandal," suggested that being gay may be socially acceptable as long as it does not appear to be scandalous. In his study of gay Dominican immigrants, Decena (2011) also observed how some interlocutors coded their unease with effeminate behaviors through the concept of "scandal."

11   Queer scholarship on the concept of "scandal" and "the scandalous" has tracked how the negative connotations of the terms can be reconfigured and re-signified as an effective strategy to contest or subvert normative structures. Ethnographers have described how LGBTQ people throughout Latin America drew on the notion of "scandal" to make novel demands and claims on others as well as on the state itself (Babb 2003; Kulick 1996; Ochoa 2014; Sosa 2014). In her study of *travestis* in Buenos Aires, Cutuli (2012) theorized scandal as both a political strategy to achieve specific

objectives and the site of communal negotiations. Cutuli argued that *travestis* re-signified scandal as an idea that "is fruitful for them to think, to make themselves visible and for them to act politically" (2012, 88). De la Barreda Solórzano (2023) reverses the direction of the scandal, positing that homophobia (and not homosexuality) is the scandal. My conceptualization of scandal further resonates with scholarship that takes excess—or "too much"—as a site of abundance that challenges the austerities often imposed on racial and sexual others (Hernandez 2020). In highlighting the spectacular, the excessive, and the extravagances of social life, excess can also subvert the idea that "too much" is unnecessary, unproductive, or not useful.

12 It is important to emphasize that my use of *scandal* is not intended to describe individuals themselves as an *escandaloso/a*, or "scandalous person." It is an adjective to describe a situated narrative practice. This does not mean that interlocutors might not have considered themselves as such at some time. As Paula indicates in the opening story of the chapter, she explicitly "threw a scandal" at the disco and would not disagree if, for example, I had said she was an *escandalosa* in the situation. In the context of HIV prevention efforts, however, I rarely encountered anyone, trans or gay, explicitly assuming or taking ownership of a scandal or being perceived as scandalous. Thus, I see *scandal* as a term that can invoke multiple layers of meaning and can be particularly context dependent. A term that works analogously to *scandal* and that has received significant critical attention in the field of queer Latin American studies is the concept of *la locura*, or "craziness." *La loca*, "the crazy person," for example, "is pathologized at the clinical level, seen as scandalous at the popular one, and celebrated as a site of knowledge and resistance in psychoanalytically inspired cultural critique" (La Fountain-Stokes 2008, 196). Like *la loca*, scandal can be used in different ways in everyday life or in critical analysis. Sívori (2004) argues that the *loca*, as invoked in everyday life, typically functions as an interpellative category. One might not say, "I am *loca*," but in the act of calling another person *loca*, one assumes reciprocity with the term. So when someone calls someone else *loca*, they are identifying themselves as such and expecting to be interpellated by others as such. Scholars across diverse disciplines have sought to challenge the negative stereotypes sometimes associated with the term by reconfiguring it as what Ochoa (2008) calls an honorific. Other examples of scholarship on the *loca* figure include Decena (2011), La Fountain-Stokes (2014), Lima (2011), Peña (2013), Perez (2011), Vidal-Ortiz (2011), and Viteri (2014). I put forward *scandal* as a key term to be in conversation with the efforts to reinvigorate and re-signify terms like *loca* as part of an expansive queer Latin American vernacular that goes beyond the conventional and globalizing terms of sexual orientation and gender identity.

13 Garro and Mattingly (2001) ask anthropologists to more closely consider anthropological approaches to the story: "In ordinary speech and in much scholarly writing, there is a certain tendency to treat a story as a 'natural' object that needs no explaining, which one can somehow just point to" (9). I situate my analytical approach to narrative and story within longer anthropological traditions that see stories and storytelling as essential sites of data that help bring readers into diverse social worlds that may sometimes be very different from their own. Looking through what she termed the spy-glass of anthropology, Zora Neale Hurston (2008 [1935]) pioneered this approach in *Mules and Men*, reproducing the stories that she encountered as she traveled back to her hometown of Eatonville, Florida, to collect the folktales that animated Black social worlds in the US South. I draw on what Hernández (1995) terms Hurston's "harmonic" literary approach that blends subjective self-reflection with the objective reproduction of the stories she collected, thereby implicating the reader (or the listener) "in the creative act by calling on a reader's subjective interpretations of the text" (Hernández 1995, 156). Debates around the elision of Hurston in the anthropological canon and the subsequent projects to recuperate her contributions speak to her continued significance to anthropology and beyond. For further interpretation, analysis, and critique of *Mules and Men* and on Hurston's legacy in anthropology, see Baker (1989), Boxwell (1992), Mikell (1983), and Wall (1989). My analytical approach is informed by Renato Rosaldo's (1989) vision of narrative as part of the remaking of anthropological social analysis. As he writes, "Rather than being merely ornamental, a dab of local color, protagonists' narratives about their own conduct merit serious attention as forms of social analysis" (Rosaldo 1989, 143). The social analysis of the scandalous stories I undertake in *Queer Emergent* is directed toward understanding an abstract and technical ambition—the "end of AIDS"—that transformed the lives of gay and transgender Peruvians over the 2010s. It is through their everyday responses, circulated in the form of exaggerated and embellished stories, that I ground the abstract in lived experiences and explore how they made sense of changing and emergent social worlds.

14 Nyong'o (2019) proposes the concept of "fabulationality" as a black, feminist, and queer mode of relationality and world-making in his study of contemporary aesthetic practices. One of the characteristics of "fabulationality" is anexactness, which means being intentionally rather than accidentally inexact. I see resonance between his discussion of the art of anexactness and the practice of scandalous storytelling. As Nyong'o (2019) does, I trace the contours of scandalous storytelling with the help of theorists of queer sensibilities and social life like Allen (2022), Halberstam (2011), Manalansan (2014), and Muñoz (2009), whose texts orient toward the experiments that go on in the everyday as people attempt to make queer

lives livable as well as a mode of storytelling as critique that draws on the feminist traditions encapsulated by scholars like Huerta (2021), Berlant and Stewart (2019), Stewart (2007), Anzaldúa (1987), and Hartman (2019).

15    My approach to scandalous storytelling is, in part, an ethnographic response to Cornejo's (2019) call for serious engagement with what he terms "the queer art of lying" as a way to make sense of *travesti* and queer life in Peru. I further engage with and extend anthropological traditions in Peru and the Andes that have emphasized the cultural significance of stories, storytelling, and creative experimentation. I draw particular inspiration from the approaches of Babb (1989), Dean (2023), García (2021), Kernaghan (2009), Mayer (2009), Theidon (2013), and Weismantel (2001). The subtitle of this book, *Scandalous Stories at the Twilight of AIDS in Peru*, riffs on the title of Mayer's (2009) elegant, hybrid ethnography *Ugly Stories of the Peruvian Agrarian Reform*. Greene's (2016) experimentation with ethnographic genre to describe the subversive potential of the subculture of punk in Peru and Gandolfo's (2009) ethnography of urban transgression in Lima offer important points of departure for my conceptualization of scandalous storytelling as queer social critique.

16    Some scholars suggest that "starting" the story of AIDS in 1981 elides the colonial and imperial structures that fundamentally lay at the center of the origins of AIDS. Starting the story in the year 1921, sixty years before the year the first cases of the syndrome that would come to be called AIDS were identified, Pepin (2011) describes how the Belgian and French colonization and administration of Central Africa led to the construction of railroads and precipitated new forms of urbanization and large-scale, labor-related migration. Colonial medical campaigns for treating malaria and sleeping sickness among these newly mobile populations, though well-intentioned, used unsterilized syringes and likely led to the amplification of HIV in the region.

17    For a more thorough periodization of Peru's response to AIDS, Cueto (2001) is the definitive historical study of the AIDS response in Peru; however, it covers only as far as the 1990s. Cáceres and Mendoza (2009) offer a concise historical periodization through the 2000s.

18    The era of the scale-up of ART has been the subject of a rich and robust ethnographic record. Ethnographic accounts of scale-up show how the impacts of treatment went far beyond the biological; significantly, the scale-up of ART engendered diverse and unanticipated political and cultural changes, all amid the intensifying neoliberal entrenchment of healthcare (Pigg and Adams 2005; Benton 2015; Decoteau 2013; Kalofonos 2014; Kenworthy 2017; Nguyen 2010). In Latin America and the Caribbean, Abadía-Barrero and Castro (2006), Biehl (2007), Frasca (2005), Gutmann (2007), Padilla (2007), Parker (2009), and Smallman (2007), to name a

few, captured the radical transformations in subjectivities and social relations that emerged right before and over the course of a decade focused on the scale-up of antiretroviral therapies. Their ethnographies, alongside those from other regions, remind us of the fallacy of a so-called magic bullet—the idea that a technological innovation itself can be a panacea. Even though lifesaving treatments were available, access to therapies and resources remained variegated and unequal.

19    This differed from the response unfolding at the time in neighboring Brazil. No sooner was combination antiretroviral therapy introduced than activists in Brazil began to pursue right-to-health litigation, demanding access to the treatment and setting the stage for the Brazilian government to assume the role of what Biehl (2004) termed an "activist state"—that is, politicizing the managerial and economic practices of the global pharmaceutical industry to negotiate better rates for patented drugs and, in theory, commit to the effort to universalize access to treatment.

20    The Global Fund was launched in 2002 to help countries reduce the impact of the three diseases primarily through grant-making and program monitoring. A multilateral funding mechanism, the Global Fund receives financial support from multiple donor countries and then directs that funding to multiple recipient countries that oversee the implementation of programming. Potential recipient countries must establish a "country coordinating mechanism" in order to solicit funding, with funding opportunities presented in rounds. The country coordinating mechanism in each country is in charge of preparing the country's proposal for funding and selecting the nongovernmental organization that will be designated as the principal recipient to carry out the implementation and programming.

21    However, as Amaya et al. (2014) suggested, the sequence of rounds did not always play out as planned. For one, tensions arose between the Ministry of Health and NGOs, as NGOs were selected to be the principal recipients of Global Fund grants and sometimes made unilateral decisions without consulting the Ministry of Health. But also, as Amaya et al. (2014) evidenced, NGOs were found to have limited technical capacity and operated without accountability or adherence to established practices of independent evaluation or self-evaluation. Accountability concerns and growing tensions would come to have significant consequences in the following decade.

22    This has been accompanied by the circulation of the slogan "Undetectable = Untransmittable," or "U = U." During my fieldwork on HIV prevention in urban Amazonian Peru in the 2010s, I did not observe messaging around "U = U." For a critical analysis of the TasP paradigm—and the enduring global inequities that it elided—see Gagliolo (2012), Nguyen, O'Malley, and Pirkle (2011), and Sandset (2021). Bor et al. (2021) track the uneven circulation of the "U = U" campaign and shifting global attitudes toward TasP.

23 Launched in 2015, the Sustainable Development Goals marked a reassess-
ment and redirection of the Millennium Development Goals, which had
been launched in 2000 and concluded in 2015. The Sustainable Development Goals codified at the level of the United Nations and World Health
Organization a version of the "post-AIDS" discourse that had in fact been
in circulation before the actual announcement of the goals. The appearance of "post-AIDS" language prominently appeared in the promotional
material and reports produced by the World Health Organization, UNAIDS,
and PEPFAR as early as at least 2010 (O'Connell 2020, 91).

24 A "concentrated epidemic" is one in which HIV prevalence is greater than
5 percent within a particular population and less than 1 percent among
the general population. The general population measurement is typically
assessed based on HIV prevalence among pregnant women in urban areas.

25 Crane's (2013) concept of "valuable inequalities" within the global health
sciences helps describe the scenario in Peru with regard to the vulnerabilities of gay and transgender Peruvians to HIV/AIDS. In her analysis of the
explosion of health research in Uganda on HIV/AIDS, Crane describes how
suffering, death, and poverty paradoxically became the conditions in which
a "resource-poor" setting like Uganda could come to be a valuable site of
research for US research institutions. Though Peru did not experience the
same level of investment in HIV/AIDS research as the contexts analyzed
by Crane, the concept is still productive for considering the "value" of gay
and transgender vulnerability. As Crane and other researchers show (Biruk
2018; McKay 2018; Nading 2014), the persistence of colonial relations
continues to shape the politics of global health knowledge. In Latin America, the traditions of social medicine and collective health pose important
critiques of global health's colonial geopolitics (Adams et al. 2019; Carter
2023; Laurens, Abadía-Barrero, and Hernández 2023; Vasquez, Perez-
Brumer, and Parker 2020; Waitzkin, Pérez, and Anderson 2021)

26 See Peru Ministry of Health, National Center for Epidemiology, Prevention, and Disease Control, "Vigilancia epidemiológica del VIH/SIDA,"
https://www.dge.gob.pe/portalnuevo/vigilancia-epidemiologica/vigilancia
-epidemiologica-del-vih-sida/.

27 Dirección General de Epidemiologia, "Situación del VIH/SIDA en el Perú:
Boletín Epidemiológico Mensual," January 31, 2010, https://www.dge.gob
.pe/vigilancia/vih/Boletin_2010/enero.pdf.

28 This study took an expansive view of the MSM category and included
subjects who identified as heterosexual, bisexual, and homosexual. It also
used the term *cross-dressers* and considered "cross-dressers" to be MSM.
Subsequent reports and proposals that invoked this particular study's data
about prevalence replaced this term with *transgender women*. The technical
terminology changed in the years between when the study was published

and when the data was used for the purposes of the Tenth Round proposal. A subsequent study (Silva-Santisteban et al. 2012) focused specifically on transgender women in Lima and determined HIV prevalence to be 30 percent.

29    The paradoxical consequences of HIV exceptionalism for low- and middle-income countries, as evidenced most tellingly in Adia Benton's (2015) ethnography of HIV/AIDS support organizations and government agencies in Sierra Leone, were that it results in the underfunding and defunding of robust, comprehensive health care systems and infrastructure. As a consequence, people living with HIV experience slightly better medical attention than their seronegative counterparts, which paradoxically can cause otherwise preventable suffering or harm.

30    See Moyer (2015) for a review of anthropological research in the "age of treatment." Rose (2007) suggests that labeling a phenomenon as problematic or suspect because it is the result of "medicalization" elides just how foundational and omnipresent medical expertise is for making us who we are. Medical expertise still sanctioned the emphasis on interventions in transactional sex and discrimination, but these were decidedly not biomedical forms of HIV prevention.

31    PrEP remained a "promise" for gay and transgender Peruvians throughout the decade, at least for those even aware of its existence. For example, Silva Torres et al. (2019) found that only 46 percent of gay male survey respondents in Peru indicated awareness of PrEP, and Tang et al. (2014) found that 57.5 percent of healthcare providers in Lima reported awareness of PrEP.

32    In pointing to how the "end of AIDS" imaginary assumes that new technologies can resolve long-standing inequalities, humanistic and social scientific inquiry has emphasized the persistence of racial disparities that have long characterized the AIDS epidemic. Advocates and scholars have revived classic declarations like "The AIDS crisis is not over" and the "Black AIDS epidemic" as a direct response to the circulation of the "end of AIDS" imaginary to underscore how even in well-resourced contexts like the United States, the "end of AIDS" universalizes the contexts and prospects of some groups (e.g., white, urban, and wealthy gay men, who may have access to medical care and PrEP) with less consideration for the realities of others (e.g., urban Black and Latinx gay men, Black women in the American South, transgender women). Insisting that the AIDS epidemic is ongoing, critical scholarship asserts that robust theories of race continue to be obligatory interventions in the dominant modes of biomedical intervention and global health measurement (Bailey and Bost 2019; Caruth et al. 1991; Cheng, Juhasz, and Shahani 2020; Gossett and Hayward 2020; Hobson and Royles 2021; Jolivette 2016; Mackenzie 2013;

Walker 2020). *Queer Emergent* engages in dialogue with this scholarship on racial disparity and HIV as it situates HIV prevention efforts in Peru within the deeply entrenched legacies of colonial ethno-racial hierarchies.

33    Further anthropological discussion of the temporalities of HIV/AIDS, and its moralizing effects, can be found in Murray (2022a, 2022b), Sangaramoorthy (2018), Thomann (2018), and Vernooij (2022).

34    Peru's administrative structure is divided into departments, provinces, and districts. Each of the twenty-four departments (and the province of Callao) has a regional government. The seat of the regional government of San Martín is in Moyobamba, its capital city. The department is divided into ten provinces. Tarapoto is the capital of the province of San Martín. San Martín province is divided into fourteen districts. The districts of Morales, La Banda de Shilcayo, and Tarapoto constitute an urban center, colloquially called Tarapoto, that had a population of approximately 143,000 inhabitants in the year 2015 (INEI 2017). I focused most research in Tarapoto (including Morales and La Banda), but also integrated fieldwork with smaller cities in the department within a day's travel from Tarapoto, including Juanjuí, Sauce, Juan Guerra, Lamas, and Chazuta.

35    I draw on the assertion of Boellstorff et al. (2012), who contend that "intersubjectivity, the dynamic flow of communication and engagement between people, is one of the foundations of the ethnographic encounter" (42).

36    Mary Weismantel's (2001) reflection on the intersubjectivity of her ethnographic claims in *Cholas and Pishtacos* is particularly apt: "My claim to the reader's trust rests not on my singular authority as eyewitness but on my ability to construct a credibly intersubjective narrative about a particular social world" (xxiv).

**Chapter 1. Stories That Scandalize**

An earlier version of chapter 1 appeared as "Peche Problems: Transactional Sex, Moral Imaginaries, and the 'end of AIDS' in Postconflict Peru" in *American Ethnologist* 49 (2): 234–48, 2022.

1    The term *peche* is part of a regional lexicon of transgender, *travesti*, and gay language varieties known as Lóxoro or Húngaro in Peru. See Rojas-Berscia (2016) for a sociolinguistic analysis of Lóxoro. In his analysis of Claudia Llosa's film *Loxoro*, Cornejo (2021) theorizes that "travesti worldmaking is intimately bound to the cultivation of the travesti language Lóxoro" (34). Fernández-Dávila et al. (2008) locate the term within homosexual social worlds and describe it as a verb: *pechar*. They write, "*Pechar* is the term used in the language of homosexual men to refer to the 'purchase' of company or sexual favors in exchange for some type of economic or mate-

rial compensation (e.g., money, clothes, shoes, food, or alcohol). *Pechar* literally refers to breastfeeding" (Fernández-Dávila et al. 2008, 358).

2　Cáceres Palacios (1998) considers the *mapero* to be a social role and discusses *maperismo* in the Amazonian port city of Iquitos as a dynamic of practices and representations rooted in the city's culture. To my knowledge, Cáceres Palacios provides the earliest scholarly reference and discussion of the term. Cáceres Palacios suggests that it is synonymous with the terms *máscara*, *fletero*, and *caquero*. Though I am unable to determine a precise etymology, interlocutors in Tarapoto considered the term *mapero* to be a euphemism. One day, while getting my hair cut by Brenda, I asked her where the term came from. She explained to me that it was a polite term that people from the region had come up with to refer to those who perform the penetrative role in anal sex. Instead of referring to them as *cacaneros*, or "shit eaters," which she said sounded vulgar, they replaced *caca* with *mapa*, which means "snot."

3　Outside of the gay and transgender communities in Peru's Amazonian region, most were unfamiliar with the language of *peches* and *maperos* and the dynamics they entailed. Even other gay and transgender people in Peru, including those from Lima, may not have used the terms in reference to their romantic and sexual lives. Cáceres Palacios's (1998) discussion of *maperismo* in Iquitos is attentive to the dynamic between gay tourists and *maperos*. During my primary fieldwork in Tarapoto, this factor was less significant, as Tarapoto typically attracted fewer international and domestic gay tourists than Iquitos.

4　There is a vast body of scholarship about the origins, development, ideology, and legacy of the Shining Path. Some of these texts include Degregori (1990, 2012), Gorriti (1999), Portocarrero (2012), Rénique and Poole (1992), and Starn and La Serna (2019). Stern (1998) is an extensive and influential edited volume that covers these themes.

5　For more on Alberto Fujimori's presidency and the legacies of Fujimorismo, see Burt (2007), Conaghan (2005), and Degregori (2001).

6　The edited collections by Degregori et al. (2015), del Pino and Yezer (2013), Denegri and Hibbett (2016), and Bedoya Forno et al. (2021) speak to the persistently unequal impacts of violence and the conflict's ongoing legacies.

7　As the MRTA established itself within Lima, it struggled to gain a foothold outside of the city. MRTA leaders believed that the San Martín department would be an ideal location to establish and mobilize a new front in the countryside. San Martín had a strong network of organized peasants, students, and teachers with a history of militancy toward the state through strikes, roadblocks, and civilian defense militias (La Serna 2020).

8    This is further reflected in the extent of scholarly literature on violence in the region. As Dean (2023) observes, "the participation of the Túpac Amaru Revolutionary Movement in the Lower and Central Huallaga Valley during the internal war (1980–2000) is poorly understood and virtually undocumented in the scholarly literature" (8).

9    This is not to say that the MRTA was insignificant. As La Serna (2020) notes, "The MRTA ranks among the formidable Latin American insurgencies of the Cold War, similar in size, scope, and impact to Uruguay's Tupamaros, Colombia's M-19, and El Salvador's FMLN" (3). Perhaps the group's highest-profile action was when it stormed the residence of the Japanese ambassador to Peru in December 1996, resulting in a hostage crisis that lasted 126 days.

10   At its 1989 congress the MRTA had approved a "crime and punishment" clause that was "designed to curb thievery, drug trafficking, and drug addiction." However, regional commanders in San Martín added homosexuality to the list of so-called immoral behaviors (La Serna 2020, 123).

11   Even though the inclusion in the CVR of acts of violence toward trans, *travesti*, and other sexual and gender dissidents during the internal armed conflict was an important step toward making visible their experiences, Almenara (2022) observed that the report listed their names as they appeared in identity documents and not their "social" names. The official record thus continued to be incomplete, as "recognition avoids remembering these people with their chosen names, their *travesti* or transgender names" (Almenara 2022, 98).

12   For examples, see Bracamonte Allain and Alvarez Chávez (2006), Campuzano (2008), Cortázar (2020), Goicochea (2017), Infante (2013), López Díaz (2016), Meza (2014), and Salazar and Garro (2023).

13   Serrano-Amaya (2018) invokes the term *chiaroscuro* as a metaphor for understanding the long-term consequences of invisibility and silence around homo- and transphobic violence during armed conflict and political transition. Drawing on the technical artistic practice of using shade and contrasts to create a sense of three dimensions on a two-dimensional canvas, Serrano-Amaya writes, "Grey areas are not just silences or empty spaces waiting to be discovered or enlightened. They are produced in order to render relevant other areas" (2018, 109). In relation to the sexual politics of homophobic violence, he means to underscore the paradox that while there can be intense fixation on some exemplary cases of political homophobia in national and international media, this can sometimes come at the expense of action on the structural causes of homo- and transphobia. Aware of the national (and international) prominence and media representation of this particular case, some gay and transgender interlocutors in Tarapoto crafted and circulated their own stories about their sexual and social lives set against the backdrop of the internal armed conflict. These stories did

not reach the national circulation of the emblematic cases recorded by the CVR, although they did circulate locally. Serrano-Amaya's invocation of *chiaroscuro* is relevant because while such stories sometimes diverged from the human rights record, they also emerged in response to this record's gray areas.

14 Interlocutors often used the term *terruco* to describe MRTA rebels in their stories. *Terruco/a* was a colloquialism for "terrorist." In national politics, the term *terrucear* refers to the accusation of being a sympathizer of terrorism, commonly hurled at leftist politicians; it played on racist stereotypes and was aligned with what Milton (2014) called the "salvation narrative" framework about the conflict. It has been wielded in a postwar context as an insult to stigmatize human rights defenders, nongovernmental organizations, victims of violence and their families, and, more generally, indigenous communities (Aguirre 2011; Bedoya Forno et al. 2021). In the everyday life of people in the countryside of Peru, the term can be, as Kernaghan (2022) observes, an off-the-cuff expression sometimes hurled in its diminutive form *tuco*, which can "carry less sting and even a tinge of endearment" (5). Although, as Dietrich (2019) contends, terrorism is no longer a significant part of internal state affairs, the figure of the terrorist "continues to haunt contemporary politics, not only during elections but in debates about national security, citizens' rights, and education" (61).

15 *Piraña* literally translates as "piranha"; however, it is also a Peruvian colloquialism that typically refers to a young gang member who may pose the risk of pickpocketing or robbery. A *piraña* was dangerous, but he could also be a potential romantic partner, or *punto*.

16 The term *maricón* can be an offensive and derogatory slur used against some gay and trans people. However, during fieldwork, I found that both gay and transgender interlocutors often used the term as a tongue-in-cheek way to refer to themselves as a collective. Others might use the term differently. I reproduce the term in the translated interview transcription to capture Karla's sense of a collective "we." Drawing on a feminist tradition of reappropriating and re-signifying terms that could be used as insults, critical scholarship has also re-signified the term as a contingent placeholder for sexual dissidence and diversity in Latin America until new categorical forms emerge (Falconí Trávez 2018).

17 In her groundbreaking essay "Thinking Sex," Gayle Rubin (1993 [1984]) outlined a conceptual toolkit for the analysis of sexuality, particularly in historical moments of social anxiety around the politics of sex. In one diagram, Rubin illustrated the social hierarchy of sexual values through two concentric circles. The inner circle, or "the charmed circle," corresponded to the characteristics associated with "good" or "normal" sexuality: married, monogamous, heterosexual, and so on. The outer circle corresponded to

characteristics associated with "bad" or "abnormal" sexuality: unmarried, promiscuous, homosexual, et cetera. Lines in the diagram paired a positive value in the charmed circle with its direct negative inverse in the outer circle. While sexual hierarchies may be more detailed than the figure suggested, and some characteristics in the outer circle may be more stigmatized than others, the general thesis was that sex in the charmed circle was socially accorded richness and complexity, while the outer circle was simply "considered utterly repulsive and devoid of all emotional nuance" (Rubin 1993 [1984], 15).

18 For some, these stories could "scandalize" in the sense that they could provoke discomfort and unease. For one, they typically aligned with the "salvation narrative" framework (Milton 2014). But they also portrayed figures who were the perpetrators of rape and sexual violence during the internal armed conflict as objects of sexual fantasy and desire (Boesten 2014; Bueno-Hansen 2015; Theidon 2013). In my consideration of the ethical dilemma that may emerge in the reproduction of the stories, I turned to queer-of-color scholars like Manalansan (2014) and Vargas (2014), who discuss the study of the messy, or *sucio*, elements of queer social life at the margins. To hear and read these stories as queer is "to locate discomfort, dissonance, and disorder as necessary and grounded experiences in the queer everyday and not as heroic acts of exceptional people" (Manalansan 2014, 97). Close attention to the stories was merited not because they were unproblematic but because they emerged as an important genre of stories in interlocutors' everyday life and because their circulation within Tarapoto (and beyond) was a meaningful way through which interlocutors sought to assert authorship over their shared experiences.

19 Anthropological research in Peru has pointed to the significance of everyday stories, rumors, and even conspiracies as repositories for experiences about political violence that have not made their way into formal archives. For example, Yezer (2008) looked beyond the testimonies collected by the CVR to show how some rural villagers in Ayacucho—the region most severely affected by violence—controlled "the shape and content of their narratives" through the circulation of everyday rumors and conspiracy theories. In his ethnography of life along the Huallaga River in Peru, Kernaghan (2009) insists that stories and storytelling are particularly suited for situations of political violence and its aftermath, "in that they provided glimpses of contemporary conditions and recent history not found in other sources such as newspaper accounts, scholarly literatures, and institutional archives" (23). To tell stories about the "curious and cruel turns" of life in the region's cocaine boom, Kernaghan's interlocutors blended fact and fiction in their stories for both ethical and pragmatic reasons. The facts and details were less important than the "affective winds that reverberate through lived events" (24).

20    Eduardo used *maricón* with tongue in cheek and as an umbrella term that included the categories "gay" and "transgender."

21    For example, see Drinot (2009), Falcón (2018), Feldman (2021), Vich (2015), Willis (2020), and Yezer (2008).

22    Even though men did not typically consider themselves *maperos* or assume the term as a social identity, this did not preclude them from participating in intergroup social dynamics between and among themselves. For example, Cáceres Palacios (1998) observed that in Iquitos, *maperos* were organized, had leaders, and frequently broke out in violence among themselves in competition over money and gifts (86).

23    Hirsch et al. (2009) explore extramarital sexuality and the risk that it can pose to married heterosexual women. The authors consider extramarital sex a secret—but widespread—social practice across the multiple cultures they surveyed. For interlocutors in Peru, a *mapero* was typically, though not always, married, and they generally understood their relationships with them as discreet and extramarital.

24    Commercial sex work was predominantly a feminized form of labor. Consequently, while the culture of *peches* often structured the romantic and sexual encounters of both gay men and transgender women with heterosexual men, in Tarapoto it was much more common for transgender women to labor as sex workers than it was for gay men to do so. Gay men more commonly sought the services of commercial sex workers. See Drinot (2020) for a history of sex work—and state efforts to regulate it—in Peru.

25    For example, nearly half of the gay male respondents of a survey in Peru indicated that taking pills every day or regularly undergoing HIV/STI testing was a barrier to PrEP adherence (Silva Torres et al. 2019). Longino et al. (2020) found a strong sense of skepticism among men who have sex with men and among transgender women sex workers in Lima around the safety and effectiveness of PrEP.

26    Applications of the category "transactional sex" certainly extend beyond discussions of HIV/AIDS. For example, Wentzell (2014) shows how men confronting erectile difficulty framed their sexual relationships as mediated by gifts and charitable support in order to perform a "good" masculinity.

27    Research on transactional sex considers the gendered dynamics between who gives the gifts and who receives them, often within broader contexts of accelerated economic stratification and gender inequality (Leclerc-Madlala 2003; Poulin 2007; Verheijen 2011; Wardlow 2020; Wyrod 2016). In Mojola's (2014) study of disparities of HIV incidence between women and men in Kenya, transaction and consumption were synonymous with modernity and characterized globalized gender inequalities. Likewise, there is a rich ethnographic record of transactional and commodified sex that draws on long-standing social scientific categories of analysis, including kinship,

exchange, and value (Canova 2020; Groes-Green 2013; Luna 2020; Meiu 2017; Padilla 2007; Smith 2017; Stout 2014).

28 Lancaster (1987) offers one of the most influential ethnographic theorizations of the *activo/pasivo* dynamic. As elaborated by Lancaster, the *activo/pasivo* framework was a theory of relations—specifically, the relation of a subject (i.e., a stigmatized or nonstigmatized subject) to a sexual role (i.e., the active role or the passive role). In doing so, Lancaster made both an ontological claim (i.e., the North American "gay" subject was fundamentally different from the Latin American *activo* or *pasivo*) and an epistemological claim (i.e., that how we come to know and understand social hierarchies and stigma is culturally specific). See Carrier (1995), Carrillo (2002), and Wright (2000) for other rich and nuanced ethnographic elaborations of Latin American sexual cultures that expanded on the *activo/pasivo* dynamic. Subsequent critiques of the *activo/pasivo* literature focused on the framework's ontological claims and the limits of its descriptive capacity. Cantú (2011), for example, argued that one of the consequences was the reification of Latin American cultures as Other, thus pathologizing Latinos as more perverse or unruly than their North American counterparts. Also see Clark et al. (2013), Decena (2011), and Nesvig (2001).

29 Carrillo (2017) theorizes the *activo/pasivo* distinction among gay Mexican migrants as one of several sexual schemas that constitute their many worlds of desire.

### Chapter 2. Collaboration on the *Cancha*

1 *Joven*, "young man" or "young person," was a common term for young adults, especially young men, in their teens and their twenties. It was also a term used for drawing the attention of service workers, such as waiters or store attendants. As young, heterosexual men married and fathered children, aging out of the category, unmarried gay men who were not fathers continued to be called *joven*, even as they progressed into their thirties and forties. I suggest that this practice of referring to adult gay men as *joven* speaks to a particular sensibility sometimes expressed in Tarapoto that sexual orientation is not necessarily permanent but rather reflects a particular stage of life to be eventually grown out of.

2 Throughout Latin America, "clientelism" and "patronage" have persisted as categories to name the social relations some poor and marginalized peoples cultivate in order to access resources, and, as Auyero (2000) describes, solve the problems of surviving the ongoing entrenchment of social welfare and state services. Specifically, they refer to the relations between a "patron," often a politician, who distributes money, resources, or opportunities, and a "client," who promises political or electoral support. Graham (1990) de-

fined patronage as "granting protection, official positions, and other favors in exchange for political and personal loyalty" (1). Such vertical relations often coexist with egalitarian ones, oriented horizontally toward kin and family, a coexistence Scheper-Hughes (1993) calls the "double ethic" of reciprocity and dependency. I specifically highlight the concept of *la colaboración* because it names a triadic relationship that is often missing from discussions of clientelism and patronage—namely, the role some gay and transgender organizers played in facilitating and creating the space for the reproduction of redistributive social relations. Though sometimes these relations may be clientelistic, this was certainly not always the case. Take, for example, the story of Ramón's visit to Nicole in Vista Alegre. This was not a cheap favor: for some, the costs of round-trip transportation could be a week's salary or more. Under a framework of clientelism, Ramón would have called me, explained the situation, and likely asked me (the foreign anthropologist with more resources) to financially support the journey to bring Nicole back to Tarapoto. I would have happily obliged. But a collaborative approach is focused not on the mediation of redistribution but on the creation of redistributive relationships. So while Ramón likely was anxious about going to a place he had never been, he was also hoping to more directly connect me with Nicole, even if it was just momentarily. So I see *la colaboración* as constituting an autonomous category of social relations, different from (though adjacent to) those specifically captured by the categories "clientelism," "patronage," or "patron-client relationship." Strickon and Greenfield's 1972 book is a classic survey of clientelism, patronage, and power across Latin America. For recent ethnographic accounts of clientelism in Latin America, see Ansell (2018), Borges Martins da Silva (2022), Diamond (2021), Hetherington (2020), and Hilgers (2012). For more on patron-client relations and the concept of the *patrón*, or patron/boss, in Peru, see Degregori (2012), Mayer (2009), and Pinedo (2017).

3    Dehne's 2016 publication in *The Lancet*, which set the tone for HIV prevention efforts in key populations in the latter half of the 2010s before the onset of the COVID-19 pandemic, specifically emphasized community empowerment and changing social norms.

4    In the case of key populations in Peru, some examples include Maiorana et al. (2016), Salazar et al. (2016), and Young et al. (2015).

5    Drawing on Fassin's (2007) discussion of the "inexpressibility" of social issues amid an AIDS controversy in South Africa, Kippax points to the pervasiveness of a tendency in HIV prevention research to acknowledge the social "without interrogating it" (Kippax 2012, 6). The effort to ethnographically flesh out the social relationships involving gay and transgender communities thus also comes from a long-standing call to give a fuller vocabulary of the social in HIV prevention.

6   Perez (2020) offers an expanded and detailed account of the historical trajectory of LGBT community-based organizations in Tarapoto.

7   Beauty pageants were frequent in Tarapoto and surrounding towns. The largest and most popular beauty pageants featured cisgender women contestants and were typically held around a municipal anniversary or patron saint celebration. As Ochoa (2014) described in her ethnography of beauty queens in Venezuela, the use of the word *miss* is derived from the English word used to describe beauty pageants. In Spanish, the term can be used to refer to the contestants themselves as well. The second part of the name of a particular beauty pageant typically used the name of the sponsoring municipality (e.g., Miss Tarapoto or Miss Morales) or of the patron saint festival (e.g., Miss San Juan). *Miss Gay* was a general term that was used to describe beauty contests that featured contestants who identified as gay, transgender, or *travesti*. Nascimento (2014) observed similar naming conventions in her ethnographic study of trans visibility and sociality in the Brazilian state of Paraíba. I suspect that in Tarapoto the term *Miss Gay* became anachronistic by the 2010s from an earlier period when *gay* was more frequently used as an umbrella term for those who might consider themselves trans or *travesti* as well as gay. Miss Gay beauty pageants also occurred around municipal anniversaries, patron saint festivities, or other occasions like seasons (e.g., Miss Gay Verano during the summer) or general themes (e.g., Miss Gay Mitológica for emphasizing figures and themes from local folklore). While miss contests were typically organized by sponsoring organizations or entities, such as a municipality, Miss Gay beauty contests were organized by individuals who carefully cultivated their reputation around specific contests, though Noleto (2014) analyzes two Miss Gay beauty contests organized by both municipal and state governments during the San Juan patron saint celebrations in the Brazilian state of Pará. Organizers and contestants themselves debated the appropriateness of the term *Miss Gay*, pointing out the fact that not all of the participants identified as gay, though many did. Some organizers in other parts of Peru switched to using the name *Miss Trans*, though the convention of using the *Miss Gay* terminology persisted in Tarapoto throughout my fieldwork. Again, interlocutors found moments for debate around categories of sexual orientation and gender identity, as a way both to inhabit them and to exceed them in everyday life.

8   Interlocutors expressed the prospect of "winning one's name" (*ganar su nombre*) as an ambiguous but worthwhile aspiration. In interviews, it was typically described retrospectively: organizers made sense of current successes or opportunities as a result of having "won their name" through organizing previous activities. What this aspiration looked like ultimately varied, but Martín's trajectory offers a good example of what interlocu-

tors meant. When he was in his teens and twenties, Martín participated in Miss Gay beauty contests and competed frequently in volleyball tournaments. He then began to organize these events. After that he began to work for the social assistance division of a municipal office in Tarapoto, where one of his primary responsibilities was organizing social events and entertainment.

9  The *pollada* is an informal, popular fundraising activity common in Peru, especially among the lower and middle classes. With roots in the urban exclaves of Andean migrants that emerged after large-scale migration to Lima in the 1960s, the practice has been linked to traditional forms of Andean reciprocity and exchange (Béjar-Rivera and Álvarez Alderete 2010; Cuberos-Gallardo 2020). A *pollada* can help cover a range of un-expected costs, typically including emergency medical costs or education expenses. A *pollada* might sometimes just involve picking up a portion of pre-purchased food. A *pollada bailable*, or danceable *pollada*, involves creating a more festive environment for those who purchased a ticket to hang out, and serving beer becomes another opportunity for fundraising through alcohol sales. Hence, the capacity to generate *la convocatoria* was key to organizing a successful *pollada*. While the recipient of funds might also be an organizer, in Tarapoto several of the gay and trans individuals who organized large activities started out by organizing *polladas*. This typifies the notion of collaboration as an aspirational ethos. The role of the organizer of a *pollada* was not just that of a broker who channeled or redistributed resources, as suggested by the concept of clientelism. Rather, the organizer was at the center of the production of new collaborative relations, drawing in and connecting, for example, anyone who reserved a ticket into a new relation of collaboration with the individual in need.

10  The popularity of team sports, especially soccer and volleyball, in part is related to how they reflect back the value of *la colaboración*. Volleyball, in particular, requires devotion by an individual to one specific role (e.g., setting), but when the roles are well coordinated, it can result in a successful and cohesive collective effort. See Perez (2011) for more on queer volleyball in Peru.

11  The most widely known example of such a scandalous episode came from the 2013 iteration of the Miss Gay San Juan beauty contest. At the end of the contest, after the winners had been announced, one contestant grabbed the wig and crown of the winner and a brief quarrel ensued. A video of a fight that broke out between two contestants onstage went viral on the internet. The clip was reedited by Peruvian television stations with exaggerated sound bites and sensationalized in national media outlets. It even circulated in English-language media outside of Peru. In one sense, popular media in Peru and around the world recognized the incident as

scandalous and—conjuring insensitive and offensive stereotypes about queer people—converted the story and footage into clickbait or daytime talk show filler. Within a few months, though, the clip was widely forgotten. But in Tarapoto, stories about Miss Gay San Juan—whether the judges were bribed, whether the runner-up was justified, or whether the whole episode was negative—persisted and circulated for years afterward.

12 *Machomenos* is a double entendre in Spanish that refers to a gay man. On the one hand, it is a portmanteau of the word *macho*, suggesting hyper- or normative masculinity, and the word *menos*, meaning "less than" or "minus." So the first meaning is something along the lines of "less than manly." On the other hand, the term sounds like the phrase *más o menos*, meaning "more or less" or "kind of." As a descriptor of a soccer tournament, the term *campeonato machomenos* plays with the idea of "kind of" or "sort of" a soccer tournament. Ramón's use of the term for the soccer tournament was tongue-in-cheek, and it was generally understood by participants and spectators as such.

13 Vaso de Leche (literally "glass of milk") is a food assistance program that provides milk to low-income families throughout Peru. The program does not have strict, income-based eligibility limits. Rather, the list of recipients is determined by the neighborhood mothers' club (or mothers' committee), which typically administers this program as well as the food assistance program called Comedor Popular (Communal Kitchen) (Brewer et al. 2021). These autonomous popular action programs are traditionally associated with the urban poor in Lima, where they emerged among base communities in the city's periphery (Davidson and Stein 1988). See Renkert (2022) for a history and critique of state food aid programs in Peru.

14 Sponsoring a soccer team for the tournament could be a significant investment, even for a successful local business owner. While advertising and publicity were certainly an incentive, the possibility of placing lucrative wagers with other local business owners was also a significant incentive for putting together a competitive team. For the *machomenos* soccer tournament, particularly enthusiastic team sponsors—like Wilmer, Claudia, and Brenda—recruited talented players from cities throughout the region, as far away as Yurimaguas and Tocache. In other instances, especially for volleyball tournaments, sponsors could recruit players from Iquitos, Pucallpa, and even Lima. A team sponsor would likely have to provide accommodations for the player throughout the duration of the tournament. During the week, players might arrange their own games of soccer or volleyball. Visiting players made (or lost) money during the week through the wagers made on their behalf during these impromptu games.

15 It is likely that, as a municipal administrator, Felix had attended several sensitivity trainings as part of the ongoing Global Fund–supported efforts

to institutionalize municipal antidiscrimination ordinances that included sexual orientation and gender identity as well as garner municipal support for HIV and STI health clinics to serve vulnerable populations. In these workshops, it was common to include the names of all of the international entities that had, in some form, supported the community-based organizations implementing the projects. So materials, posters, and other workshop ephemera featured the names and logos of entities such as the European Union, the United States Department of State, the United States Agency for International Development, the Global Fund, and a range of nongovernmental organizations. In his interactions with Felix, Ramón encountered two consequences of these workshops. First, Felix expressed the common critique that gay and transgender organizers focused too much on HIV/AIDS among their communities, both at the expense of other issues and at the expense of HIV/AIDS in other communities. This misconception was so frequently expressed that Ramón already had a prepared response to it. A less anticipated consequence, though, was the perception that gay and transgender communities in Tarapoto had huge budgets from the European Union and the US government. Though this was a more subtle perception, it certainly affected Felix's and the city council's willingness to give municipal money to support the soccer tournament. This particular misconception could be found even among other gay and transgender individuals not directly involved in administering Global Fund programs, as they typically overestimated how much money was actually sent to Tarapoto for HIV prevention.

16     The invitation to participate in the municipal anniversary parade felt consequential for Ramón and others. As further analyzed in Perez (2020), it was precisely the effort to be included in a municipal anniversary parade nearly a decade earlier that many in Tarapoto remembered as having been the origin of their collective advocacy.

17     See Friedman (2017) for the role that internet technologies played in transforming feminist and queer counterpublics in Latin America. Focusing on the robust and contentious debates and dialogues that emerged over listservs, forums, message boards, and other virtual spaces, Friedman explains how virtual spaces could "serve as arenas for internal development and debate, where movement participants articulate their identities, build their communities, and hone their strategies" (16).

18     These debates coexist alongside broader conversations in health promotion and HIV prevention about practices and limits of categories and classification. See Boellstorff (2011), Boyce (2007), Calazans and Facchini (2022), Parker (2019), Parker, Aggleton, and Perez-Brumer (2016).

19     It is likely that preexisting debates influenced the perceptions and positions of many of the participants. Many, for example, were familiar with

the Brazilian volleyball athlete Tiffany Abreu. Tiffany is a trans woman who played in the premier professional women's volleyball league in Brazil, and whose inclusion generated national and international debate about gender, bodies, and ideas of heteronormativity in sport (Sant'Ana 2022). She has a very popular following among volleyball fans in Latin America, especially gay and transgender fans, and was often the subject of informal conversation among interlocutors during my fieldwork.

20 In naming the upcoming game something both so absurd and so serious as War of the Salons, Veronica epitomized the queer camp sensibility that David Halperin, in describing Esther Newton's *Mother Camp*, described as "the deliberate refusal of self-exemption from the mockery [she] directs at the larger social world" (2012, 202). For even as Veronica took seriously the chance for her team to win the soccer game, she included herself in her derision of the earnestness of the game.

21 "Luis Neira habla del baño que se dio Carlos Philco en laguna," Via Televisión, March 27, 2015, https://viatelevision.pe/7546/luis-neira-habla-bano -dio-carlos-philco-laguna.

22 "Discoteca Anaconda denunciará a Carlos Philco por abuso de autoridad," *Voces*, July 31, 2017, www.diariovoces.com.pe/85904/discoteca-anaconda -denunciara-carlos-philco-abuso-autoridad.

23 "Mónica Guevara: 'Actitud de alcalde Carlos Philco es una payasada,'" *Voces*, April 10, 2018, https://diariovoces.com.pe/103940/monica-guevara -actitud-alcalde-carlos-philco-payasada.

24 "Las promesas incumplidas de campana de Carlos Philco," *Voces*, May 16, 2017, https://www.diariovoces.com.pe/80928/promesas-incumplidas -campana-carlos-philco.

25 "Confirman sentencia de 4 años de prisión para el ex alcalde de Morales Carlos Philco, ayer no se presentó a lectura de sentencia," Radio Tropical, December 12, 2019, https://radiotropical.pe/confirman-sentencia-de -4-anos-de-prision-para-el-ex-alcalde-de-morales-carlos-philco-ayer-no -se-presento-a-lectura-de-sentencia/.

### Chapter 3. Scandal at the Disco

An earlier version of chapter 3 appeared as "Scandalous Denouncement: Discrimination, Difference, and Queer Scandal in Urban Amazonian Peru" in *Latin American and Caribbean Ethnic Studies* 17 (1): 78–98, 2022.

1 Since early on, HIV/AIDS has been considered an "epidemic of discrimination" (Farmer 1992). Cáceres, Aggleton, and Galea (2008) and Thomas et al. (2017) acutely synthesize the recommendation for comprehensive and inclusive HIV prevention programs that directly attend to the social

exclusion of and discrimination toward gay, transgender, and MSM populations. By focusing on the key steps in the process of controlling HIV and/
or achieving viral suppression, the HIV care continuum model oriented
public health data collection toward the key indicators of the 90-90-90
goals (i.e., that 90 percent of people living with HIV know their status,
90 percent of those who know their status receive treatment, and 90 percent
of those on treatment reach viral suppression). Chow et al. (2016) use the
HIV care continuum model to offer a snapshot of Peru's HIV epidemic in
the mid-2010s.

2   For example, see Clark et al. (2020), Perez-Brumer et al. (2017), and Salazar et al. (2016) for empirical evidence directly connecting discrimination,
stigma, and HIV among vulnerable populations in Peru.

3   The System of Community Protection (also sometimes called the System of Community Vigilance) was a cornerstone of the Tenth Round's
intervention.

4   Falcón (2016) describes intersectionality as an increasingly universal paradigm "that acknowledges—rather than flattens—differences that can be at-
tributed to structural, institutional, systematic, geopolitical, and individual
factors" (156). Though originally developed to draw attention to the blind
spots that emerged amid the legal application of normative categories of
race and gender in the United States, in Peru intersectional perspectives
and sensibilities have connected feminist advocacy with issues around
human rights, democracy, and racial discrimination (Bueno-Hansen 2015;
Cox Hall, Alcalde, and Babb 2022; Ewig 2010; Falcón 2016). For an application of an intersectional perspective toward health equity in Amazonian
Peru, see Shannon et al. (2017).

5   Parker and Aggleton (2003) and Castro and Farmer (2005) note how discrimination and stigma have been either misinterpreted as static and devoid of social context or simply used as a shorthand for eliding complex
social inequalities when applied to the global HIV epidemic, and they call
for deeper theorizations of the concepts.

6   This was during Alberto Fujimori's second presidential term and part of a
broader period of health policy shifts in Peru that Christina Ewig (2010)
terms "second-wave neoliberalism." While Fujimori's government allocated
very little to HIV treatment and prevention during its first term (1990–95),
its second term (1995–2000) saw an expansion of resources dedicated to the
rapidly expanding HIV epidemic in the country. As Marcos Cueto (2001)
notes, this was marked through the creation of PROCETSS, the National
Program for the Control of Sexually Transmitted Infections and AIDS, and
through a congressional law that obligated the Ministry of Health to coordinate a plan to implement national STI and HIV control efforts and to
promote collaboration with international organizations such as the newly

created UNAIDS. Even with an increased budget, it appeared as though resources were inequitably allocated between Lima and the rest of the country, nor was the budget nearly enough to ensure universal coverage of ART.

7    While Via Libre, the first NGO in Peru focused on the issue of AIDS, was established in Lima in 1990, it is important to underscore the severity of the internal armed conflict at the time (Cueto and Palmer 2015). The widespread violence resulting from the internal armed conflict deterred foreign tourism and consequently slowed the spread of HIV to areas impacted by the violence (Cueto 2001, 40).

8    Founded in 1982, the Movimiento Homosexual de Lima (MHOL) is one of the earliest organizations for LGBT advocacy and liberation in Peru. The naming of the Movimiento Homosexual de Tarapoto follows the naming conventions established by MHOL. For essays by two of MHOL's founders, see Ugarteche (1997) and Miró Quesada (2022). For a history of the development of MHOL, see Marreros Núñez (2021). Over the 2010s, MHOL activists maintained a close relationship with the members of MHOTA and, subsequently, DISAM. The renowned and influential activist Gio Infante maintained strong connections with DISAM and other members of LGBT communities throughout the Amazonian region. He visited and consulted with DISAM on several occasions over the period of my fieldwork. For more on the legacy and impact of Gio Infante, see Cornejo (2023).

9    The development and implementation of this proposal coincided with two rounds of project funding from the Global Fund: the Fifth and Sixth Rounds. Compared with prior rounds of funding, which emphasized the scale-up of treatment, the Fifth Round (2006–10) and Sixth Round (2007–11) were increasingly oriented toward HIV prevention activities. This included sex education and syndromic management in the general population, peer health promotion activities and regular screening and checkups among vulnerable populations, and the promotion of a favorable sociopolitical environment that supported human rights and reduced discrimination and stigma (Cáceres et al. 2013).

10   Golash-Boza (2010) argues that the passage of antidiscrimination laws and ordinances indicates how the recognition of racism and discrimination have become part of national debates. Antidiscrimination laws that explicitly include sexual orientation and gender identity, however, did not exist at the national level in Peru during the time of my fieldwork. Rights advocates have interpreted the prohibition of discrimination on the basis of origin, race, sex, language, religion, opinion, economic status, or "any other status" (*cualquiera otra índole*) to include sexual orientation and gender identity.

11   By 2016, there existed ordinances across Peru that specifically named or included sexual orientation and/or gender identity as protected categories.

These ordinances existed at the levels of districts, provinces, and regions across several departments, including but not limited to Apurímac, Arequipa, Ayacucho, Cajamarca, Callao, Huancavelica, Junín, Lambayeque, Lima, Loreto, Piura, San Martín, and Ucayali. In Lima, because there was no citywide antidiscrimination ordinance that included sexual orientation and gender identity, "antidiscrimination ordinances [we]re instituted in some districts while not in others, and the types of discrimination included in these ordinances var[ied]" (Alcalde 2018, 125). Also see Kogan et al. (2013) and Sanborn (2012).

12    In an ethnography of medical training in Mexico, Smith-Oka (2021) suggests that medical professionals evoke culturalist explanations to describe the challenges of providing care to underserved, low-income, or indigenous populations. Culture, she writes, embeds intersecting forms of ethno-racial, class, and gender difference, and thus becomes a way to ascribe blame for "why the country is the way it is" (Smith-Oka 2021, 130). I found resonance with the way the culture concept could be used as shorthand for making sense of the complicated confluence of social and health inequalities.

13    The terms *cholo* and *chola* are quite dynamic and traverse cultural and scholarly fields across the Americas. In the Andean worlds of Ecuador, Bolivia, and Peru, as Weismantel (2001) observes, the category of *chola* draws on a legacy of gendered and racial meanings, typically referring to market women who sell produce and evoking images of the traditional skirt, or *pollera*, and bowler hat that have been associated with market women. The international popularity of the *chola luchadores* (professional wrestlers) in Bolivia has become another site for the reworking and refashioning of the category, through a process that Haynes (2013) terms "strategic essentialism." The category takes on a completely different meaning among Latino and Chicano urban subcultures in the United States, evoking another distinct aesthetic style fashioned amid different sexual cultures and regimes of racialization.

14    Heckert (2018), Howe (2009), and Perez (2017) show how emblematic cases can translate abstract concepts such as discrimination or homophobia into popular discourse, in turn shaping narratives about how discrimination affects people living with HIV/AIDS and other vulnerable communities. As Heckert (2018) writes in her analysis of Magaly, the first person living with HIV in Bolivia to successfully bring a case of medical negligence in the courts, an exemplary case such as Magaly's offers "a window into understanding the systematic discrimination and humiliation that HIV-positive patients in Bolivia experience" (53). And emblematic cases have consequences both intended and unintended. For example, they can productively set legal precedent and result in systematic change, as Magaly's case did in Bolivia. If enough people know about an emblematic case, like

Godfrey's case in Peru, then those cases can be used in everyday instances to contest discriminatory practices.

15    In some television reports about the incident, Godfrey self-identified with the term *transsexual*. My analysis focuses on the circulation of Godfrey's story, particularly how and why it was used within the context of HIV prevention workshops to promote the cultivation of a culture of denouncement. I rarely, if ever, encountered this particular term voiced by interlocutors to refer either to Godfrey or to themselves. When Godfrey's story was recounted by project coordinators or technical assistants, Godfrey was referred to as *trans* or *travesti*.

16    Throughout the 2000s, Peruvian media popularized several cases in which nightclubs in Lima and Cusco were fined for discriminating on the basis of physical appearance (Golash-Boza 2010). The dissemination of these emblematic cases of racial discrimination had established a precedent and a capacious media narrative surrounding nightlife and discos that could include incidents of discrimination on the basis of sexual orientation and gender identity.

17    "Cuarto Poder: Esta es la historia de Godfrey y su triunfo ante la discoteca 'Gótica," YouTube, posted by América Noticias, September 1, 2013, https:// youtu.be/5dHEMfvyDGY.

18    Moodie (2010) describes the term "entextualization" as referring to "the movements of detached fragments of texts (stories and bits of stories that are retold) through transformations in genre (from one kind of situation to another)" (8). Yesika's insistence on the denouncement of the injustice she experienced emerged as a result of the ongoing entextualization of Godfrey's emblematic case. The basic components of the story—experiencing discrimination at the entrance to a nightclub—circulated across the country, yet as the story moved across regions and was used for different ends, it had varying effects. At a capacity-building workshop, it worked as a parable for how to build one's capacities and denounce discrimination. In this instance, it was used to discourage Yesika's denouncement.

19    Kulick (1996), for example, described "throwing a scandal" as a strategy for *travesti* sex workers in Brazil to compel clients to pay them. Instead of resisting hegemonic descriptions of them as scandalous, they used this depiction to their advantage by enveloping and imbricating their unmarked, heterosexual clients into the sphere of the scandalous. Vasquez del Aguila (2012), riffing on the popular saying "God forgives the sin, but not the scandal," found that gay Peruvian migrants in New York positioned themselves away from scandal through the active management of the "open secret" about their sexual identity.

20    Ahmed summarizes the double bind that those who file formal complaints encounter when she writes that "to become a complainer is to become the

location of a problem" (2021, 3). Though her statement is attuned to the institutional university context, I find this observation to resonate deeply with Yesika's experience with denouncement. Rather than the problem being systematic discrimination against trans women at the nightclub, by denouncing discrimination she became the de facto problem for being "too scandalous."

21 Dr. Leguía is a pseudonym. I include the title "Dr." to show how some individuals were accorded this honorific as a sign of respect. It was common in Tarapoto for engineers and some state authorities to be called *doctór*, even if they did not hold an academic doctorate.

22 The social scientific encounter with "homosexual social worlds" that emerged during the 1950s through the 1970s played a crucial role in reframing "deviance" from an intrinsic and individual trait toward a dynamic social and relational experience (Love 2021; Rubin 2002). Many of the foundational ethnographic texts from this period emphasized the centrality of commercial establishments, especially bars, as social institutions (Achilles 1967; Hooker 1967; Newton 1972). As Maskovsky (2002) observed, this emphasis on consumption in the study of sexual subcultures often elided the labor practices and racial hierarchies of bars as themselves places of work that often relied on exploitation. Scholarship on queer nightlife has expanded the focus on commercial establishments to include the varying spaces where "queer people congregate to get relief from the pressures of everyday life" (Adeyemi, Khubchandani, and Rivera-Servera 2021, 3). Despite their limits as exclusionary, commercial spaces like discos, bars, and nightclubs persist both as practical sites to ground ethnographic participant observation of queer social livelihoods and, more significantly, as sites of queer possibility, imagination, and sociality across the ethnographic record (e.g., Allen 2022; Russo Garrido 2020; Valentine 2007; Vargas 2014; Wilson 2004). In invoking the term *nightscape*, I suggest that nightclubs and discos can be considered as part of, but not completely isomorphic with, the many ways gay and trans people in Tarapoto inhabit a nocturnal social world.

23 Kernaghan (2012) shows how the infrastructure and maintenance of the highway itself has long been a site of intense political contestation and the exercise of state power in the region.

24 *La farándula* refers to the world of popular entertainment or show business. Due to coverage in popular media and tabloids, there is an intrinsic interest in and fascination with the personal lives of *farándula* celebrities that does not necessarily extend to all famous or renowned individuals. Over the 2010s, prominent members of the *farándula* were typically professional athletes or appeared in competition-based reality shows that focused intensely on the romantic storylines among the competitors (e.g., *Esto es Guerra* and *Combate*).

25 The Spanish term *el ambiente* can mean "air," "atmosphere," "milieu," or "environment." In many queer subcultures across Latin America and in parts of the United States, the term typically refers to queer spaces generally known exclusively to and inhabited by queer people. As Russo Garrido (2020) notes, "*El ambiente* only exists in the hands of the people who make it happen" (21). As such, *el ambiente* can encompass varying spaces, including bars, internet cabins, street corners, parks, political organizations, and community centers. Motta (1999) describes how young people created an *ambiente* in Lima. In Tarapoto, there was a popular bar known as Bunker Space that was generally considered a gay nightclub, but it was by no means exclusively gay. While interlocutors in Tarapoto were aware of the term, they understood it as a dynamic that existed in Lima; they did not typically use it to describe their social worlds in Tarapoto. This was likely because many of the central sites of gay and transgender sociality were not known exclusively to them.

### Chapter 4. When Projects End

1 Kaulard (2018) describes the process through which the Peruvian state came to reassert economic control over the San Martín department of Peru through alternative development models in the aftermath of the region's cocaine boom. Kaulard noted that some of the technical experts—known colloquially as *tigres*, or tigers—assumed new levels of expertise on agricultural products like coffee and cacao and thus played an important role in the continuity of economic development. Ethnographically, I never heard the term *tigre* applied to HIV prevention project specialists, though I am not surprised that new terms emerged in adjacent sectors of human rights and economic development in the region to make sense of the new kinds of expertise required to participate in *la cooperación internacional*. Of the project specialists profiled in this chapter, Anderson was the only one who held a postsecondary degree. Ramón was in the process of obtaining a degree in psychology at a local private university. Norma was the only trans project specialist involved with Global Fund projects in Tarapoto.

2 H. Alvear, "Presentan propuesta sobre orientación sexual e identidad," *Diario Hoy*, June 28, 2013, 4.

3 Mariscal Cáceres is a province in the San Martín department. The principal city of the province is Juanjuí, which is located approximately eighty-five miles from Tarapoto.

4 Global Fund, "The Framework Document," 2001, www.theglobalfund.org /media/6019/core_globalfund_framework_en.pdf.

5 "Introduction to the Global Fund and CCMs," YouTube, posted by the Global Fund, March 15, 2012, https://youtu.be/qOPU9f6MM0E.

6     Corresponsales Clave, "Perú cierra proyecto de ronda 10 y apuesta por una nota conceptual," January 29, 2015, https://corresponsalesclave.org/peru-cierra-proyecto-de-ronda-10-y-apuesta-por-una-nota-conceptual/.

7     Corresponsales Clave, "Perú cierra proyecto de ronda 10."

8     Considering the wide circulation of stories about discrimination at the disco in Tarapoto, there was a significant intertextual element to Norma's composite story. Norma was acutely aware of how the accusation of scandal makes it difficult for someone to proceed with a formal discrimination grievance. Thus, as opposed to stories like the one told by Paula (see chapter 3) about inciting a scandal when encountering discrimination, Norma encouraged a different approach. In her composite story of discrimination, she leaves the nightclub immediately and the very next day begins the process of filing a formal grievance.

9     The original grievance form coded HIV status without ever explicitly mentioning it through the phrase *esa enfermedad*, or "that disease." In some contexts, interlocutors preferred to reference HIV/AIDS through coded phrases and colloquialisms. One of these colloquialisms was the term *bu*. The term *bu* was likely a shortening of the term *buses*, which I described previously (see chapter 1) as a term meant to warn others of possible danger and to proceed with caution or discretion. Giancarlo Cornejo (personal correspondence) describes the term *buses* as originating in *travesti* culture as a term of admonition.

10    Project specialists were aware of the gossip and speculation about them. It is important to acknowledge ethnographically the existence of speculation about their administration of the Tenth Round projects in the region. On the one hand, the speculation was a function of the temporality of the Tenth Round's problems. Ellen Moodie, for example, writes about the "early versions of events." The news of an event can incite a "fecund flow" of speculation and rumors about it in its early stages, as the details are not yet confirmed or determined (Moodie 2006, 64). Regarding the news of the closure of the Tenth Round, at the point in time described here interlocutors were still making sense of what actually happened, and speculation about robbery and fraud were part of the "early version" of stories. It is of equal importance to consider how the wielding of the language of corruption among some interlocutors can also be a reflection of a broader cultural milieu characterized by widespread political dissatisfaction and societal disapproval of state institutions (Carrión 2022; Levitsky 2014). Political and social crisis in the latter half of the 2010s intensified this dissatisfaction and disapproval. For example, over the tumultuous six-year period 2016–22 the country had seven different presidents and experienced a seemingly unending series of revelations and allegations of graft and corruption (Cox Hall, Alcalde, and Babb 2022; McClintock 2019;

Muñoz 2021). It is therefore not surprising that community participants in HIV prevention programming viewed or discussed their frustrations or misgivings about project specialists in the "early version" of accounts of the discontinuation of the Tenth Round through the language of corruption, even if there were not specific or documented instances of it.

11 See Cornejo (2023) for a discussion of the legacy of Peruvian scholar-activist Gio Infante.

12 US Department of State, "Global Equity Fund," n.d., www.state.gov/global-equality-fund/.

13 Biehl and Locke's formulation of an anthropology of becoming inspires my approach to Anderson's stories. That is, I see the stories as, at once, a reckoning "with the overdetermined constraints and resources of the worlds into which [he] is thrown," while also a reflection of his tremendous ability "to imagine worlds and characters that do not—but may yet—exist" (Biehl and Locke 2017, 9). Anderson confronted and navigated the adversities and limitations of the world that surrounded him, ranging from a disapproving familial context to his experience of active discouragement by the educational system. He confronted the limited applicability of the terms and categories insisted on by the donors and funders of the Global North to the contours of his community, even as he tried to identify new sources of support of advocacy and antidiscrimination. And yet, as he storied the structural failures of HIV prevention and the Tenth Round, he imagined an emergent version of queer advocacy at the margins of these structural limitations.

14 The "concept note" is the most important document for any given country's application to the Global Fund. It outlines a country's overall health plan, makes a case for how the Global Fund's disease-specific support will fill in critical gaps, and is closely evaluated by the Global Fund's technical review panels.

15 As Sandset (2021) affirms, the launch of the 90-90-90 targets at a UNAIDS summit in October 2014 was "perhaps the most important pillar in the work toward the end of AIDS" (32–33). I underscore the stark contrast at this moment between how global enthusiasm for the ending of AIDS was formalized and how gay and transgender communities in Peru were experiencing the failures of an HIV prevention project oriented toward the goal of controlling the epidemic in the country.

16 UNAIDS, "Pandemic Triad: HIV, Covid-19, and Debt in Developing Countries," October 11, 2022, www.unaids.org/en/resources/documents/2022/pandemic-triad-HIV-COVID19-debt-in-developing-countries.

1    Adams (2016) refers to a broader context within the field of global health that insists on data and metrics produced from randomized controlled trials, or RCTs. Considered the gold standard in global health and evidence-based medicine, Adams points to how the ends can sometimes elide the means: in other words, specific interventions can be justified only on the grounds of data from RCTs. However, RCTs have their limits. For one, as Valdez (2022) explains in the case of pregnancy interventions, they can involve diverse sets of risks and ethics. Furthermore, "they are primarily designed and funded in the Global North, which creates an uneven distribution of knowledge production and global health policy influence" (Valdez 2022, 39). Adams (2016) thus suggests that "data deprivation" may be a fate "even more tragic than lacking health" because it can mean the contraction of investments or the withdrawal of interventions not because they do not work, but because there is not the "right" kind of data to justify them.

2    As Adams notes, "Another outcome of the use of scientific metrics is that every kind of health behavior (from latrine use to breastfeeding, use of bed nets, or voucher programs) is now identified as a problem that can be measured in the same way as experiments produce data" (2016, 34).

3    This includes Jaime Ballero (2009a, 2009b, 2010), Otsuka Salinas and Arriagáda Barrera (2012), Silva Ticllacuri (2013), Meza Caballero (2014), Dador and Saldaña (2015), and Otsuka et al. (2016). The annual reports on LGBT human rights published by PROMSEX are available at https://promsex .org/publicaciones/#diversidad-sexual-osig.

4    The Yogyakarta Principles were first drafted in 2006 by human rights experts outlining legal standards regarding sexual orientation and gender identity. The full text of the Yogyakarta Principles is available at https:// yogyakartaprinciples.org/.

5    I was often talked about as *gringa* by interlocutors, especially those (like Anderson) whom I accompanied closely throughout fieldwork. Though I spoke about myself in the grammatical masculine, the term was used in a playful manner, which allowed interlocutors a way to acknowledge some significant social differences (of nationality and class, in particular) while also forging a connection by playfully speaking to or about me in the grammatical feminine. Likewise, Anderson's question about where to find volleyball was typical. While it was common knowledge that groups of gay men, and some trans women, played volleyball every afternoon and evening, it was hard to know exactly *where* the popular place was to play at any given time. The specific parks and streets that drew the best players and largest spectators were constantly in flux. A park in the Morales district might be popular for a couple of months, and then a street in the

Banda de Shilcayo district might overtake it in popularity. Unless one went to watch or play volleyball consistently, it did require some research or asking around to know where the most popular site was on any given day.

6    On afternoon volleyball games at popular parks such as this one, each team could be betting upward of 1,000–2,000 soles, or $300–$600.

7    In 2013, DISAM activists in Tarapoto brokered a significant and groundbreaking agreement between the provincial government of San Martín (Municipalidad Provincial de San Martín), the Ministry of Labor's social security health program (EsSalud), and DISAM. The tripartite agreement created a medical post with the specific goal of serving vulnerable populations through reducing the transmission of HIV and other STIs and improving the care of people living with HIV. The provincial government agreed to pay up to 1,750 soles monthly to subsidize the rent of the medical post, and EsSalud agreed to staff it with medical personnel. The intention was to establish continuity and continued care after the eventual withdrawal of the Global Fund. At the time the agreement was first negotiated, Manuel Nieves, a gay man and LGBT activist, was the lieutenant mayor of the provincial government. Though DISAM had a key ally in the municipal government at the time, the agreement persisted through successive provincial administrations. Certain days were designated for service to "sex workers" and other days were designated for service to gay men, trans women, and men who have sex with men ("vulnerable populations"). I was unclear about the reason behind these distinctions; however, in practice, gay men and trans women who might also engage in sex work sought services on the days designated for gay men and trans women. During periods of my fieldwork when the medical post was operational, staffing and services were infrequent and experiences like the one described by Axel were typical.

8    Ten soles was equivalent to approximately $3.

9    For example, in a survey of trans women's access to hospital care in Tarapoto, Hidalgo (2023) found that while nearly all individuals surveyed were knowledgeable about their right to health, nearly 75 percent of those surveyed experienced some form of discrimination or exclusion at the hospital.

10   Tuesdays and Thursdays were intended to provide specialized attention for "vulnerable populations" (i.e., gay, transgender, and MSM individuals), while Mondays and Wednesdays were intended for "sex workers." Again, while these were, of course, not mutually exclusive categories, they were for the purposes of seeking HIV and STI testing and services and represented the kinds of social categories that queer people in Tarapoto navigated in their everyday lives.

11   A listserv is an electronic mailing list. See Friedman (2017) for a discussion of feminist and queer counterpublic formation in Latin America through internet technologies like email listservs.

12    Callao is part of the greater Lima metropolitan area, but it is a separate administrative region and province from Lima. It is the primary port for Lima as well as the location of Peru's primary airport.

13    This relationship extends as far back as 2008, when I was an undergraduate exchange student in Peru. I conducted a senior thesis project on street volleyball among gay and transgender volleyball players in Callao (Perez 2011). Several interlocutors from that project were members of a community-based organization selected to implement programming for the Tenth Round of the Global Fund in Callao.

14    The demonym for Callao is *chalaco* or *chalaca*.

15    See Machuca Rose, Cocchella Loli, and Gallegos Dextre (2016, 253) for a reproduction of the final version of this form.

16    Dr. Enriquez is a pseudonym. I include the title "Dr." to note one of several hierarchies with which Anderson contended in this situation. Dr. Enriquez was a medical doctor, but it was common for some individuals, like engineers, to be referred to as *doctór* as well.

17    In comparing his ethnographic data on the number of AIDS-related deaths among people living on the streets of Salvador, Brazil, with the official state databases, Biehl (2007) found that nearly three-quarters of those who had died were never registered. He called this an "invisible epidemic": social factors, such as informal or unspoken procedures for intake at hospitals, made it so that the poorest and most marginalized could not access care. As a result, those in the margins often went unnoticed (or noticed, but unaccounted for) by official registries and statistics. Consequently, because social factors conditioned the incompleteness of the data, if the social roots were not addressed, no amount of statistical techniques or analysis could overcome those absences. Biehl showed not only that people can be accounted for in terms of categories and numbers, but also that these very technologies of categorization and counting produce absences and invisibility. In a parallel fashion, Anderson was aware of the absences in official statistics about HIV/AIDS in Peru. And though he, too, was not necessarily able to produce verifiable epidemiological and demographic data, he could produce authoritative data about discrimination that could in some ways stand in as a proxy for the purposes of HIV prevention advocacy.

18    Treichler (1999) theorizes the AIDS epidemic as an "epidemic of signification." Originally posed in the early 1990s, Treichler's call for an "epidemiology of signification" was responding to a call for the cultural analysis of the AIDS crisis among scholars. Because so much was still unknown about the virus, scholars brought a critical eye to the representations of AIDS that influenced scientists, politicians, bureaucrats, laypeople, and the individuals and communities living with and dying from HIV/AIDS (Altman 1986; Sontag 1990). Anderson's use of the PROMSEX reports in this context

suggests that knowledge and data about HIV prevention, too, continue to emerge in symbolic terrains. In a context of data deprivation, Anderson invoked the PROMSEX *informe* to make an authoritative point about the epidemic to experts who might otherwise have dismissed his assertions.

19  Scholarship on people living with HIV/AIDS has noted how the medical fixation on numerical metrics has had the effect of creating new subjectivities based on these numbers (Cormier McSwiggin 2017; Miller 2016; O'Daniel 2014). In her ethnography on HIV/AIDS in South Florida among Haitian migrants, Thurka Sangaramoorthy observed clients introducing themselves and assuming an identity based on their viral load and CD4 counts. She calls this way of articulating one's self and one's understanding of others based on numbers, categories, and disease status "numerical subjectivity" (Sangaramoorthy 2014, 38). I am adapting this concept to describe how the management and wielding of numerical data further create a new form of subjectivity among project specialists involved in HIV prevention.

**Afterword**

1  As early as the mid-2000s, studies indicated rising rates of HIV in certain indigenous Amazonian communities in Peru, particularly in the Loreto and Amazonas departments. For example, a study of a small community of 162 persons in Loreto found HIV prevalence in adults to be 7.5 percent (Zavaleta et al. 2007). Structural factors, including but not limited to underinvestment in intercultural health services, little support for comprehensive or preventive healthcare, and long travel distances to hospitals, resulted in vulnerability to a range of infectious disease in addition to HIV/AIDS. Coordinating and arranging travel to hospitals, in fact, had become an important part of the provision of intercultural health care in the Peruvian Amazon (Del Mastro N. 2022). A study on the structural factors that contribute specifically to HIV/AIDS vulnerability among indigenous Amazonians further pointed to factors such as opportunities for transactional sex as a result of riverine commercial activity, the lack of knowledge about access to HIV treatment, and a preference for traditional healing practices (Orellana et al. 2013). AS HIV prevention projects are expanded and reoriented toward indigenous Amazonians, and as health science researchers apply standard technical frameworks like "transactional sex" to determine the sites of vulnerability, I hope this research engages with *Queer Emergent* to consider a more robust and contextual approach to the social worlds of indigenous Amazonians and take seriously their practices of storytelling and world-making.

2  In the years since my primary period of fieldwork (2014–15), Anderson began her gender transition and assumed a new social, lived name. In

*Queer Emergent*, both the names "Anderson" and "Leyla" are pseudonyms. In consultation with Leyla, I determined to leave "Anderson" as the pseudonym for the majority of the book, as the name reflected the gendered dimensions of the former name it stood in for.

3   In this moment, it appeared as though the bodies coordinating the proposal were not considering how these categories might intersect.

4   For example, the work of Garcia et al. (2018), which was published after this conversation with Leyla, referenced the 2014 spectrum data as a baseline for the 90-90-90 targets in Peru; it did not use the 2011 sentinel data. The authors found that, of the estimated 72,000 people living with HIV/AIDS in 2014, 64 percent were diagnosed, 46 percent were receiving ART, and 36 percent had achieved viral suppression. These were lower than what I had written in my notes from that afternoon's presentation (78 percent diagnosed, 68 percent on ART, and 43 percent with viral suppression).

5   Ministry of Health, "Norma técnica de salud 'Prevención combinada del virus de la inmunodeficiencia humana para poblaciónes en alto riesgo' (NTS NO 204-MINSA/DGIESP-2023)," 2023, http://bvs.minsa.gob.pe/local /MINSA/6345.pdf.

6   Serodiscordant couples are couples in which one partner is living with HIV and the other is not.

## REFERENCES

Abadía-Barrero, César Ernesto, and Arachu Castro. 2006. "Experiences of Stigma and Access to HAART in Children and Adolescents Living with HIV/AIDS in Brazil." *Social Science and Medicine* 62, no. 5: 1219–28.

Achilles, Nancy. 1967. "The Development of the Homosexual Bar as an Institution." In *Sexual Deviance*, edited by John Gagnon and William Simon, 228–44. New York: Harper and Row.

Adams, Vincanne. 2016. "Metrics of the Global Sovereign: Numbers and Stories in Global Health." In *Metrics: What Counts in Global Health*, edited by Vincanne Adams, 19–54. Durham, NC: Duke University Press.

Adams, Vincanne, Dominique Behague, Carlo Caduff, Ilana Löwy, and Francisco Ortega. 2019. "Re-imagining Global Health through Social Medicine." *Global Public Health* 14, no. 10: 1383–400.

Adams, Vincanne, Nancy J. Burke, and Ian Whitmarsh. 2013. "Slow Research: Thoughts for a Movement in Global Health." *Medical Anthropology* 33, no. 3: 179–97.

Adeyemi, Kemi, Kareem Khubchandani, and Ramón H. Rivera-Servera. 2021. "Introduction." In *Queer Nightlife*, edited by Kemi Adeyemi, Kareem Khubchandani, and Ramón H. Rivera-Servera, 1–18. Ann Arbor: University of Michigan Press.

Aguirre, Carlos. 2011. "Terruco de m . . . Insulto y stigma en la guerra sucia peruana." *Histórica* 35, no. 1: 103–39.

Ahmed, Sara. 2021. *Complaint!* Durham, NC: Duke University Press.

Alcalde, M. Cristina. 2018. *Peruvian Lives across Borders: Power, Exclusion, and Home*. Urbana: University of Illinois Press.

Allen, Jafari S. 2022. *There's a Disco Ball between Us: A Theory of Black Gay Life*. Durham, NC: Duke University Press.

Almenara, Erika. 2022. *The Language of the In-Between: Travestis, Post-Hegemony, and Writing in Contemporary Chile and Peru*. Pittsburgh: University of Pittsburgh Press.

Altman, Dennis. 1986. *AIDS in the Mind of America: The Social, Political and Psychological Impact of a New Epidemic*. Garden City, NY: Anchor.

Alvarez, Sonia. 2014. "Beyond NGOization? Reflections from Latin America." In *Theorizing NGOs: States, Feminisms, and Neoliberalism*, edited by Victoria Bernal and Inderpal Grewal, 285–300. Durham, NC: Duke University Press.

Amaya, Ana B., Carlos Cáceres, Neil Spicer, and Dina Balabanova. 2014. "After the Global Fund: Who Can Sustain the HIV/AIDS Response in Peru and How?" *Global Public Health* 9, nos. 1–2: 176–97.

Anamaria, Pablo, Alfonso Silva-Santisteban, and María José Bustamante. 2018. *Informe final: Índice de estigma y discriminación hacia las personas con VIH en Perú*. Lima: Consorcio de Organizaciones de Personas con VIH en el Perú.

Anderson, Benedict. 1983. *Imagined Communities: Reflections on the Origin and Spread of Nationalism*. New York: Verso.

Ansell, Aaron. 2018. "Clientelism, Elections, and the Dialectic of Numerical People in Northeast Brazil." *Current Anthropology* 59, suppl. 18: S128–S137.

Anteparra, Hugo. 2019. "Por caso 'Las Gardeñas' citan a la fiscalía a cinco emerretistas." *Diario Voces*, May 30. https://www.diariovoces.com.pe/134142/caso -gardenas-citan-fiscalia-exemerretistas.

Anzaldúa, Gloria. 1987. *Borderlands/La Frontera: The New Mestiza*. San Francisco: Aunt Lute Books.

Auyero, Javier. 2000. *Poor People's Politics: Peronist Survival Networks and the Legacy of Evita*. Durham, NC: Duke University Press.

Babb, Florence. 1989. *Between Field and Cooking Pot*. Austin: University of Texas Press.

Babb, Florence. 2003. "Out in Nicaragua: Local and Transnational Desires after the Revolution." *Cultural Anthropology* 18, no. 3: 304–28.

Bailey, Marlon M., and Darius Bost. 2019. "Guest Editors' Note: The Black AIDS Epidemic." *Souls* 21, nos. 2–3: 97–106.

Baker, Lee D. 1989. *From Savage to Negro: Anthropology and the Construction of Race, 1896–1954*. Berkeley: University of California Press.

Bedoya Forno, Ricardo, Dorothée Delacroix, Valérie Robin Azevedo, and Tania Romero Barrios, eds. 2021. *La violencia que no cesa: Huellas y persistencias del conflicto armado en el Perú contemporáneo*. Lima: Punto Cardinal.

Béjar Rivera, Héctor, and Magno Antenor Álvarez Alderete. 2010. "Las polladas: Una estrategia de sobrevivencia en época de crisis económica y política. Lima, 1980–2003." *Investigaciones Sociales* 14, no. 24: 259–83.

Benton, Adia. 2015. *HIV Exceptionalism: Development through Disease in Sierra Leone*. Minneapolis: University of Minnesota Press.

Benton, Adia, and Thurka Sangaramoorthy. 2021. "Exceptionalism at the End of AIDS." *AMA Journal of Ethics* 23, no. 5: E410–E417.

Benton, Adia, Thurka Sangaramoorthy, and Ippolytos Kalofonos. 2017. "Temporality and Positive Living in the Age of HIV/AIDS." *Current Anthropology* 58, no. 4: 454–76.

Berg, Ulla. 2015. *Mobile Selves: Race, Migration, and Belonging in Peru and the U.S.* New York: New York University Press.

Berkins, Lohana. 2007. *Cumbia, copeteo y lágrimas: Informe nacional sobre la situación de las travestis, transexuales y transgéneros*. Buenos Aires: Ediciones Madres de Plaza de Mayo.

Berkins, Lohana, and Josefina Fernández. 2005. *La gesta del nombre propio: Informe sobre la situación de la comunidad travesti en la Argentina*. Buenos Aires: Ediciones Madres de Plaza de Mayo.

Berlant, Lauren, and Kathleen Stewart. 2019. *The Hundreds*. Durham, NC: Duke University Press.

Biehl, João. 2004. "The Activist State: Global Pharmaceuticals, AIDS, and Citizenship in Brazil." *Social Text* 22, no. 3: 105–32.

Biehl, João. 2007. *Will to Live: AIDS Therapies and the Politics of Survival*. Princeton, NJ: Princeton University Press.

Biehl, João. 2008. "Pharmaceuticalization: AIDS Treatment and Global Health Politics." *Anthropological Quarterly* 80, no. 4: 1083–126.

Biehl, João, Byron Good, and Arthur Kleinman. 2007. "Introduction: Rethinking Subjectivity." In *Subjectivity: Ethnographic Investigations*, edited by João Biehl, Byron Good, and Arthur Kleinman, 1–23. Berkeley: University of California Press.

Biehl, João, and Peter Locke. 2017. "Ethnographic Sensorium." In *Unfinished: The Anthropology of Becoming*, edited by João Biehl and Peter Locke, 1–38. Durham, NC: Duke University Press.

Biehl, João, and Adriana Petryna. 2013. "Critical Global Health." In *When People Come First: Critical Studies in Global Health*, edited by João Biehl and Adriana Petryna, 1–20. Princeton, NJ: Princeton University Press.

Biruk, Crystal. 2018. *Cooking Data: Culture and Politics in an African Research World*. Durham, NC: Duke University Press.

Boellstorff, Tom. 2003. "Dubbing Culture: Indonesian *Gay* and *Lesbi* Subjectivities and Ethnography in an Already Globalized World." *American Ethnologist* 30, no. 2: 225–42.

Boellstorff, Tom. 2005. *The Gay Archipelago: Sexuality and Nation in Indonesia*. Princeton, NJ: Princeton University Press.

Boellstorff, Tom. 2007. "Queer Studies in the House of Anthropology." *Annual Review of Anthropology* 36: 17–35.

Boellstorff, Tom. 2009. "Nuri's Testimony: HIV/AIDS in Indonesia and Bare Knowledge." *American Ethnologist* 36, no. 2: 351–63.

Boellstorff, Tom. 2011. "But Do Not Identify as Gay: A Proleptic Genealogy of the MSM Category." *Cultural Anthropology* 26, no. 2: 287–312.

Boellstorff, Tom, Bonnie Nardi, Celia Pearce, and T. L. Taylor. 2012. *Ethnography and Virtual Worlds: A Handbook of Method*. Princeton, NJ: Princeton University Press.

Boesten, Jelke. 2014. *Sexual Violence during War and Peace: Gender, Power, and Post-Conflict Justice in Peru*. New York: Palgrave Macmillan.

Boesten, Jelke. 2018. *Desigualdades interseccionales: Mujeres y política social en el Perú, 1990–2000*. Lima: Instituto de Estudios Peruanos.

Bor, Jacob, Charlie Fischer, Mirva Modi, Bruce Richman, Cameron Kinker, Rachel King, Sarah K. Calabrese, Idah Mokhele, Tembeka Sineke, Thembelihle Zuma, Sydney Rosen, Till Bärnighausen, Kenneth H. Mayer, and Dorina Onoya. 2021. "Changing Knowledge and Attitudes towards HIV Treatment-as-Prevention and 'Undetectable = Untransmittable': A Systematic Review." *AIDS and Behavior* 25: 4209–24.

Borges Martin da Silva, Mariana. 2022. "Weapons of Clients: Why Do Voters Support Bad Patrons? Ethnographic Evidence from Rural Brazil." *Latin American Politics and Society* 65, no. 1: 22–46. https://doi.org/10.1017/lap.2022.49.

Bórquez, Annick, Juan Vicente Guanira, Paul Revill, Patricia Caballero, Alfonso Silva-Santisteban, Sherrie Kelly, Ximena Salazar, Patricia Bracamonte, Percy Minaya, Timothy B. Hallet, and Carlos F. Cáceres. 2019. "The Impact and Cost-Effectiveness of Combined HIV Prevention Scenarios among Transgender Women Sex-Workers in Lima, Peru: A Mathematical Modelling Study." *Lancet Public Health* 4, no. 3: e127–e136.

Boxwell, D. A. 1992. "'Sis Cat' as Ethnographer: Self-Presentation and Self-Inscription in Zora Neale Hurston's *Mules and Men*." *African American Review* 26, no. 4: 605–17.

Boyce, Paul. 2007. "'Conceiving *Kothis*': Men Who Have Sex with Men in India and the Cultural Subject of HIV Prevention." *Medical Anthropology* 26, no. 2: 175–203.

Bracamonte Allaín, Jorge, and Roland Alvarez Chávez. 2006. *Informe annual 2005: Situación de los derechos humanos de lesbianas, trans, gays y bisexuales en el Perú*. Lima: Movimiento Homosexual de Lima.

Brewer, J. D., M. P. Santos, M. A. Lopez, V. A. Paz-Soldan, and M. P. Chaparro. 2021. "Use of Formal and Informal Food Resources by Food Insecure Families in Lima, Peru: A Mixed-Method Analysis." *Journal of Community Health* 46: 1069–77.

Brier. Jennifer. 2009. *Infectious Ideas: U.S. Political Responses to the AIDS Crisis*. Chapel Hill: University of North Carolina Press.

Briggs, Charles L., and Clara Mantini-Briggs. 2003. *Stories in the Time of Cholera: Racial Profiling during a Medical Nightmare*. Berkeley: University of California Press.

Brown, Wendy. 1995. *States of Injury: Power and Freedom in Late Modernity*. Princeton, NJ: Princeton University Press.

Bueno-Hansen, Pascha. 2015. *Feminist and Human Rights Struggles in Peru: De-colonizing Transitional Justice*. Urbana: University of Illinois Press.

Bueno-Hansen, Pascha. 2018. "The Emerging LGBTI Rights Challenge to Transitional Justice in Latin America." *International Journal of Transitional Justice* 12, no. 1: 126–45.

Burt, Jo-Marie. 2007. *Political Violence and the Authoritarian State in Peru: Silencing Civil Society*. New York: Palgrave Macmillan.

Butler, Judith. 1993. *Bodies That Matter: On the Discursive Limits of "Sex."* London: Routledge.

Cáceres, Carlos F., Peter Aggleton, and Jerome Galea. 2008. "Sexual Diversity, Social Inclusion, and HIV/AIDS." *AIDS* 22: S45–S55.

Cáceres, Carlos F., Ana B. Amaya, Clara Sandoval, and Rocío Valverde. 2013. "A Critical Analysis of Peru's HIV Grant Proposals to the Global Fund." *Global Public Health* 8, no. 10: 1123–37.

Cáceres, C. F., J. Maziel Girón, C. Sandoval, R. López, R. Valverde, J. Pajuelo, P. Vásquez, A. M. Rosasco, A. Chirinos, and A. Silva-Santisteban. 2010. "Implementation Effects of GFATM-Supported HIV/AIDS Projects on the Health Sector, Civil Society, and Affected Communities in Peru, 2004–2007." *Global Public Health* 5, no. 3: 247–65.

Cáceres, Carlos F., and Walter Mendoza. 2009. "The National Response to the HIV/AIDS Epidemic in Peru: Accomplishments and Gaps—A Review." *Journal of Acquired Immune Deficiency Syndrome* 51, suppl. 1: S60–S66.

Cáceres Palacios, Carlos. 1998. *SIDA en el Perú: Imagenes de diversidad—situación y perspectivas de la epidemia en Chiclayo, Cusco e Iquitos*. Lima: Universidad Peruana Cayetano Heredia and REDESS Jóvenes.

Calazans, Gabriela, and Regina Facchini. 2022. "'But the Category of Exposure Also Has to Respect Identity': MSM, Classifications and Disputes in AIDS Policy." *Ciencia y Saúde Colectiva* 27, no. 10: 3913–22.

Campuzano, Giuseppe. 2008. *Museo travesti del Perú*. Lima: IDS.

Canova, Paula. 2020. *Frontier Intimacies: Ayoreo Women and the Sexual Economy of the Paraguayan Chaco*. Austin: University of Texas Press.

Cantú, Lionel. 2011. "Entre Hombres/Between Men: Latino Masculinities and Homosexualities." In *Gay Latino Studies: A Critical Reader*, edited by Michael Hames-Garcia and Ernesto Javier Martinez, 147–67. Durham, NC: Duke University Press.

Carrier, Joseph. 1995. *De los Otros: Intimacy and Homosexuality Among Mexicans*. New York: Columbia University Press.

Carrillo, Héctor. 2002. *The Night Is Young: Sexuality in Mexico in the Time of AIDS*. Chicago: University of Chicago Press.

Carrillo, Héctor. 2017. *Pathways of Desire: The Sexual Migration of Mexican Gay Men*. Chicago: University of Chicago Press.

Carrión, Julio F. 2022. "Takeoff and Turbulence in Modernizing Peru." *Latin American Research Review* 54, no. 2: 499–508.

Carter, Eric D. 2023. *In Pursuit of Health Equity: A History of Latin American Social Medicine*. Chapel Hill: University of North Carolina Press.

Caruth, Cathy, Thomas Keenan, Gregg Bordowitz, Douglas Crimp, and Laura Pinsky. 1991. "'The AIDS Crisis Is Not Over': A Conversation with Gregg Bordowitz, Douglas Crimp, and Laura Pinsky." *American Imago* 48, no. 4: 539–56.

Castro, Arachu, and Paul Farmer. 2005. "Understanding and Addressing AIDS-Related Stigma: From Anthropological Theory to Clinical Practice in Haiti." *American Journal of Public Health* 95, no. 1: 53–59.

Cheng, Jih-Fei, Alexandra Juhasz, and Nishant Shahani, eds. 2020. *AIDS and the Distribution of Crises*. Durham, NC: Duke University Press.

Chow, Jeremy Y., Kelika A. Konda, Annick Borquez, Patricia Caballero, Alfonso Silva-Santisteban, Jeffrey D. Klausner, and Carlos F. Cáceres. 2016. "Peru's HIV Care Continuum among Men Who Have Sex with Men and Transgender Women: Opportunities to Optimize Treatment and Prevention." *International Journal of STD and AIDS* 27, no. 12: 1039–48.

Clark, J. L., A. G. Perez-Brumer, S. L. Reisner, X. Salazar, S. McLean, L. Huerta, A. Silva-Santisteban, K. M. Moriarty, M. J. Mimiaga, J. Sanchez, K. H. Mayer, and J. R. Lama. 2020. "Social Network Organization, Structure, and Patterns of Influence within a Community of Transgender Women in Lima, Peru: Implications for Biomedical HIV Prevention." *AIDS and Behavior* 24: 233–45.

Clark, Jesse, Javier Salvatierra, Eddy Segura, Ximena Salazar, Kelika Konda, Amaya Perez-Brumer, Eric Hall, Jeffrey Klausner, Carlos Cáceres, and Thomas Coates. 2013. "*Moderno* Love: Sexual Role-Based Identities and HIV/STI Prevention among Men Who Have Sex with Men in Lima, Peru." *AIDS and Behavior* 17: 1313–28.

Conaghan, Catherine M. 2005. *Fujimori's Peru: Deception in the Public Sphere*. Pittsburgh: University of Pittsburgh Press.

Cormier McSwiggin, Chelsea. 2017. "Moral Adherence: HIV Treatment, Undetectability, and Stigmatized Viral Loads among Haitians in South Florida." *Medical Anthropology* 36, no. 8: 714–28.

Cornejo, Giancarlo. 2014. "Las Políticas Reparativas del Movimiento LGBT Peruano: Narrativas de Afectos Queer." *Revista Estudos Feministas* 22, no. 1: 257–75.

Cornejo, Giancarlo. 2019. "Travesti Dreams Outside in the Ethnographic Machine." *GLQ: A Journal of Gay and Lesbian Studies* 25, no. 3: 457–82.

Cornejo, Giancarlo. 2021. "Thinking Travesti Tears: Reading *Loxoro*." *Camera Obscura* 36, no. 3: 33–59.

Cornejo, Giancarlo. 2023. "Las *otras memorias* de Gio Infante: Repensar la homotransfobia y la violencia política en el Perú contemporáneo." *Revista de Estudios Sociales* 83, no. 1: 121–37.

Cortázar, Juan Carlos. 2020. *Como si nos tuvieran miedo*. Lima: Estación La Cultura S.A.C.

Cox Hall, Amy, M. Christina Alcalde, and Florence E. Babb. 2022. "Revisiting Race and Ethnicity in Peru: Intersectional and Decolonizing Perspectives." *Journal of Latin American and Caribbean Ethnic Studies* 17, no. 1: 1–11.

Coxshall, Wendy. 2005. "From the Peruvian Reconciliation Commission to Ethnography: Narrative, Relatedness, and Silence." *POLAR: Political and Legal Anthropology Review* 28, no. 2: 203–22.

Crane, Johanna Tayloe. 2013. *Scrambling for Africa: AIDS, Expertise, and the Rise of American Global Health Science.* Ithaca, NY: Cornell University Press.

Cuberos-Gallardo, Francisco J. 2020. "La pollada peruana en Buenos Aires: Migración y comportamiento étnico en un context de conflicto urbano." *Latin American and Caribbean Ethnic Studies* 16, no. 4: 374–91.

Cuenca, Ricardo. 2014. "Historias, trayectorias y contextos: La formación de profesionales indigenas en Bolivia y Perú." In *Etnicidades en construcción: Identidad y acción social en contextos de desigualdad,* edited by Ricardo Cuenca, 167–216. Lima: Instituto de Estudios Peruanos.

Cueto, Marcos. 2001. *Culpa y coraje: Historia de las políticas sobre el VIH/SIDA en el Perú.* Lima: Universidad Peruana Cayetano Heredia.

Cueto, Marcos, and Steven Palmer. 2015. *Medicine and Public Health in Latin America: A History.* Cambridge: Cambridge University Press.

Cutuli, Soledad. 2012. "Resisting, Demanding, Negotiating and Being: The Role of Scandals in the Everyday Lives of Argentinean Travestis." *Jindal Global Law Review* 4, no. 1: 71–88.

CVR (Comisión de la Verdad y Reconciliación). 2003. *Informe final.* Lima: CVR.

Dador, María Jennie, and Marivel Saldaña. 2015. *Informe anual sobre derechos humanos de personas trans, lesbianas, gays y bisexuales en el Perú 2014–15.* Lima: PROMSEX and Red Peruana TLGB.

Davidson, Judith R., and Steve Stein. 1988. "Economic Crisis, Social Polarization, and Community Participation in Health Care." In *Health Care in Peru: Resources and Policy,* edited by Dieter Z. Zschock, 53–77. Boulder, CO: Westview Press.

Dean, Bartholomew. 2023. *The End of the Future: Trauma, Memory, and Reconciliation in Peruvian Amazonia.* Nashville, TN: Vanderbilt University Press.

de Belaunde, Alberto. 2017. *Más allá del arcoiris.* Lima: Editorial Planeta.

Decena, Carlos Ulises. 2011. *Tacit Subjects: Belonging and Same-Sex Desire among Dominican Immigrant Men.* Durham, NC: Duke University Press.

Decoteau, Claire Laurier. 2013. *Ancestors and Antiretrovirals: The Biopolitics of HIV/AIDS in Post-Apartheid South Africa.* Chicago: University of Chicago Press.

Degregori, Carlos Iván. 1990. *El surgimiento de Sendero Luminoso: Ayacucho, 1969–1979.* Lima: Instituto de Estudios Peruanos.

Degregori, Carlos Iván. 2001. *La década de la antipolítica: Auge y huida de Alberto Fujimori y Vlademiro Montesinos.* Lima: Instituto de Estudios Peruanos.

Degregori, Carlos Iván. 2012. *How Difficult It Is to Be God: Shining Path's Politics of War in Peru, 1980–1999,* edited by Steve J. Stern, translated by Nancy Appelbaum. Madison: University of Wisconsin Press.

Degregori, Carlos Iván. 2015. "Sobre la Comisión de la Verdad y Reconciliación en el Perú." In *No hay mañana sin ayer: Batallas por la memoria y consolidación democrática en el Perú*, edited by Carlos Iván Degregori, Tamia Portugal Teillier, Gabriel Salazar Borja, and Renzo Aroni Sulca, 27–70. Lima: Instituto de Estudios Peruanos.

Degregori, Carlos Iván, Tamia Portugal Teillier, Gabriel Salazar Borja, and Renzo Aroni Sulca, eds. 2015. *No hay mañana sin ayer: Batallas por la memoria y consolidación democrática en el Perú*. Lima: Instituto de Estudios Peruanos.

Dehne, Karl L. 2016. "HIV Prevention 2020: A Framework for Delivery and a Call for Action." *Lancet* 3: E323–E332.

de la Barreda Solórzano, Luis. 2023. *El escándalo de la homophobia: Crónica de una repression milenaria*. Mexico City: Trilce Ediciones.

de la Cadena, Marisol. 2000. *Indigenous Mestizos: The Politics of Race and Culture in Cuzco, Peru, 1919–1991*. Durham, NC: Duke University Press.

del Mastro N., Irene. 2022. "Providing Culturally Competent and Universal Health Care in the Peruvian Amazon: The Role of Medical Authority." *Social Science and Medicine* 315: 115556.

del Pino, Ponciano, and Caroline Yezer, eds. 2013. *Las formas del recuerdo: Etnografías de la violencia política en el Perú*. Lima: Instituto de Estudios Peruanos.

Denegri, Francesca, and Alexandra Hibbett, eds. 2016. *Dando cuenta: Estudios sobre el testimonio de la violencia política en el Perú (1980–2000)*. Lima: Fondo Editorial de la Universidad Católica del Perú.

Diamond, Alex. 2021. "Pork Belly Politics: The Moral and Instrumental Reasons Clients Donate to Patrons in a Rural Colombian Mayoral Election." *Qualitative Sociology* 44: 151–73.

Dietrich, Martha-Cecilia. 2019. "Pursuing the Perpetual Conflict: Ethnographic Reflections on the Persistent Role of the 'Terrorist Threat' in Contemporary Peru." *History and Memory* 31, no. 1: 59–86.

Díez, Jordi. 2015. *The Politics of Gay Marriage in Latin America: Argentina, Chile, and Mexico*. Cambridge: Cambridge University Press.

Di Pietro, Pedro José Javier. 2016. "Decolonizing *Travesti* Space in Buenos Aires: Race, Sexuality and Sideways Relationality." *Gender, Place, and Culture* 23, no. 5: 677–93.

Dominguez Ruvalcaba, Héctor. 2016. *Translating the Queer: Body Politics and Transnational Conversations*. London: Zed Books.

Dorr, Kirstie A. 2018. *On Site, in Sound: Performance Geographies in América Latina*. Durham, NC: Duke University Press.

Drinot, Paulo. 2009. "For Whom the Eye Cries: Memory, Monumentality, and the Ontologies of Violence in Peru." *Journal of Latin American Cultural Studies* 18, no. 1: 15–32.

Drinot, Paulo. 2020. *The Sexual Question: A History of Prostitution in Peru, 1850s–1950s*. New York: Cambridge University Press.

Epstein, Steven. 1996. *Impure Science: AIDS, Activism, and the Politics of Knowledge*. Berkeley: University of California Press.

Ewig, Christina. 2010. *Second-Wave Neoliberalism: Gender, Race, and Health Sector Reform in Peru*. University Park: Pennsylvania State University Press.

Falcón, Sylvanna. 2016. *Power Interrupted: Antiracist and Feminist Activism inside the United Nations*. Seattle: University of Washington Press.

Falcón, Sylvanna. 2018. "Intersectionality and the Arts: Counterpublic Memory-Making in Postconflict Peru." *International Journal of Transitional Justice* 12, no. 1: 26–44.

Falconí Trávez, Diego. 2013. "La leyenda negra marica: Una crítica comparatista desde el Sur a la teoría queer hispana." In *Resentir lo queer en América Latina: Diálogos desde/con el Sur*, edited by Diego Falconí Trávez, Santiago Castellanos, and María Amelia Viteri, 81–116. Barcelona: Egales Editorial.

Falconí Trávez, Diego. 2018. "Inflexión marica: Escrituras del descalabro gay en América Latina." In *Inflexión Marica: Escrituras del descalabro gay en América Latin*, edited by Diego Falconí Trávez. Barcelona: Egales Editorial.

Falconí Trávez, Diego, Santiago Castellanos, and María Amelia Viteri, eds. 2013. *Resentir lo queer en América Latina: Diálogos desde/con el Sur*. Barcelona: Egales Editorial.

Fan, Elsa. 2017. "Counting Results: Performance-Based Financing and HIV Testing among MSM in China." *Critical Public Health* 27, no. 2: 217–27.

Farmer, Paul. 1992. *AIDS and Accusation: Haiti and the Geography of Blame*. Berkeley: University of California Press.

Fassin, Didier. 2007. *When Bodies Remember: Experiences and Politics of AIDS in South Africa*. Berkeley: University of California Press.

Fauci, Anthony, and Hilary Marston. 2013. "Achieving an AIDS-Free World: Science and Implementation." *Cell* 155, no. 4: 733–34.

Feldman, Joseph P. 2012. "Exhibiting Conflict: History and Politics at the Museo de la Memoria de ANFASEP in Ayacucho, Peru." *Anthropological Quarterly* 85, no. 2: 487–518.

Feldman, Joseph. 2021. *Memories before the State: Postwar Peru and the Place of Memory, Tolerance, and Social Inclusion*. New Brunswick, NJ: Rutgers University Press.

Fernández-Dávila, Percy, Ximena Salazar, Carlos F. Cáceres, Andre Maiorana, Susan Kegeles, Thomas J. Coates, and Josefa Martinez. 2008. "Compensated Sex and Sexual Risk: Sexual, Social and Economic Interactions between Homosexually- and Heterosexually-Identified Men of Low Income in Two Cities of Peru." *Sexualities* 11, no. 3: 352–74.

Foucault, Michel. 1990 (1976). *The History of Sexuality, Vol. 1: An Introduction*. New York: Vintage Books.

Frasca, Tim. 2005. *AIDS in Latin America*. New York: Palgrave Macmillan.

Friedman, Elisabeth Jay. 2017. *Interpreting the Internet: Feminist and Queer Counterpublics in Latin America*. Oakland: University of California Press.

Gagliolo, Agostina. 2012. "All the Other Stuff: Treatment as Prevention and the Embodiment of Undetectability." *Medical Anthropology* 40, no. 8: 759–71.

Gandolfo, Daniella. 2009. *The City at Its Limits: Taboo, Transgression, and Urban Renewal in Lima.* Chicago: University of Chicago Press.

Garcia, Jonathan, Amaya G. Perez-Brumer, Robinson Cabello, and Jesse L. Clark. 2018. "'And Then Break the Cliché': Understanding and Addressing HIV Vulnerability through Development of an HIV Prevention *Telenovela* with Men Who Have Sex with Men and Transwomen in Lima, Peru." *Archives of Sexual Behavior* 47: 1995–2005.

García, María Elena. 2021. *Gastropolitics and the Specter of Race: Stories of Capital, Culture, and Coloniality in Peru.* Oakland: University of California Press.

Garcia-Fernandez, Lisset, Rommy Novoa, Byelca Huaman, and Carlos Benites. 2018. "Continuo de la atención de personas que viven con VIH y brechas para el logro de las metas 90-90-90 en Perú." *Revista Peruana de Medicina Experimental y Salud Pública* 35, no. 3: 491–96.

Garro, Linda C., and Cheryl Mattingly. 2001. "Narrative as Construct and Construction." In *Narrative and the Cultural Construction of Illness and Healing*, edited by Cheryl Mattingly and Linda C. Garro, 1–49. Berkeley: University of California Press.

Gill, Lyndon K. 2018. *Erotic Islands: Art and Activism in the Queer Caribbean.* Durham, NC: Duke University Press.

Global Fund. 2017. "Peru: Overview." https://www.theglobalfund.org/en/portfolio/country/?k=6a5d3eb0-0d70-4b68-a767-12ce2b302bbd&loc=PER.

Goicochea, Juan Carlos. 2017. "El pecado social: Avance de investigación." YouTube. Posted by Micromuseo Perú, August 6, 2017. https://youtu.be/_ncZSUT11g4.

Goicochea, Pedro, and Orlando Montoya. 2014. "Implementing Biomedical HIV Prevention Advances in Ecuador and Peru." In *Biomedical Advances in HIV Prevention*, edited by L. A. Easton and S. C. Kalichman, 251–66. New York: Springer.

Golash-Boza, Tanya. 2010. "'Had They Been Polite and Civilized, None of This Would Have Happened': Discourses of Race and Racism in Multicultural Peru." *Latin American and Caribbean Ethnic Studies* 5, no. 3: 317–30.

Gomez, Gabriela B., Annick Borquez, Carlos F. Cáceres, Eddy R. Segura, Robert M. Grant, Geoff P. Garnett, and Timothy B. Hallett. 2012. "The Potential Impact of Pre-Exposure Prophylaxis for HIV Prevention among Men Who Have Sex with Men and Transwomen in Lima, Peru: A Mathematical Modelling Study." *PLoS Medicine* 9, no. 10: e1001323.

González, Olga M. 2011. *Unveiling Secrets of War in the Peruvian Andes.* Chicago: University of Chicago Press.

Gorriti, Gustavo. 1999. *The Shining Path: A History of the Millenarian War in Peru*, trans. Robin Kirk. Chapel Hill: University of North Carolina Press.

Gossett, Che, and Eva Hayward. 2020. "Trans in the Time of HIV/AIDS." *TSQ: Transgender Studies Quarterly* 7, no. 4: 527–53.

Graham, Richard. 1990. *Patronage and Politics in Nineteenth-Century Brazil*. Stanford, CA: Stanford University Press.

Greene, Shane. 2016. *Punk and Revolution: 7 More Interpretations of Peruvian Reality*. Durham, NC: Duke University Press.

Groes-Green, Christian. 2013. "'To Put Men in a Bottle': Eroticism, Kinship, Female Power, and Transactional Sex in Maputo, Mozambique." *American Ethnologist* 40, no. 1: 102–17.

Guerra-Reyes, Lucia. 2019. "Numbers That Matter: Right to Health and Peruvian Maternal Strategies." *Medical Anthropology* 38, no. 6: 478–92.

Gutmann, Matthew. 2007. *Fixing Men: Sex, Birth Control, and AIDS in Mexico*. Berkeley: University of California Press.

Halberstam, Jack. 2011. *The Queer Art of Failure*. Durham, NC: Duke University Press.

Halperin, David. 2012. *How to Be Gay*. Cambridge, MA: Harvard University Press.

Hanssmann, Christoph. 2020. "Epidemiological Rage: Population, Biography, and State Responsibility in Trans-Health Activism." *Social Science and Medicine* 247: 112808.

Haraway, Donna J. 2016. *Staying with the Trouble: Making Kin in the Chthulucene*. Durham, NC: Duke University Press.

Hartman, Saidiya. 2008. "Venus in Two Acts." *Small Axe* 12, no. 3: 1–14.

Hartman, Saidiya. 2019. *Wayward Lives, Beautiful Experiments: Intimate Histories of Riotous Black Girls, Troublesome Women, and Queer Radicals*. New York: W. W. Norton.

Haynes, Nell. 2013. "Global Cholas: Reworking Tradition and Modernity in Bolivian Lucha Libre." *Journal of Latin American and Caribbean Anthropology* 18, no. 3: 432–46. https://doi.org/10.1111/jlca.12040.

Heckert, Carina. 2018. *Fault Lines of Care: Gender, HIV, and Global Health in Bolivia*. New Brunswick, NJ: Rutgers University Press.

Heckert, Carina. 2019. "*Travesti* Subjectivity and HIV Care: The Collision of the Global LGBT Rights and Evangelical Ex-Gay Movements in Bolivia." *Journal of Latin American and Caribbean Anthropology* 24, no. 2: 406–23. https://doi.org/10.1111/jlca.12401.

Hernández, Graciela. 1995. "Multiple Subjectivities and Strategic Positionality: Zora Neale Hurston's Experimental Ethnographies." In *Women Writing Culture*, edited by Ruth Behar and Deborah A. Gordon, 148–65. Berkeley: University of California Press.

Hernandez, Jillian. 2020. *Aesthetics of Excess: The Art and Politics of Black and Latina Embodiment*. Durham, NC: Duke University Press.

Hetherington, Kregg. 2020. *The Government of Beans: Regulating Life in the Age of Monocrops*. Durham, NC: Duke University Press.

Hidalgo, Florentina. 2023. "Vulneración del derecho al acceso a los servicios de salud de la comunidad trans." *Revista Científica Ratio Iure* 3, no. 1: e483. https://doi.org/10.51252/rcri.v3i1.483.

Hilgers, Tina, ed. 2012. *Clientelism in Everyday Latin American Politics*. New York: Palgrave Macmillan.

Hirsch, Jennifer S., Holly Wardlow, Daniel Jordan Smith, Harriet M. Phinney, Shanti Parikh, and Constance Nathanson. 2009. *The Secret: Love, Marriage, and HIV*. Nashville, TN: Vanderbilt University Press.

Hobson, Emily K., and Dan Royles. 2021. "Editor's Introduction: The AIDS Crisis Is Not Over." *Radical History Review* 140: 1–8.

Hooker, Evelyn. 1967. "The Homosexual Community." In *Sexual Deviance*, edited by John Gagnon and William Simon, 167–83. New York: Harper and Row.

Howe, Cymene. 2009. "The Legible Lesbian: Crimes of Passion in Nicaragua." *Ethnos* 74: 261–378.

Huayhua, Margarita. 2014. "Racism and Social Interaction in a Southern Peruvian Combi." *Ethnic and Racial Studies* 37, no. 13: 2399–417.

Huerta, Monica. 2021. *Magical Habits*. Durham, NC: Duke University Press.

Hurston, Zora Neale. 2008 (1935). *Mules and Men*. New York: Harper Perennial Modern Classics.

INEI (Instituto Nacional de Estadistica e Informatica). 2017. "Población 2000 a 2015." http://proyectos.inei.gob.pe/web/poblacion/.

Infante, Gio. 2013. "Las Otras Memorias: Persecución, Tortura y Muerte de Homosexuales durante el Conflict Armado Interno." August 28, 2013. https://gioinfante.lamula.pe/2013/08/28/las-otras-memorias/gioinfante/.

Jagose, Annamarie. 2013. *Orgasomology*. Durham, NC: Duke University Press.

Jaime Ballero, Martín. 2009a. *Informe anual sobre derechos humanos de personas trans, lesbianas, gays y bisexuales en el Perú 2009*. Lima: PROMSEX and Red Peruana TLGB.

Jaime Ballero, Martín. 2009b. *Informe anual sobre derechos humanos de personas trans, lesbianas, gays y bisexuales en el Perú 2008*. Lima: PROMSEX and Red Peruana TLGB.

Jaime Ballero, Martín. 2010. *Informe anual sobre derchos humanos de personas trans, lesbianas, gays y bisexuales en el Perú 2010*. Lima: PROMSEX and Red Peruana TLGB.

Jolivette, Andrew J. 2016. *Indian Blood: HIV and Colonial Trauma in San Francisco's Two-Spirit Community*. Seattle: University of Washington Press.

Kalofonos, Ippolytos Andreas. 2014. "'All They Do Is Pray': Community Labour and the Narrowing of Care during Mozambique's HIV Scale-Up." *Global Public Health* 9, nos. 1–2: 7–24.

Kaulard, Anke. 2018. "Sinergias e incrustación del estado en la sociedad: La política económica alternativa del Gobierno Regional de San Martín." *Debates en Sociología* 47: 41–71.

Kenworthy, Nora. 2017. *Mistreated: The Political Consequences of the Fight against AIDS in Lesotho*. Nashville, TN: Vanderbilt University Press.

Kenworthy, Nora J., and Richard Parker. 2014. "HIV Scale-Up and the Politics of Global Health." *Global Public Health* 9, nos. 1–2: 1–6. https://doi.org/10.1080/17441692.2014.880727.

Kenworthy, Nora, Matthew Thomann, and Richard Parker. 2018. "From a Global Crisis to the 'End of AIDS': New Epidemics of Signification." *Global Public Health* 13, no. 8: 960–71. https://doi.org/10.1080/17441692.2017.1365373.

Kernaghan, Richard. 2009. *Coca's Gone: Of Might and Right in the Huallaga Post-Boom*. Stanford, CA: Stanford University Press.

Kernaghan, Richard. 2012. "Furrows and Walls, or the Legal Topography of a Frontier Road in Peru." *Mobilities* 7, no. 4: 501–20.

Kernaghan, Richard. 2022. *Crossing the Current: Aftermaths of War along the Huallaga River*. Stanford, CA: Stanford University Press.

Kippax, Susan. 2012. "Effective HIV Prevention: The Indispensable Role of Social Science." *Journal of the International AIDS Society* 15. http://dx.doi.org/10.7448/IAS.15.2.17357.

Kippax, Susan, and Niamh Stephenson. 2016. *Socializing the Biomedical Turn in HIV Prevention*. London: Anthem Press.

Kogan, Liuba, Ros María Fuchs Ángeles, and Patricia Lay Ferrato. 2013. *No pero sí: Discriminación en empresas de Lima metropolitana*. Lima: Universidad del Pacífico.

Krueger, Evan A., ChingChe J. Chiu, Luis A. Menacho, and Sean D. Young. 2016. "HIV Testing among Social Media–Using Peruvian Men Who Have Sex with Men: Correlates and Social Context." *AIDS Care* 28, no. 10: 1301–5.

Kulick, Don. 1996. "Causing a Commotion: Public Scandal as Resistance among Brazilian Transgendered Prostitutes." *Anthropology Today* 12, no. 6: 3–7.

La Fountain-Stokes, Lawrence. 2008. "Trans/Bolero/Drag/Migration: Music, Cultural Translation, and Diasporic Puerto Rican Theatricalities." *WSQ: Women's Studies Quarterly* 36, nos. 3–4: 190–209.

La Fountain-Stokes, Lawrence. 2014. "Epistemología de la loca: Localizando a la transloca en la transdiáspora." In *Resentir lo queer en América Latina: Diálogos desde/con el Sur*, edited by Diego Falconí Trávez, Santiago Castellanos, and María Amerlia Viteri, 133–45. Barcelona: Egales Editorial.

Lancaster, Roger. 1987. "Subject Honor and Object Shame: The Construction of Male Homosexuality and Stigma in Nicaragua." *Ethnology* 27, no. 2: 111–25.

Landes, Ruth. 1940. "A Cult Matriarchate and Male Homosexuality." *Journal of Abnormal and Social Psychology* 35, no. 3: 386–97.

Larson, Brooke. 2004. *Trials of Nation Making: Liberalism, Race, and Ethnicity in the Andes, 1810–1910*. Cambridge: Cambridge University Press.

La Serna, Miguel. 2020. *With Masses and Arms: Peru's Tupac Amaru Revolutionary Movement*. Chapel Hill: University of North Carolina Press.

Laurens, Vivian, César Abadía-Barrero, and Mario Hernández. 2023. "Latin American Social Medicine in Colombia: Violence, Neoliberalism, and *Buen*

*Vivir."* *Journal of Latin American and Caribbean Anthropology* 28, no. 2: 93–105.

Leclerc-Madlala, Suzanne. 2003. "Transactional Sex and the Pursuit of Modernity." *Social Dynamics* 29, no. 2: 213–33.

Leinius, Johanna. 2022. *The Cosmopolitics of Solidarity: Social Movement Encounters across Difference.* Cham, Switzerland: Springer.

Lemebel, Pedro. 2002. *Tengo miedo torero.* Barcelona: Editorial Seix Barral.

León Almenara, Juan Pablo. 2014. "Tarapoto aún vive intolerancia a 23 años de matanza homofóbica." *El Comercio*, June 28. https://elcomercio.pe/peru/san -martin/tarapoto-vive-intolerancia-25-anos-matanza-homofobica-335106 -noticia/.

Levi, Jacob, Alice Raymond, Anton Pozniak, Pietro Vernazza, Philipp Kohler, and Andrew Hill. 2016. "Can the UNAIDS 90-90-90 Target Be Achieved? A Systematic Analysis of National HIV Treatment Cascades." *BMJ Global Health* 1: e000010.

Levitsky, Steven. 2014. "First Take: Paradoxes of Peruvian Democracy—Political Bust amid Economic Boom?" *ReVista: Harvard Review of Latin America* 14, no. 1: 2–6. https://revista.drclas.harvard.edu/first-take-paradoxes-of-peruvian -democracy-revista/.

Levitt, Peggy, and Sally Merry. 2009. "Vernacularization on the Ground: Local Uses of Global Women's Rights in Peru, China, India and the United States." *Global Networks* 9, no. 4: 441–61. https://doi.org/10.1111/j.1471-0374.2009.00263.x.

Lima, Lázaro. 2011. "Locas al Rescate: The Transnational Hauntings of Queer Cubanidad." *Journal of Transnational American Studies* 3, no. 2: 79–103.

Liu, Albert, David V. Glidden, Peter L. Anderson, K. R. Amico, Vanessa McMahan, Megha Mehrotra, Javier R. Lama, John MacRae, Juan Carlos Hinojosa, Orlando Montoya, Valdilea G. Veloso, Mauro Schechter, Esper G. Kallas, Suwat Chariyalerstak, Linda-Gail Bekker, Kenneth Mayer, Susan Buchbinder, and Robert Grant. 2014. "Patterns and Correlates of PrEP Drug Detection among MSM and Transgender Women in the Global iPrEx Study." *Journal of Acquired Immune Deficiency Syndromes* 67, no. 5: 528–37.

Longino, August, Michalina A. Montano, Hugo Sanchez, Angela Bayer, Jorge Sanchez, Kathy Tossas-Milligan, Ann Duerr, and Yamilé Molina. 2020. "Increasing PrEP Uptake and Adherence among MSM and TW Sex Workers in Lima, Perú: What and Whom Do Different Patients Trust?" *AIDS Care* 32, no. 2: 255–60.

López Díaz, Antonio. 2016. "Los indeseables de Tarapoto." *El País*, April 4. https:// elpais.com/elpais/2016/04/01/planeta_futuro/1459513097_580273.html.

Love, Heather. 2021. *Underdogs: Social Deviance and Queer Theory.* Chicago: University of Chicago Press.

Ludescher, Monika. 2001. "Instituciones y prácticas coloniales en la Amazonía peruana: Pasado y presente." *Indiana* 17–18: 313–59.

Luna, Sarah. 2020. *Love in the Drug War: Selling Sex and Finding Jesus on the Mexico-U.S. Border.* Austin: University of Texas Press.

Machuca, Malú, and Rodolfo Cocchella. 2014. *Estado de violencia: Diagnóstico de la situación de personas lesbianas, gays, bisexuales, transgénero, intersexuales y queer en Lima metropolitana.* Lima: No Tengo Miedo.

Machuca Rose, Malú. 2019. "Giuseppe Campuzano's Afterlife: Toward a Travesti Methodology for Critique, Care, and Radical Resistance." *TSQ: Transgender Studies Quarterly* 6, no. 2: 239–53.

Machuca Rose, Malú, Rodolfo Cocchella Loli, and Adriana Gallegos Dextre. 2016. *Nuestra voz persiste: Diagnóstico de la situación de personas lesbianas, gays, bisexuales, transgénero, intersexuales y queer en el Perú.* Lima: No Tengo Miedo.

Mackenzie, Sonja. 2013. *Structural Intimacies: Sexual Stories in the Black AIDS Epidemic.* New Brunswick, NJ: Rutgers University Press.

Maiorana, Andres, Susan Kegeles, Ximena Salazar, Kelika Konda, Alfonso Silva-Santisteban, and Carlos Cáceres. 2016. "'Proyecto Orgullo,' and HIV Prevention Empowerment and Community Mobilization Intervention for Gay Men and Transgender Women in Callao/Lima, Peru." *Global Public Health* 11, nos. 7–8: 1076–92.

Manalansan, Martin F., IV. 2003. *Global Divas: Filipino Gay Men in the Diaspora.* Durham, NC: Duke University Press.

Manalansan, Martin F., IV. 2014. "The 'Stuff' of Archives: Mess, Migration, and Queer Lives." *Radical History Review*, no. 120: 94–107.

Mangham, Lindsay J., and Kara Hanson. 2010. "Scaling Up in International Health: What Are the Key Issues?" *Health Policy and Planning* 25: 85–96.

Manrique, Nelson. 1995. "Political Violence, Ethnicity and Racism in Peru in Time of War." *Journal of Latin American Cultural Studies* 4, no. 1: 5–18.

Marreros Núñez, Joaquín. 2021. "Los orígenes y los desarrollos del Movimiento Homosexual de Lima en la década de 1980." Thesis for professional license, Pontifical Catholic University of Peru.

Maskovsky, Jeff. 2002. "Do We All 'Reek of Commodity'? Consumption and the Erasure of Poverty in Lesbian and Gay Studies." In *Out in Theory: The Emergence of Lesbian and Gay Anthropology*, edited by Ellen Lewin and William L. Leap, 264–86. Urbana: University of Illinois Press.

Mayer, Enrique. 2009. *Ugly Stories of the Peruvian Agrarian Reform.* Durham, NC: Duke University Press.

Mayer, Kenneth. 2013. "Thinking about an AIDS End Game." *Lancet* 382, no. 9903: 1462–64.

McClintock, Cynthia. 2019. "Peru's Cleavages, Conflict, and Precarious Democracy." In *Oxford Research Encyclopedias, Politics.* Online. https://doi.org/10.1093/acrefore/9780190228637.013.1706.

McCullough, Rachel. 2016. "¿Puede ser travesti el pueblo? Testimonio subalterno y agencia marica en la memoria del conflict armado." In *Dando cuenta: Estudios sobre el testimonio de la violencia política en el Perú (1980–2000)*, edited by Francesca Denegri and Alexandra Hibbett, 121–53. Lima: Fondo Editorial Pontificia Universidad Católica del Perú.

McKay, Ramah. 2018. *Medicine in the Meantime: The Work of Care in Mozambique*. Durham, NC: Duke University Press.

McLean, Sarah, Jerome T. Galea, Holly J. Prudden, Gino Calvo, Hugo Sánchez, and Brandon Brown. 2016. "Association between Sexual Role and HIV Status among Peruvian Men Who Have Sex with Men Seeking an HIV Test: A Cross-Sectional Analysis." *International Journal of STD and AIDS* 27, no. 9: 783–89.

Meinert, Lotte, and Susan Reynolds Whyte. 2014. "Epidemic Projectification: AIDS Responses in Uganda as Event and Process." *Cambridge Journal of Anthropology* 32, no. 1: 77–94.

Meiu, George Paul. 2017. *Ethno-Erotic Economies: Sexuality, Money, and Belonging in Kenya*. Chicago: University of Chicago Press.

Méndez, Cecilia G. 1996. "Incas Sí, Indios No: Notes on Peruvian Creole Nationalism and Its Contemporary Crisis." *Journal of Latin American Studies* 28: 197–225.

Mendoza, Zoila S. 2000. *Shaping Society through Dance: Mestizo Ritual Performance in the Peruvian Andes*. Chicago: University of Chicago Press.

Mentore, Laura. 2017. "The Virtualism of 'Capacity Building' Workshops in Indigenous Amazonia." *HAU: Journal of Ethnographic Theory* 7, no. 2: 279–307.

Merry, Sally Engle. 2008. "Transnational Human Rights and Local Activism: Mapping the Middle." *American Anthropologist* 108, no. 1: 38–51.

Meza, Amanda. 2014. "Testigos del horror: Las víctimas LGBTI del conflicto armado en Perú." http://sinetiquetas.org/2014/11/07/testigos-del-horror-las -victimas-lgbti-del-conflicto-armado-en-peru/.

Meza Caballero, Carla. 2014. *Informe anual sobre derechos humanos de personas trans, lesbianas, gays y bisexuales en el Perú 2013–2014*. Lima: PROMSEX and Red Peruana TLGB.

Mikell, Gwendolyn. 1983. "The Anthropological Imagination of Zora Neale Hurston." *Western Journal of Black Studies* 7, no. 1: 27–35.

Miller, Casey James. 2016. "Dying for Money: The Effects of Global Health Initiatives on NGOs Working with Gay Men and HIV/AIDS in Northwest China." *Medical Anthropology Quarterly* 30, no. 3: 414–30.

Milton, Cynthia. 2014. "Introduction: Art from Peru's Fractured Past." In *Art from a Fractured Past: Memory and Truth-Telling in Post-Shining Path Peru*, edited by Cynthia Milton, 1–34. Durham, NC: Duke University Press.

Miró Quesada, Roberto. 2022. *Lo popular viene del futuro: Escritos escogidos (1981–1990)*. Edited by Mijail Mitrovic. Lima: La Siniestra Ensayos.

Mojola, Sanyu A. 2014. *Love, Money, and HIV: Becoming a Modern Woman in the Age of AIDS*. Oakland: University of California Press.

Montaner, Julio S. G. 2011. "Treatment as Prevention—A Double Hat-Trick." *Lancet* 378, no. 9787: 208–9.

Moodie, Ellen. 2006. "Microbus Crashes and Coca-Cola Cash: The Value of Death in 'Free-Market' El Salvador." *American Ethnologist* 33, no. 1: 63–80.

Moodie, Ellen. 2010. *El Salvador in the Aftermath of Peace: Crime, Uncertainty, and the Transition to Democracy.* Philadelphia: University of Pennsylvania Press.

Motta, Angelica. 1999. "El 'ambiente': Jóvenes homosexuales construyendo identidades en Lima." In *Juventud: Sociedad y cultura*, edited by Aldo Panfichi and Marcel Valcárcel, 429–69. Lima: Red para el desarrollo de las ciencias sociales en el Perú.

Motta, Angelica. 2011. "La 'charapa ardiente' y la hipersexualización de las mujeres amazónicas en el Perú: Perspectivas de las mujeres locales." *Sexualidad, Salud y Sociedad: Revista Latinoamericana* 9: 29–60.

Moyer, Eileen. 2015. "The Anthropology of Life after AIDS: Epistemological Continuities in the Age of Antiretroviral Treatment." *Annual Review of Anthropology* 44: 259–75.

Moyer, Eileen, and Anita Hardon. 2014. "A Disease unlike Any Other? Why HIV Remains Exceptional in the Age of Treatment." *Medical Anthropology* 33, no. 4: 263–69.

Muñoz, José Esteban. 1999. *Disidentifications: Queers of Color and the Performance of Politics.* Minneapolis: University of Minnesota Press.

Muñoz, José Esteban. 2009. *Cruising Utopia: The Then and There of Queer Futurity.* New York: New York University Press.

Muñoz, Paula. 2021. "Latin America Erupts: Peru Goes Populist." *Journal of Democracy* 32, no. 3: 48–62.

Muñoz-Laboy, Miguel. 2004. "'Beyond MSM': Sexual Desire among Bisexually-Active Latino Men in New York City." *Sexualities* 7, no. 1: 55–80.

Muñoz-Laboy, Miguel, Richard Parker, Ashley Perry, and Jonathan Garcia. 2013. "Alternative Frameworks for Examining Latino Male Bisexuality in the Urban Space: A Theoretical Commentary Based on Ethnographic Research in Rio de Janeiro and New York." *Sexualities* 16, nos. 5–6: 501–22.

Murray, David A. B. 2022a. "Anachronic: Viral Socialities and Project Time among HIV Support Groups in Barbados." *Medical Anthropology Quarterly* 36, no. 3: 350–66.

Murray, David A. B. 2022b. "Opting Out: Aging Gays, HIV/AIDS and the Bio-Politics of Queer Viral Time." *Journal of Homosexuality* 69, no. 6: 967–84.

Nading, Alex M. 2014. *Mosquito Trails: Ecology, Health, and the Politics of Entanglement.* Oakland: University of California Press.

Nascimento, Silvana de Souza. 2014. "Variações do feminino: Circuitos do universo trans na Paraíba." *Revista de Antropologia* 57, no. 2: 377–411. https://doi .org/10.11606/2179-0892.ra.2014.89117.

Nesvig, Martin Austin. 2001. "The Complicated Terrain of Latin American Homosexuality." *Hispanic American Historical Review* 81, nos. 3–4: 689–729.

Newton, Esther. 1972. *Mother Camp: Female Impersonators in America*. Chicago: University of Chicago Press.

Nguyen, Vinh-Kim. 2010. *The Republic of Therapy: Triage and Sovereignty in West Africa's Time of AIDS*. Durham, NC: Duke University Press.

Nguyen, Vinh-Kim, Jeffrey O'Malley, and Catherine M. Pirkle. 2011. "Remedicalizing an Epidemic: From HIV Treatment as Prevention to HIV Treatment Is Prevention." *AIDS* 25: 291–93.

Noleto, Rafael da Silva. 2014. "'Brilham estrelas de São João!': Notas sobre os concursos de 'Miss Caipira Gay' e 'Miss Caipira Mix' em Belem (PA)." *Sexualidad, Salud y Sociedad: Revista Latinoamericana* 18: 74–110.

No Tengo Miedo. 2016. *Nuestra voz persiste*. Lima: Tránsito–Vías de Comunicación Escénica.

Nyong'o, Tavia. 2019. *Afro-Fabulations: The Queer Drama of Black Life*. New York: New York University Press.

Ochoa, Marcia. 2008. "Perverse Citizenship: Divas, Marginality, and Participation in 'Loca-lization.'" *WSQ: Women's Studies Quarterly* 36, nos. 3–4: 146–69.

Ochoa, Marcia. 2014. *Queen for a Day: Transformistas, Beauty Queens, and the Performance of Femininity in Venezuela*. Durham, NC: Duke University Press.

Ochs, Elinor, and Lisa Capps. 1996. "Narrating the Self." *Annual Review of Anthropology* 25: 19–43.

Ochs, Elinor, and Lisa Capps. 2001. *Living Narrative: Creating Lives in Everyday Storytelling*. Cambridge, MA: Harvard University Press.

O'Connell, Gráinne. 2020. "Introduction: Framing 'Post-AIDS' and Global Health Discourses in 2015 and Beyond." *Journal of Medical Humanities* 41: 89–94.

O'Daniel, Alyson. 2014. "'They Read [the Truth] in Your Blood': African American Women and Perceptions of HIV Health." *Medical Anthropology* 33, no. 4: 318–34.

Orellana, E. Roberto, Issac E. Alva, Cesar P. Cárcamo, and Patricia J. Garcia. 2013. "Structural Factors That Increase HIV/STI Vulnerability among Indigenous People in the Peruvian Amazon." *Qualitative Health Research* 23, no. 9: 1240–50.

Otsuka, Liurka, Karen Anaya, Alberto Hidalgo, and Manuel Forno. 2016. *Informe anual sobre derechos humanos de personas trans, lesbianas, gays y bisexuales en el Perú 2015–2016*. Lima: PROMSEX and Red Peruana TLGB.

Otsuka Salinas, Liurka, and Soledad Arriagáda Barrera. 2012. *Informe anual sobre derechos humanos de personas trans, lesbianas, gays y bisexuales en el Perú 2011*. Lima: PROMSEX and Red Peruana TLGB.

Padilla, Mark. 2007. *Caribbean Pleasure Industry: Tourism, Sexuality, and AIDS in the Dominican Republic*. Chicago: University of Chicago Press.

Parker, Richard. 1999. *Beneath the Equator: Cultures of Desire, Male Homosexuality, and Emerging Gay Communities in Brazil*. New York: Routledge.

Parker, Richard. 2009. "Civil Society, Political Mobilization, and the Impact of HIV Scale-Up on Health Systems in Brazil." *Journal of Acquired Immune Deficiency Syndromes* 52, suppl. 1: S49–S51.

Parker, Richard. 2019. "Beyond Categorical Imperatives: Making Up MSM in the Global Response to HIV and AIDS." *Medicine Anthropology Theory* 6, no. 4: 265–75.

Parker, Richard. 2020. "AIDS Crisis and Brazil." In *Oxford Research Encyclopedia of Latin American History*, edited by Lauren Derby et al. Online. https://doi .10.1093/acrefore/9780199366439.013.865.

Parker, Richard. 2024. "Epidemics of Signification and Global Health Policy: From the End of AIDS to the End of Scale-Up of the Global AIDS Response." *Global Public Health* 19, no. 1: 2327523. https://doi.org/10.1080/17441692.2024 .2327523.

Parker, Richard, and Peter Aggleton. 2003. "HIV and AIDS-Related Stigma and Discrimination: A Conceptual Framework and Implications for Action." *Social Science and Medicine* 57, no. 1: 13–24.

Parker, Richard, Peter Aggleton, and Amaya G. Perez-Brumer. 2016. "The Trouble with 'Categories': Rethinking Men Who Have Sex with Men, Transgender and Their Equivalents in HIV Prevention and Health Promotion." *Global Public Health* 11, nos. 7–8: 819–23.

Peinado, Jesus, Steven M. Goodreau, Pedro Goicochea, Jorge Vergara, Nora Ojeda, Martin Casapia, Abner Ortiz, Victoria Zamalloa, Rosa Galvan, and Jorge R. Sanchez. 2007. "Role Versatility among Men Who Have Sex with Men in Urban Peru." *Journal of Sex Research* 44, no. 3: 233–39.

Peña, Susana. 2013. *Oye Loca: From the Mariel Boatlift to Gay Cuban Miami*. Minneapolis: University of Minnesota Press.

Pepin, Jacques. 2011. *The Origins of AIDS*. New York: Cambridge University Press.

Perez, Justin. 2011. "Word Play, Ritual Insult, and Volleyball in Peru." *Journal of Homosexuality* 58, nos. 6–7: 834–47.

Perez, Justin. 2017. "Virtual Hagiography and Sexual Rights: The Case of Daniel Zamudio." In *Sexual Diversity and Religious Systems: Transnational Dialogues in the Contemporary World*, edited by Martín Jaime, 249–63. Lima: CMP Flora Tristán, UNMSM.

Perez, Justin. 2020. "Global LGBT Politics at Scale: Memory and Rights in Early Twenty-First Century Peru." In *The Oxford Handbook of Global LGBT and Sexual Diversity Politics*, edited by Michael J. Bosia, Sandra M. McEvoy, and Momin Rahman, 89–102. New York: Oxford University Press.

Perez-Brumer, Amaya G., Sari L. Reisner, Sarah A. McLean, Alfonso Silva-Santisteban, Leyla Huerta, Kenneth H. Mayer, Jorge Sanchez, Jesse L. Clark, Mathew J. Mimiaga, and Javier R. Lama. 2017. "Leveraging Social Capital: Multilevel Stigma, Associated HIV Vulnerabilities, and Social Resilience Strategies among Transgender Women in Lima, Peru." *Journal of the International AIDS Society* 20: 21462.

Petryna, Adriana. 2017. "Horizoning: The Work of Projection in Abrupt Climate Change." In *Unfinished: An Anthropology of Becoming*, edited by João Biehl and Peter Locke, 243–66. Durham, NC: Duke University Press.

Pierce, Joseph M. 2020. "I Monster: Embodying Trans and *Travesti* Resistance in Latin America." *Latin American Research Review* 55, no. 2: 305–21.

Pigg, Stacy Leigh, and Vincanne Adams. 2005. "Introduction: The Moral Object of Sex." In *Sex in Development: Science, Sexuality, and Morality in Global Perspective*, edited by Vincanne Adams and Stacy Leigh Pigg, 1–38. Durham, NC: Duke University Press.

Pinedo, Danny. 2017. "The Making of the Amazonian Subject: State Formation and Indigenous Mobilization in Lowland Peru." *Latin American and Caribbean Ethnic Studies* 12, no. 1: 2–24.

Plemons, Eric. 2017. *The Look of a Woman: Facial Feminization Surgery and the Aims of Trans-Medicine*. Durham, NC: Duke University Press.

Pollock, Lealah, Alfonso Silva-Santisteban, Jae Sevelius, and Ximena Salazar. 2016. "'You Should Build Yourself Up as a Whole Product': Transgender Female Identity in Lima, Peru." *Global Public Health* 11, nos. 7–8: 981–93.

Poole, Deborah. 1997. *Vision, Race, and Modernity: A Visual Economy of the Andean Vision World*. Princeton, NJ: Princeton University Press.

Portocarrero, Gonzalo. 2007a. "Introducción: Hacía una comprensión del racismo en el Perú." In *Racismo y mestizaje y otros ensayos*, 13–26. Lima: Fondo Editorial del Congreso del Perú.

Portocarrero, Gonzalo. 2007b (1990). "El silencio, la queja y la acción." In *Racismo y mestizaje y otros ensayos*, 229–52. Lima: Fondo Editorial del Congreso del Perú.

Portocarrero, Gonzalo. 2007c. *Racismo y mestizaje y otros ensayos*. Lima: Fondo Editorial del Congreso del Perú.

Portocarrero, Gonzalo. 2012. *Profetas del odio: Raíces culturales y líderes de Sendero Luminoso*. Lima: Fondo Editorial de la Pontificia Universidad Católica del Perú.

Poulin, Michelle. 2007. "Sex, Money, and Premarital Partnerships in Southern Malawi." *Social Science and Medicine* 65, no. 11: 2383–93.

Prieur, Annick. 1998. *Mema's House, Mexico City: On Transvestites, Queens, and Machos*. Chicago: University of Chicago Press.

Quijano, Aníbal. 2007. "El 'Movimiento Indígena,' la democracia y los asuntos pendientes en América Latina." In *Colonialidad y crítica en América Latina: Bases para un debate*, edited by Carlos A. Jáuregui and Mabel Moraña, 299–335. Puebla, Mexico: Universidad de las Américas Puebla.

Ravasi, Giovanni, Beatriz Grinsztejn, Ricardo Baruch, Juan Vicente Guanira, Ricardo Luque, Carlos F. Cáceres, and Massimo Ghidinelli. 2016. "Towards a Fair Consideration of PrEP as Part of Combination HIV Prevention in Latin America." *Journal of the International AIDS Society* 19, no. 6: 21113.

Rénique, Gerardo, and Deborah Poole. 1992. *Peru: Time of Fear*. London: Latin America Bureau.

Renkert, Sarah Rachelle. 2022. "False Generosity: A Freirean Reflection on Food Aid in Lima's *Comedores Populares*." *Latin American Perspectives* 50, no. 6: 224–38. https://doi.org/10.1177/0094582X221128792.

Reyes, Carlos Alberto Leal. 2016. "Sobre las dimensiones del pensamiento queer en Latinoamérica: Teoría y política."*Aposta. Revista de Ciencias Sociales* 70: 170–86.

Rizki, Cole. 2019. "Latin/x American Trans Studies: Toward a *Travesti*-Trans Analytic." *TSQ: Transgender Studies Quarterly* 6, no. 2: 145–55.

Rofel, Lisa. 2007. *Desiring China: Experiments in Neoliberalism, Sexuality, and Public Culture*. Durham, NC: Duke University Press.

Rojas-Berscia, Luis Miguel. 2016. "Lóxoro, Traces of a Contemporary Peruvian Genderlect." *Borealis—An International Journal of Hispanic Linguistics* 5, no. 1: 157–70.

Rosaldo, Renato. 1989. *Culture and Truth: The Remaking of Social Analysis*. Boston: Beacon Press.

Rose, Nikolas. 2007. "Beyond Medicalisation." *Lancet* 369, no. 9562: 700–702.

Rubin, Gayle. 1993 (1984). "Thinking Sex: Notes for a Radical Theory of the Politics of Sexuality." In *The Lesbian and Gay Studies Reader*, edited by Henry Abelove, Michele Aina Barale, and David Halperin, 3–44. New York: Routledge.

Rubin, Gayle. 2002. "Studying Sexual Subcultures: Excavating the Ethnography of Gay Communities in Urban North America." In *Out in Theory: The Emergence of Lesbian and Gay Anthropology*, edited by Ellen Lewin and William L. Leap, 17–68. Urbana: University of Illinois Press.

Russo Garrido, Anahi. 2020. *Tortilleras Negotiating Intimacy: Love, Friendship, and Sex in Queer Mexico City*. New Brunswick, NJ: Rutgers University Press.

Salazar, Elizabeth, and Marco Garro. 2023. "Los crímenes silenciados: Discursos y delitos de odio contra personas LGBTI en la Amazonía peruana." https://crimenes-silenciados.com.

Salazar, Ximena, Arón Núñez-Curto, Jana Villayzán, Regina Castillo, Carlos Benites, Patricia Caballero, and Carlos F. Cáceres. 2016. "How Peru Introduced a Plan for Comprehensive HIV Prevention and Care for Transwomen." *Journal of the International AIDS Society* 19, suppl. 32: 20790.

Salazar Borja, Gabriel. 2015. "Sin debate no hay campo de estudios sobre memoria y violencia política en el Perú." In *No hay mañana sin ayer: Batallas por la memoria y consolidación democrática en el Perú*, edited by Ponciano del Pino, 239–79. Lima: Instituto de Estudios Peruanos.

Sanborn, Cynthia A. 2012. "La discriminación en el Perú: Introducción." In *La discriminación en el Perú: Balance y desafíos*, edited by Cynthia A. Sanborn, 11–25. Lima: Universidad del Pacífico.

Sanchez, Jorge, Javier Lama, Lourdes Kusunoki, Hugo Manrique, Pedro Goicochea, Aldo Lucchetti, Manuel Rouillon, Monica Pun, Luis Suarez, Silvia Montano, Jose L. Sanchez, Stephen Tabet, James P. Hughes, and Connie Celum. 2007. "HIV-1 Sexually Transmitted Infections, and Sexual Behavior Trends among Men Who Have Sex with Men in Lima, Peru." *JAIDS: Journal of Acquired Immune Deficiency Syndromes* 44, no. 5: 578–85.

Sancho Ordóñez, Fernando. 2011. "Locas y fuertes: Cuerpos precarios en el Guayaquil del siglo XXI." *Íconos: Revista de Ciencias Sociales* 39: 97–110.

Sandset, Tony. 2021. *"Ending AIDS" in the Age of Biopharmaceuticals: The Individual, the State, and the Politics of Prevention.* London: Routledge.

Sangaramoorthy, Thurka. 2012. "Treating the Numbers: HIV/AIDS Surveillance Subjectivity and Risk." *Medical Anthropology* 31, no. 4: 292–309.

Sangaramoorthy, Thurka. 2014. *Treating AIDS: Politics of Difference, Paradox of Prevention.* New Brunswick, NJ: Rutgers University Press.

Sangaramoorthy, Thurka. 2018. "Chronicity, Crisis, and the 'End of AIDS.'" *Global Public Health* 13, no. 8: 982–96.

Sangaramoorthy, Thurka, and Adia Benton. 2012. "Introduction: Enumeration, Identity, and Health." *Medical Anthropology* 31, no. 4: 287–91.

Sant'Ana, Guilherme. 2022. "Corpos dissonantes: O ingress da atleta transexual Tiffany na Superliga feminine de vôlei e a desestabilização da unidade corporal." *Cadernos Pagu* 64: 2226422.

Santana, M. Myrta Leslie. 2022. *"Transformista, Travesti, Transgénero*: Performing Sexual Subjectivity in Cuba." *Small Axe* 26, no. 2: 46–59.

Scheper-Hughes, Nancy. 1993. *Death without Weeping: The Violence of Everyday Life in Brazil.* Berkeley: University of California Press.

Seligman, Linda. 1989. "To Be in Between: The *Cholas* as Market Women." *Comparative Study of Society and History* 31, no. 4: 694–721.

Serrano-Amaya, José Fernando. 2018. *Homophobic Violence in Armed Conflict and Political Transition.* Cham, Switzerland: Palgrave Macmillan.

Shannon, Geordan D., Angelica Motta, Carlos F. Cáceres, Jolene Skordis-Worrall, Diana Bowie, and Audrey Prost. 2017. "¿Somos Iguales? Using a Structural Violence Framework to Understand Gender and Health Inequities from an Intersectional Perspective in the Peruvian Amazon." *Global Health Action* 10, suppl. 2: 1330458.

Silva, Joseli Maria, and Marcio Jose Ornat. 2015. "Intersectionality and Transnational Mobility between Brazil and Spain in *Travesti* Prostitution Networks." *Gender, Place, and Culture* 22, no. 8: 1073–88.

Silva Santana, Dora. 2019. *"Mais Viva!* Reassembling Transness, Blackness, and Feminism." *TSQ: Transgender Studies Quarterly* 6, no. 2: 210–22.

Silva-Santisteban, Alfonso, H. Fisher Raymond, Ximena Salazar, Jana Villayzan, Segundo Leon, Willi McFarland, and Carlos F. Cáceres. 2012. "Understanding the HIV/AIDS Epidemic in Transgender Women of Lima, Peru: Results from a Sero-Epidemiological Study Using Respondent Driven Sampling." *AIDS and Behavior* 16: 872–81.

Silva Ticllacuri, Cynthia. 2013. *Informe anual sobre derechos humanos de personas trans, lesbianas, gays y bisexuales en el Perú 2012.* Lima: PROMSEX and Red Peruana TLGB.

Silva Torres, Thiago, Kelika A. Konda, E. Hamid Vega-Ramirez, Oliver A. Elorreaga, Dulce Diaz-Sosa, Brenda Hoagland, Steven Diaz, Cristina Pimenta, Marcos

Benedetti, Hugo Lopez-Gatell, Rebeca Robles-Garcia, Beatriz Grinsztejn, Carlos Cáceres, and Valdilea G. Veloso. 2019. "Factors Associated with Willingness to Use Pre-Exposure Prophylaxis in Brazil, Mexico, and Peru: Web-Based Survey among Men Who Have Sex with Men." *JMIR Public Health and Surveillance* 5, no. 2: e13771.

Silverstein, Sydney M. 2017. "Inside a Uniform Imaginary: Gender, Politics, and Aesthetics in Peruvian Technical Education." *Journal of Latin American and Caribbean Anthropology* 22, no. 3: 578–97.

Sívori, Horacio Federico. 2004. *Locas, chongos y gays: Sociabilidad homosexual masculina durante la década de 1990*. Buenos Aires: Antropofagia.

Smallman, Shawn. 2007. *The AIDS Pandemic in Latin America*. Chapel Hill: University of North Carolina Press.

Smith, Daniel Jordan. 2017. *To Be a Man Is Not a One-Day Job: Masculinity, Money, and Intimacy in Nigeria*. Chicago: University of Chicago Press.

Smith-Oka, Vania. 2021. *Becoming Gods: Medical Training in Mexican Hospitals*. New Brunswick, NJ: Rutgers University Press.

Sontag, Susan. 1990. *Illness as Metaphor* and *AIDS and Its Metaphors*. New York: Picador.

Sosa, Joseph Jay. 2014. "'Marijuana Is a Crime, but Homophobia Is Just Fine': The Scandalous Logics of Queer Solidarity." In *Queering Paradigms IV: South-North Dialogues on Queer Epistemologies, Embodiments and Activisms*, edited by Elizabeth Sara Lewis, Rodrigo Borba, Branca Falabella Fabrício, and Diana de Souza Pinto, 215–36. London: Peter Lang.

Sosa, Joseph Jay. 2023. "Epistemic Doubt and Affective Uncertainty: Counting Homotransphobia in Brazil." *Theory and Society* 52: 95–117.

Sprungli, Marie Francoise. 2007. "Trust: The Key to Democratic Participation in a Multisectorial Experience (The Case of CONAMUSA)." CEP Alforja. http://www.cepalforja.org/sistem/documentos/cuso/pdf/cuso152-165.pdf.

Starn, Orin. 1991. "Missing the Revolution: Anthropologists and the War in Peru." *Cultural Anthropology* 6, no. 1: 63–91.

Starn, Orin, and Miguel La Serna. 2019. *The Shining Path: Love, Madness, and Revolution in the Andes*. New York: W. W. Norton.

Stern, Steve J., ed. 1998. *Shining and Other Paths: War and Society in Peru, 1980–1995*. Durham, NC: Duke University Press.

Stewart, Kathleen. 2007. *Ordinary Affects*. Durham, NC: Duke University Press.

Storeng, Katerini, and Dominique P. Béhague. 2014. "'Playing the Numbers Game': Evidence-Based Advocacy and the Technocratic Narrowing of the Safe Motherhood Initiative." *Medical Anthropology Quarterly* 28, no. 2: 260–79.

Stout, Noelle M. 2014. *After Love: Queer Intimacy and Erotic Economies in Post-Soviet Cuba*. Durham, NC: Duke University Press.

Strickon, Arnold, and Sidney M. Greenfield, eds. 1972. *Structure and Process in Latin America: Patronage, Clientage, and Power Systems*. Albuquerque: University of New Mexico Press.

Tabet, Stephen, Jorge Sanchez, Javier Lama, Pedro Goicochea, Pablo Campos, Manuel Rouillon, Jose Luis Cairo, Lucia Ueda, Douglas Watts, Connie Celum, and King K. Holmes. 2002. "HIV, Syphilis and Heterosexual Bridging among Peruvian Men Who Have Sex with Men." *AIDS* 16, no. 9: 1271–77.

Tang, Eric C., Magdalena E. Sobieszczyk, Eileen Shu, Pedro Gonzales, Jorge Sanchez, and Javier R. Lama. 2014. "Provider Attitudes toward Oral Preexposure Prophylaxis for HIV Prevention among High-Risk Men Who Have Sex with Men in Lima, Peru." *AIDS Research and Human Retroviruses* 30, no. 5: 416–24.

Theidon, Kimberly. 2013. *Intimate Enemies: Violence and Reconciliation in Peru*. Philadelphia: University of Pennsylvania Press.

Thomann, Matthew. 2018. "'On December 1, 2015, Sex Changes. Forever': Pre-Exposure Prophylaxis and the Pharmaceuticalisation of the Neoliberal Sexual Subject." *Global Public Health* 13, no. 8: 997–1006.

Thomas, Rebekah, Frank Pega, Rajat Khosla, Annette Verster, Tommy Haba, and Lale Say. 2017. "Ensuring an Inclusive Global Health Agenda for Transgender People." *Bulletin of the World Health Organization* 95, no. 2: 154–56.

Thurner, Mark. 1995. "'Republicanos' and 'La Comunidad de Peruanos': Unimagined Political Communities in Postcolonial Andean Peru." *Journal of Latin American Studies* 27, no. 2: 191–318.

Treichler, Paula. 1999. *How to Have Theory in an Epidemic: Cultural Chronicles of AIDS*. Durham, NC: Duke University Press.

Ugarteche, Oscar. 1997. *India bonita (o del amor y otras artes): Ensayos de cultura gay en el Perú*. Lima: Movimiento Homosexual de Lima.

Valdez, Natali. 2022. *Weighing the Future: Race, Science, and Pregnancy Trials in the Postgenomic Era*. Oakland: University of California Press.

Valentine, David. 2003. "'The Calculus of Pain': Violence, Anthropological Ethics, and the Category Transgender." *Ethnos* 68: 27–48.

Valentine, David. 2007. *Imagining Transgender: An Ethnography of a Category*. Durham, NC: Duke University Press.

Valenzuela, Carla, Cesar Ugarte-Gil, Jorge Paz, Juan Echevarria, Eduardo Gotuzzo, Sten H. Vermund, and Aaron M. Kipp. 2015. "HIV Stigma as a Barrier to Retention in HIV at a General Hospital in Lima, Peru: A Case-Control Study." *AIDS and Behavior* 19, no. 2: 235–45.

Vargas, Deborah. 2014. "Ruminations on Lo Sucio as a Latino Queer Analytic." *American Quarterly* 66, no. 3: 715–26.

Vartabedian, Julieta. 2018. *Brazilian Travesti Migrations: Gender, Sexualities and Embodiment Experiences*. Cham, Switzerland: Palgrave Macmillan.

Vasquez, Emily E., Amaya Perez-Brumer, and Richard Parker, eds. 2020. *Social Inequities and Contemporary Struggles for Collective Health in Latin America*. New York: Routledge.

Vasquez del Aguila, Ernesto. 2012. "God Forgives the Sin but Not the Scandal: Coming Out in a Transnational Context—Between Sexual Freedom and Cultural Isolation." *Sexualities* 15, no. 2: 207–24.

Verheijen, Janneke. 2011. "Complexities of the 'Transactional Sex' Model: Non-Providing Men, Self-Providing Women, and HIV Risk in Rural Malawi." *Annals of Anthropological Practice* 35, no. 1: 116–31.

Vernooij, Eva. 2022. "HIV Support Groups and the Chronicities of Everyday Life in eSwatini." *Medical Anthropology* 41, no. 3: 287–301.

Vich, Victor. 2015. *Poéticas del duelo: Ensayos sobre arte, memoria y violencia política en el Perú.* Lima: Instituto de Estudios Peruanos.

Vidal-Ortiz, Salvador. 2011. "'Maricón,' 'Pájaro,' and 'Loca': Cuban and Puerto Rican Linguistic Practices, and Sexual Minority Participation, in U.S. Santería." *Journal of Homosexuality* 58, nos. 6–7: 901–18.

Vidal-Ortiz, Salvador, Carlos Decena, Héctor Carrillo, and Tomás Almaguer. 2010. "Revisiting *Activos* and *Pasivos*: Toward New Cartographies of Latino/Latin American Male Same-Sex Desire." In *Latina/o Sexualities: Probing Powers, Passions, Practices, and Policies,* edited by Marysol Asencio, 253–73. New Brunswick, NJ: Rutgers University Press.

Viteri, María-Amelia. 2014. *Desbordes: Translating Racial, Ethnic, Sexual, and Gender Identities across the Americas.* Albany: State University of New York Press.

Viteri, María Amelia, José Fernando Serrano, and Salvador Vidal-Ortiz. 2011. "¿Cómo se piensa lo queer?" *Íconos: Revista de Ciencias Sociales* 39: 47–60.

Waitzkin, Howard, Alina Pérez, and Matthew Anderson. 2021. *Social Medicine and the Coming Transformation.* New York: Routledge.

Walker, Charles. 1987. "El uso oficial de la selva en el Perú republicano." *Revista Amazonía Peruana* 8, no. 14: 61–89.

Walker, Liz. 2020. "Problematising the Discourse of 'Post-AIDS.'" *Journal of Medical Humanities* 45: 95–105.

Wall, Cheryl A. 1989. "*Mules and Men* and Women: Zora Neale Hurton's Strategies of Narrations and Visions of Female Empowerment." *Black American Literature Forum* 23, no. 4: 661–80.

Wardlow, Holly. 2006. *Wayward Women: Sexuality and Agency in a New Guinea Society.* Berkeley: University of California Press.

Wardlow, Holly. 2020. *Fencing in AIDS: Gender, Vulnerability, and Care in Papua New Guinea.* Oakland: University of California Press.

Wayar, Marlene. 2018. *Travesti: Una teoría lo suficientemente buena.* Buenos Aires: Editorial Muchas Nueces.

Weismantel, Mary. 2001. *Cholas and Pishtacos: Stories of Race and Sex in the Andes.* Chicago: University of Chicago Press.

Wentzell, Emily. 2014. "'I Help Her, She Helps Me': Mexican Men Performing Masculinity through Transactional Sex." *Sexualities* 17, no. 7: 856–71.

Weston, Kath. 1993. "Lesbian/Gay Studies in the House of Anthropology." *Annual Review of Anthropology* 22: 339–67.

Willis, Daniel. 2020. "Scratched from Memory: The 1987 Prison Massacres and the Limits of Acceptable Memory Discourse in Post-Conflict Peru." *Journal of Latin American Cultural Studies* 29, no. 2: 231–50.

Wilson, Ara. 2004. *The Intimate Economies of Bangkok: Tomboys, Tycoons, and Avon Ladies in the Global City.* Berkeley: University of California Press.

Wolfgang, Simone, and Denise Portinari. 2019. "The PrEP Recommendation: The Inscribed Disease in a Healthy Body." *Social Medicine* 12, no. 3: 272–79.

World Health Organization. 2004. *An Approach to Rapid Scale-Up: Using HIV/ AIDS Treatment and Care as an Example.* Geneva: WHO. https://www.who.int /3by5/publications/documents/scaleup/en/.

Wright, Timothy. 2000. "Gay Organizations, NGOs, and the Globalization of Sexual Identity: The Case of Bolivia." *Journal of Latin American Anthropology* 5, no. 2: 89–111.

Wyrod, Robert. 2016. *AIDS and Masculinity in the African City: Privilege, Inequality, and Modern Manhood.* Oakland: University of California Press.

Yates-Doerr, Emily. 2020. "Reworking the Social Determinants of Health: Responding to Material-Semiotic Indeterminacy in Public Health Interventions." *Medical Anthropology Quarterly* 34, no. 3: 378–97.

Yezer, Caroline. 2008. "Who Wants to Know? Rumors, Suspicions, and Opposition to Truth-Telling in Ayacucho." *Latin American and Caribbean Ethnic Studies* 3, no. 3: 271–89. https://doi.org/10.1080/17442220802462386.

Young, Rebecca M., and Ilan H. Meyer. 2005. "The Trouble with 'MSM' and 'WSW': Erasure of the Sexual-Minority Person in Public Health Discourse." *American Journal of Public Health* 95, no. 7: 1144–49.

Young, Sean D., William G. Cumberland, Roch Nianogo, Luis A. Menacho, Jerome T. Galea, and Thomas Coates. 2015. "The HOPE Social Media Intervention for Global HIV Prevention in Peru: A Cluster Randomised Controlled Trial." *Lancet HIV* 2, no. 1: e27–e32.

Zavala, Virginia, and Roberto Zariquiey. 2009. "'I Segregate You Because Your Lack of Education Offends Me': An Approach to Racist Discourse in Contemporary Peru." In *Racism and Discourse in Latin America*, edited by Teun A. Van Dijk, 259–90. Lanham, MD: Lexington Books.

Zavaleta, Carol, Connie Fernández, Kelika Konda, Yadira Valderrama, Sten H. Vermund, and Eduardo Gotuzzo. 2007. "Short Report: High Prevalence of HIV and Syphilis in a Remote Native Community of the Peruvian Amazon." *American Journal of Tropical Medicine and Hygiene* 76, no. 4: 703–5.

# INDEX

*Italic text identifies figures*

Abreu, Tiffany, 79, 200n19
*la acogida* (warmth/welcoming), 70
*activo/pasivo framework*, 57–58,
    194nn28–29
Adams, Vincanne, 35, 39, 146, 148,
    209nn1–2
*adinerado* (wealth), 30
Aggleton, Peter, 31, 199n18, 200n1, 201n5
Ahmed, Sarah, 34, 92, 204n20
AHOMA (Homosexual Association of
    Mariscal Cáceres), 120–21
AIDS. *See* HIV/AIDS
Alcalde, M. Cristina, 181n10, 201n4,
    203n11
Allen, Jafari S., 183n14
Almenara, Erika, 42, 190n11
Alvarez Chávez, Roland, 148
Las Amazonas (community-based
    organization): antidiscrimination
    efforts, 96, 105–6; collecting cases
    with, 157–60; culture of denounce-
    ment at, 114–16; office, 134; System
    of Community Protection and, 94,
    126; Tenth Round funding and, 26,

136–37; violence toward transgender
    women and, 125
*el ambiente* (queer space, term for),
    206n25
La Anaconda (disco), 2–5, 86, 105, 110,
    112–13, 114, 179n1
Anderson: author and, 124, 135, 154–55;
    Axel and, 155–56; discrimination
    cases (collection of), 125–26, 154–60,
    165, 167; Global Fund and, 124,
    133–40, 153–54; life, 137–38, 153,
    206n1, 209n5, 212n2; pseudonym,
    213n2; public health work, 92, 96–97,
    167–68, 169, 208n13, 211n18
Anderson, Benedict, 12
Angel, 154
Annabella, 156–57, 160
antidiscrimination efforts, 32, 89–90, 115,
    117, 137, 151, 202n10, 202nn10–11
antiretroviral therapy (ART): equitable
    distribution of, 19; ethnography on,
    25, 184n18; global investment in,
    6, 18, 55; goals for providing, 21;
    highly active antiretroviral therapy

antiretroviral therapy (continued)
(HAART), 19; introduction of, 18;
90-90-90 targets and, 145; Peruvian
state and, 171; scaling up, 19–20; universal access, 20
Anzaldúa, Gloria, 184n14
Argentina, 147
Arturo, 129, 132, 134, 138, 141, 151–53, 169
authorship, communal, 16
Auyero, Javier, 194n2
Axel: Anderson and, 155–56; author and,
29, 51–52, 154, 155, 158–60, 165–66;
capacity-building workshops and,
154–55; on scandal, 81; stories told
by, 52–53

beauty contests: overview, 28, 171, 196n7;
collaborative redistribution and,
119–20, 129, 130; Miss Gay, 138; Miss
Gay Carnival, 69; Miss Gay San Juan,
74, 75, 76, 197n11; Olaf and, 131;
organizers, 74; recruitment and, 75;
scandalousness and, 71
Benton, Adia, 24, 25, 148, 186n29
Berg, Ulla, 100–101
Berkins, Lohana, 147
Berlant, Lauren, 184n14
bicycles, 37, 48
Biehl, João: on the activist state, 185n19;
on anthropology of becoming, 11,
208n13; on the invisible epidemic,
211n17; on subjectification, 10
biomedical interventions, 175
Boellstorff, Tom: on the category MSM, 9,
58, 199n18; on enumeration, 39; on
intersubjectivity and ethnography,
188n35; on subject positions, 11–12,
188n35
Bolivia, 203nn13–14
Bor, Jacob, 185n22
Bracamonte Allaín, Jorge, 148
Brazil, 147–48, 156, 185n19
Brenda, 43, 189n2, 198n14
Briggs, Charles L., 168–69
Buenos Aires, 69, 181n11

Cáceres Palacios, Carlos F., 146, 184n17,
189nn2–3, 193n22, 200n1

Callao (Peru), 28, 161, 166, 211nn12–13
Cantú, Lionel, 194n28
capacity-building workshops: armed conflict and, 48; author's involvement as
participant, 28; Axel and, 154–55;
importance of, 142, 171; Norma and,
115, 120; photographs of, 10, 107;
recruitment, 120; storytelling in,
101; System of Community Protection and, 129, 154–55; transgender
women's exclusion from, 115
Capps, Lisa, 17, 181n9
Carlos, 52–53
carnet (identification card), 162–63,
163
Carrillo, Héctor, 194n29
Castro, Arachu, 201n5
catharsis from storytelling, 147
causa (appetizer), 161, 166
CEDISA (Center for Amazonian Development): archives, 125, 128; office, 154,
174; Tenth Round and, 122, 124, 133,
136, 138, 173
Centro de Promoción y Defensa de los
Derechos Sexuales y Reproductivos
(PROMSEX), 50, 149–50, 152, 168,
209n3
la chacra (small farm), 73
la chanfainita (potato and cow stew),
161
charapa, use of term, 14, 98
Chiclayo (Peru), 28, 129
cholera, 19, 168–69
cholo/a, 98, 203n13
Claudia, 80, 81, 198n14
clientelism, 33, 65, 73, 133, 194n2. See also
patronage
cocaine trade, 40
la colaboración (collaboration, concept
of), 65, 69, 70, 71, 129, 195n2; community through, 87–88; as distinct
from clientelism, 33, 73, 172, 197n9;
ethos of, 119, 139–40, 143, 144, 147,
169–70; fragmentation and, 129–33,
143–44; as idealized social order,
15–16, 65; sponsorship as multiplying,
71–73
communal authorship, 16

community: defining, 66; "imagined" national community (Anderson), 12; social relations in, 66, 69–71, 73, 84–87; through collaboration, 87–88

community-based organizations (CBOS): formation of, 17; Global Fund and, 123, 129, 131, 133; interventions for HIV/AIDS and, 23; other references to, 125, 131; support of, 21; workshops, 105–6. *See also* Las Amazonas (community-based organization); DISAM (Diversidad San Martinense)

complaint. *See also* denouncements

complaint books, 3–4, 5, 103

CONAMUSA, 20, 122, 123, 131, 137

conversion, as concept, 35

*la convocatoria* (convocation), 70, 71, 73, 87, 130, 142

Cornejo, Giancarlo, 184n14, 188n1

COVID-19 pandemic, 141, 177

Crane, Johanna Tayloe, 186n25

cross-dressers, as research term, 186n28

Cueto, Marcos, 18, 20, 184n17, 201n6, 202n7

*cuir* theory, 9

culture (as concept): difference and, 97, 98, 203n12; ethno-racial hierarchies and, 91

culture of denouncement. *See* denouncement, culture of

*cumbia* music, 77

curfews, 43, 44

Cutuli, Soledad, 181n11

data: deprivation, 35, 146, 148, 151–53, 169–70, 209n1; discrimination and, 147–50; ethnography and, 31; gaps in, 35; hegemony and, 148; inconsistencies in, 146, 167–68, 169

Dean, Bartholomew, 41, 190n8

Decena, Carlos Ulises, 181n10

Defensoría del Pueblo, 105–6, *107*, 108, 125

Degregori, Carlos Iván, 50

de la Cadena, Marisol, 12, 97

denouncements: culture of, 90–91, 95, 96–97, 98–99, 114–16, 118, 128, 135, 156, 158, 159; emblematic, 99–101; emblematic vs. scandalous, 34, 91, 117; for gay men vs. transgender women, 114; of nightclubs, 100; scandalous, 101–5; storytelling and, 108, 109. *See also* complaint

*Diario Hoy* (periodical), 120, 121

difference: ethnic and racial, 97–98, 117; gender and, 114; hierarchies of, 12, 97; intersectionality and, 7, 92; reproduction of, 117, 203n12

DISAM (Diversidad San Martinense, community-based organization), 93, 105–6, 114, 134, 136, 137, 153, 158, 167, 173, 202n8, 210n7

discos. *See* nightlife

discretion: code words for, 51–52; Martín's story of, 112–14; as moral obligation, 47–50

discrimination: cases (specific), 154–59; data and, 147–50; as determinant, 90; emblematic cases, 124–25, 203n14; funding and, 155–56; grievances system, 90; individualized, 107; mitigation of, 89; narrativizing, 158–59, 165; nightlife and, 2–3, 91–92, 112–13; quantification of, 151–52, 166, 167, 169, 170; racial discrimination, 204n16; scandal as, 105–9; in schools, 121; stories about, 112; in Tarapoto (specific cases), 153–57; against transgender women, 101–2. *See also* grievance filings

drag performances, 111

drug trade, 40, 126

Eduardo, 48–50, 193n20

effeminate mannerisms, 29

egalitarian perspectives on sex, 58, 59

emblematic denouncements: overview, 34, 99–101, 105–9; cases, 42, 92, 95, 104, 124, 128, 129, 136, 190n13; consequences of, 203n14, 204n16; culture of denouncement and, 118; project specialists and, 143; vs. scandalous denouncements, 34, 91–92, 117

"End of AIDS" (as notion): as concept, 169, 187n32; exceptionalism and, 24; Global Fund and, 121–22, 143; lived experience of, 25–26, 34, 172, 183n13; as moral imaginary, 35, 39, 56–57, 59–61; 90-90-90 targets, 34–35, 145–46, 175, 208nn15–16; PrEP and, 177; scandalous storytelling and, 17; setbacks to, 144, 173; sexual subjectification and, 7; social transformation and, 7; targets, 21–22, 34–35, 145; transactional sex and, 38–39; as unfinished project, 140–41; vulnerable populations and, 61

enumeration, 11–12

Epstein, Steven, 167

*el escándalo* (scandalous episode), 14–15, 71; with author, 29, 161; at La Anaconda, 1–5, 112–14; at La Mega, 101–9; at Miss Gay Suan Juan, 197n11; at soccer tournament, 77–84; as strategic tool, 105; with the Tenth Round, 137–41. *See also* scandalousness; scandalous storytelling

EsSalud (social security health system), 158, 159

ethnocartography (Weston), 180n5

ethnography: experimentation and, 184n15; gaze of, 30, 147; of HIV/AIDS, 24–26; intersectionality and, 26–32; reflexivity in, 30–31

ethno-racial hierarchies, 34, 91, 97, 107. *See also* race and racism

Ewig, Christina, 201n6

exceptionalism, 24, 187n29

fabulationality (Nyong'o), 183n14

Falcón, Sylvanna, 201n3

*la farándula* (entertainment, form of), 110, 205n24

Farmer, Paul, 200n1, 201n5

Fassin, Didier, 195n5

Feldman, Joseph, 40

Felix, 76, 198n15

Fernandez, Josephina, 147

Fernández-Dávila, Percy, 188n1

following up (*el seguimiento*), 94–96, 125

forms: for ID card activity, 162–63, 164–65; participation in filling out, 165; System of Community Protection and, 90, 124–28, *125*, 151–52, 155, 164, 166–67, 170

fragmentation and collaboration, 129–33, 143–44

fraud, 127, 129–30

Freud, Sigmund, 57

Friedman, Elisabeth Jay, 199n17, 210n11

Fujimori, Alberto, 19, 20, 40, 50, 201n6

funding. *See* Global Fund; Tenth Round (funding)

fundraising, 70–71, 84, 93, 127, 130, 133, 161, 166. See also *polladas* (fundraisers)

Galea, Jerome T., 200n1

Gandolfo, Daniella, 184n15

García, María Elena, 12

Las Gardenias (bar), 41–42, 48

Garro, Linda C., 181n8, 183n13

gay men and gayness: collective life, 26; denouncement and, 114; discrimination against, 127–28; gay, as term, 10; Global Fund's tenth round and, 180n6; in Lima, 53; as being Mary Magdalene, 54; salons as good business for, 36, 42–43; scandal and, 181n10, 204n19; terms for, 194n1; violence against, 45

gaze of ethnography, 30, 147

gifts. See *peches* (gifts)

Global Equity Fund, 135–36, 138

Global Fund: overview, 20–21; Anderson and, 124, 133–40, 153–54; antidiscrimination ordinances and, 90; closure and freezing of Tenth Round, 34, 122, 129, 141, 154, 164, 173; community-based organizations and, 123, 129, 131, 133; concept note and, 208n14; DISAM and, 93; extensions to funding (attempts for), 173–75; Fifth Round, 20, 132, 202n9; funding support, 185n20; origins, 185n20; other references to, 28, 97, 121–22; programming, 102, 115, 122–24, 166; projects in Tarapoto, 67, 120; scandalous storytelling and, 34;

Sixth Round, 20, 202n9; support for, 21–22; System of Community Protection and, 93–95; target groups, 180n6. *See also* Tenth Round (funding)

Godfrey, 92, 99–100, 101, 104–5, 106, 108, 204n18

Golash-Boza, Tanya, 202n10

Gótica (nightclub), 100

Graham, Richard, 194n2

Greene, Shane, 184n15

grievance filings, 90, 116, 124–28, *125*, 126–28, 151–52, 155, 164, 166–67, 170, 207n9. *See also* complaint books; System of Community Protection (Sistema de Defensorías Comunitarias)

*gringa/gringo* identity, 29, 31, 161, 176, 209n5

Grundel, Walter, 93

Guzman, Abimael, 40

hair treatment as *peche*, 47, 48

Halberstam, Jack, 183n14

Halperin, David, 200n20

Hanssmann, Christoph, 147, 150

Hartman, Saidiya, 140, 184n14

Haynes, Nell, 203n13

hearing (Ahmed), 34, 92

Heckert, Carina, 203n14

Hernández, Jillian, 183n13

heteronormative violence, 42

heterosexual men, 49, 54. See also *maperos*; *peches* (gifts)

Hidalgo, Florentina, 210n9

highly active antiretroviral therapy (HAART), 19. *See also* antiretroviral therapy (ART)

Hirsch, Jennifer S., 193n23

HIV/AIDS: overview, 18–23; categories in research vs. in reality, 39; colonialism and, 184n16; discrimination due to, 5, 32, 87, 200n1; extortion after death, 127–28; funding for treatment, 6, 20–22; Global Fund, 20–21, 22–23; global response to, 24; vs. internal armed conflict, 32–33, 38; origins of "story" of, 184n16; periods within epidemic, 18; programming, 141; re-medicalization of, 24–25; scaling up care, 19–21; sexual roles and, 58–59; size of epidemic, 211n18; social conditions and, 66; statistics, 186n24; storying, 18–19; testing for, 67; transmission risks, 56; universal access to treatment, 19; World AIDS Day, 167. *See also* Tenth Round (funding); treatment

Homosexual Association of Mariscal Cáceres (Asociación Homosexual Mariscalence, AHOMA), 120–21

Howe, Cymene, 203n14

Huayco (Tarapoto, neighborhood), 43–44, 157

Huerta, Monica, 184n14

Hugo, 74, 75–77, 86–87, 88

human rights memory, 50

humor: in scandalous storytelling, 29–30, 37–38, 45; trauma and, 46–47

Hurston, Zora Neale, 183n13

INDECOPI (National Institute of the Defense of Competition . . . Intellectual Property), 4, 5–6, 94, 96, 100, 125, 127

indigenous languages, 40

individualized discrimination, 107

Infante, Gio, 132, 190n12, 202n8, 208n11

INPPARES, 123

insurgency groups, 19, 37, 40–41

internal armed conflict (1980–2000), 16–17, 32–33, 38, 42–50, 51

intersectionality, 7, 92, 162, 201n4

intersubjectivity and ethnography, 26–32

Iquitos (Peru), 28, 132, 134, 138, 140, 141, 152, 153. *See also* Arturo

La Jarrita (bar), 160–61

Jefferson, 93–96, 102, 125–26, 127

Jorge, 154

*joven* (young man/person), 194n1

*juane* (snack), 154, *155*

Juan Guerra (Peru), 115

Juanjuí (Peru), 94, 96, 206n3. *See also* AHOMA (Homosexual Association of Mariscal Cáceres)

Juan Manuel, 160–61, 162–63, 165, 166, 174

Karla, 36–37, 46–47, 48–50, 191n16
Kenworthy, Nora, 24
Kernaghan, Richard, 191n14, 192n19, 205n23
Kippax, Susan, 195n5
Kulick, Don, 204n19

Lancaster, Roger, 194n28
land use, 13
La Serna, Miguel, 41
legal personhood (*personaria juridica*), 120
Leyla, 174, 175–77, 213n2
*libro de reclamaciones*. *See* complaint books
*loca* (crazy person), 162, 182n12
Locke, Peter, 11, 208n13
Lóxoro (language variety), 188n1

*machomenos* soccer games, 74, 75, 76, 78, 79, 86–88, 101, 198n12, 198n14
Manalansan, Martin F., IV, 183n14, 192n18
Mantini-Briggs, Clara, 168–69
Manuel, 81–82
*maperos*: overview, 37, 51, 180n6; discretion and, 50; marriage and, 193n23; in Martín's story about armed forces, 45–46; *peches* and, 49, 50, 52, 53, 54, 66; sexual roles, 57–58; social roles, 189n2, 193n22; unequal relationships with, 54. *See also* MSM (men who have sex with men); *puntos*
maps: Peru, 8; San Martín department, 27
Mariana, 133, 134–36, 137, 138, 174
*maricón* (slur), 49, 191n16, 193n20
Maritza, 157, 158, 159
Martín: author and, 54; community reputation, 69, 196n8; discrimination story, 112–14; luck of, 140; stories told by, 29, 44–46, 92; story about Axel and author, 29
martyrdom, 100
Mary Magdalene (biblical figure), 54
Maskovsky, Jeff, 205n22
Mattingly, Cheryl, 181n8, 183n13
mediation vs. multiplicity, 33
La Mega (disco), 101–4, *103*, 105, 108, 110, 157–58

Meinert, Lotte, 121
Melissa (obstetrician), 167–68
memorialization, 42
Méndez, Cecilia G., 12
Mendoza, Zoila S., 184n17
*mestizaje* (myth of race mixing), 12, 97–98, 107
metrics: in global health, 17, 21, 145, 148, 169, 209n2, 212n19; randomized controlled trials and, 209n1; social, 69–71
MHOL (Movimiento Homosexual de Lima), 132
MHOTA (Movimiento Homosexual de Tarapoto), 92, 93
Millenium Development Goals (United Nations), 19–20, 21
Milton, Cynthia, 191n14, 192n18
Miss Gay beauty contest, 11, 138, 196n7
Miss Gay Carnival, 69
Miss Gay San Juan, 74, 75, 76, 197n11
Mojola, Sanyu A., 193n27
Moodie, Ellen, 91, 204n18, 207n10
Morales (district), 67, 72
morality: discretion as obligation, 47–50; "End of AIDS" and, 35, 39, 56–57, 59–61; transactional sex and, 60
Motta, Angelica, 206n25
Movimiento Homosexual de Lima (MHOL), 132, 148, 149, 202n8
Movimiento Homosexual de Tarapoto (MHOTA), 92, 93
Movimiento Homosexual de Tarapoto (MHOTA), 92
Moyer, Eileen, 187n30
MRTA (insurgency group): crime and punishment clause, 190n10; killings of *travestis* and others, 41–42; location for, 189n7; political theater, 41; vs. Shining Path, 40–41; size, 190n9; stories about, 37, 43–44, 47–48, 50, 191n14
MS (men who have sex with men): as category, 9; community-based organizations for, 134; Global Fund's tenth round and, 180n6; HIV/AIDS's concentration among, 22–23; other references to, 33; scholarship on,

186n28; sexual roles and, 57–58.
See also *maperos*
multisectoral health governance, 122
municipality, collaboration with, 75–76,
80, 85–87, 115, 159, 196n7, 210n7
Muñoz, José Esteban, 183n14

narrative, 17, 147, 150, 165, 181n8, 182n12,
183n13, 188n36
Nascimento, Silvana de Souza, 196n7
neoliberalism, 201n6
Nicole, 64–66
Nieves, Manuel, 93
nightlife: use of term, 205n22; clothing
and, 112–13; discrimination and, 2–3,
91, 92, 100, 101–5, 106–7, 110, 112–14,
126–27, 157–58; importance, 109;
photographs of, *111*; *recreos* serving as,
72; in stories, 2, 44, 52; in Tarapoto,
109–11; transgender women and,
101–7, 111, 128, 157–58
90-90-90 targets, 34–35, 145–46, 175,
208nn15–16
Noleto, Rafael da Silva, 196n7
Norma: Las Amazonas and, 114–15, 116,
134, 136, 137; capacity-building workshops and, 115, 120; discrimination
cases and, 125–27, 136, 157–59; Global
Fund and, 120, 206n1; scandalous
storytelling, 92, 207n8; War of the
Salons and, 81
No Tengo Miedo (activist collective), 150,
161–65
Nyong'o, Tavia, 183n14

Ochoa, Marcia, 182n12, 196n7
Ochs, Elinor, 17, 181n9
Olaf, 120, 129, 131–32
oral sex, 44–45
otherness vs. *travesti*/trans, 12–13

La Pachanga (disco), 110
Pamela, 92, 115–16
Papua New Guinea, 56
Parker, Richard, 18, 24, 201n5
PARSALUD (Support Program for Health
Sector Reform), 123, 124
*pasinja meri* (passenger women), 56

passenger women (*pasinja meri*), 56
patronage, 194n2. *See also* clientelism
Paula: discrimination against at La Anaconda, 2–5, 14, 105, 207n8; life, 1–2, 5,
179n2, 179nn1–2; scandal and, 182n12;
volleyball playing, 3, 154
*peches* (gifts): overview, 37–39, 47–48,
51–55, 188n1; imaginative potential
of, 60–62; as interpretive device, 33;
*maperos* and, 49, 50, 52, 53, 54, 66;
negativity towards, 53; perspectives
on, 53–54; as problem, 55–60; as
"real" relationships or not, 53;
relationships mediated through,
48–49, 58, 60; signification and,
61; social status and, 52–53, 59;
stories about, 46, 47–48, 50, 52–53;
transactional sex and, 33, 39, 47, 52,
53, 61
peer community health promoters
(*promotores*), 132–33
peer health resources, 92
penetrative role in sex, 57
Pepin, Jacques, 184n16
Perez, Justin: photographs of, *10*
*personaria juridica* (legal personhood),
120
personhood, legal, 120
Peruvian Communist Party—Shining
Path (Sendero Luminoso), 40
Philco, Carlos, 74, 85–87
photography projects, 162–64, *163*
Pigg, Stacy Leigh, 39
*piraña*, 191n15
policing, 115–16, 126, 157, 167. See also
*serenazgo* (auxiliary municipal
police)
political theater, 41
politicians, social relations with, 33, 74,
85–87
*polladas* (fundraisers): overview, 70–71,
197n9; Anderson and, 93–94; author
and, 161; collaboration and, 70–71,
143; Ramón and, 127–28; Rogerio
and, 130; after Tenth Round funding
termination, 130, 133, 160, 161, 173
Portocarrero, Gonzalo, 98–99, 100, 101,
107, 116

poverty, 20
power, coloniality of, 12
PrEP (pre-exposure prophylaxis): adherence to, 193n25; Peru and, 55–56, 59–60, 175, 177, 187n31; re-medicalization of AIDS epidemic and, 24–25; transactional sex and, 57, 175
prevention: culture of denouncement and, 91; Lima and, 141; mitigating discrimination and stigma and, 89; obligations due to, 171–72; pharmaceuticalization of, 24; treatment as, 6, 21; in urban Amazonian Peru, 66; vulnerable populations and, 112, 151. *See also* PrEP (pre-exposure prophylaxis)
Pride parades, 12, *13*, 69
project specialists: challenges for, 172; culture of denouncement and, 124–25, 135; data and, 169–70; gossip about, 207n10; perceptions of, 129–30; as role, 120, 121, 131, 132, 143, 146; System of Community Protection and, 128, 151; Tenth Round funding and, 122–24, 128, 143–44, 173
*promotores* (peer community health promoters), 132–33
PROMSEX (Centro de Promoción y Defensa de los Derechos Sexuales y Reproductivos), 149–50, 168, 211n18
public space, 26, 71, 77–78
Pucallpa (Peru), 28, 131–32, 153. *See also* Olaf
*puntos* (heterosexual partners), 37–38. *See also* maperos

quantification, 148, 151; of discrimination, 151–52, 166, 167, 169, 170
Quechua (language), 40
queer life and experience: terminology, 9, 11, 146, 150, 151, 180n6, 182n12, 206n25; camp sensibility, 200n20; emergence, 11, 17, 147, 169, 170; messy, 192n18; persistence, 121–22, 173; relationality, 88, 183n14; social critique, 184n15; world-making, 7, 178, 205n22

Quijano, Aníbal, 12
quinceañeras, 72

race and racism: AIDS disparities and, 187n32; culture and, 91, 203n12, 203n13; differentiation, 12, 13, 97–98, 107; discrimination, 201n4, 204n16; ethno-racial hierarchies, 34, 91, 97, 107, 172, 178, 188n32, 205n22; hierarchy of, 14, 17, 117, 166; individualization and, 14, 60, 97, 105, 107, 181n7; whitening, 13. *See also* mestizaje (myth of race mixing)
Ramón: author and, 102; community involvement, 72, 127–28, 199n15, 199n16; death of young gay man and, 127–28; on experience living with HIV, 76; Hugo and, 74, 76–77, 86–87, 88; life, 63–65, 67–69, 72, 206n1; scandal and, 78–79; soccer tournament and, 66–67, 69, 71–81, 84, 85, 86–88; visit to Nicole, 195n2; Yesika and, 101–2, 104, 105, 106, 108–9
randomized controlled trials, 209n1
reciprocity, 158
*recreos* (recreational facilities), 72
redistributive activities, 33, 119–20, 129. *See also* polladas (fundraisers)
Red Peruana de Trans, Lesbianas, Gays y Bisexuales (Red Peruana TLGB), 149–50
redress, 166
reflexivity, 30
"right" vs. "wrong" categories, 79
Rogerio, 129, 130, 132
Rosaldo, Renato, 183n13
Rose, Nikolas, 187n30
Rubin, Gayle, 191n17

Salomé, 69
salons: activities at, 28; other references to, 50; photographs of, *43*; storytelling in, 1–2, 14, 36–37, 42–45; War of the Salons, 80–84, *82*, 85
salvation memory, 50, 191n14, 192n18
Sandset, Tony, 208nn15–16
Sangaramoorthy, Thurka, 24, 25, 148, 188n33, 212n19

San Martín department, 27, 40–41, 189n7, 206n1

scandalousness: overview, 14–17, 105; use of term, 15, 182n12; avoiding, 103–4, 106–7; beauty contests and, 71; community relations and, 71; differentiation and, 107–8; as discrimination, 105–9; emblematic vs. scandalous denouncements, 34; excess and, 84; gay and transgender people and, 83–84; gay men and, 181n10, 204n19; importance of, 5; injustice as justifying, 83; in Paula's disco story, 3, 4–5, 6, 14; queer social world-making and, 7; "right" vs. "wrong" categories and, 79; scholarship on, 181n11; as storytelling genre, 7, 14–15; trans women and, 118; use of term, 15. See also *el escándalo* (scandalous episode)

scandalous storytelling: overview, 14–17, 32, 71, 181n8; agency and, 90; author's involvement in, 29, 31; differentiation in, 92; exaggeration and embellishment in, 29, 33; flies in, 29, 161; Global Fund's Tenth Round and, 34; humor in, 29–30, 37–38, 45; the "I"/protagonist of, 16; as life made livable through, 47; other references to, 51; *peches* in, 60; scholarship on, 183n14; social determinants of health framework and, 31; social outcomes and, 33–34; as structure for this text, 11; in Tarapoto, 29; Tenth Round and, 137–41; about unfinished projects, 137–41; "wink" at end of story, 16, 42. See also *el escándalo* (scandalous episode)

Scheper-Hughes, Nancy, 195n2

schools, discrimination in, 121

*el seguimiento* (following up), 94–96, 125

Seguro Integral de Salúd (SIS), 65

self-defense, 156

selfhood, 7, 9, 11, 12, 80, 150

*la selva* (Amazonian jungle region, Peru): national imagination and, 13

*el serenazgo* (auxiliary municipal police), 115–16, 126, 167

Serrano-Amaya, José Fernando, 190n13

sexuality, western terminology for, 56

sexually transmitted infections (STI): management in Peru, 20

sexual positions, 57–58

sexual subjectification: as system of power, 10; terminology for, 9

sexual violence, 126

sex work, 115, 156, 193n24, 210n7

Shining Path (insurgency group), 19, 40, 50, 189n4

Sierra Leone, 187n29

silence to suffering, 98–99, 100, 116

Silverstein, Sydney M., 98

Sistema de Defensorías Communitarias (System of Community Protection), 90, 91, 92–96

Sívori, Horacio Federico, 182n12

Smith-Oka, Vania, 202n12

snakes, 45

soccer playing: *la colaboración* and, 197n10; collaborative redistribution and, 119–20, 129, 130; lesbians and, 11, 78–79, 80, 164; other references to, 171; photographs of, 82; Ramón and, 66–67, 69, 71–81, 84, 85, 86–88; scandalousness and, 71, 77–79, 80–83, 84, 88; team of lesbian mothers, 11, 78–79, 80; tournaments, 66–67, 69, 164, 198n14

social cleansing, 41

social determinants of health, 31, 90

sociality. See *la colaboración* (collaboration, concept of)

social metrics, 69–71

social relations, 66, 69–71, 73; reimagining, 6–7

Sosa, Joseph Jay, 147–48, 156

sports tournaments, 28, 34, 79, 130. See also soccer; volleyball

Stewart, Kathleen, 184n14

stigma: as determinant, 66, 90, 201n2; misinterpretation of, 31, 201n5; mitigation of, 21–24, 28, 32, 87, 89–90, 98–99, 117, 128, 135–36, 202n9; as social force or problem, 9, 16, 25, 151, 171, 194n28. See also discrimination stories and storytelling: affective possibilities and, 49; in capacity-building workshops, 101; catharsis from, 147; competing with each other, 50; denouncements and, 108, 109; everyday narrative practices, 17; flourishes added to, 5; as knowledge building site, 7; "near-misses" in, 44; questions to listener during, 2; retelling of, 16, 17, 29–30, 36–37; in salons, 1–2, 14, 36–37, 42–45; twists in, 37. *See also* narrative

subjectivities, 11

subject positions, 11

success abroad (*triunfo en el exterior*), 101

Support Program for Health Sector Reform (PARSALUD), 123

Sustainable Development Goals, 186n23

System of Community Protection (Sistema de Defensorías Comunitarias): overview, 92–96; Las Amazonas and, 115–16; continuation of, 136; development of, 91, 175; formal grievance process through, 90, 124–28, *125*, 151–52, 155, 164, 166–67, 170; implementation, 101, 105–6, 114, 150; Ramón and, 102; Tenth Round and, 93, 135, 143, 154, 201n2; Yesika and, 102

Tang, Eric C., 187n31

Tarapoto (Peru): discrimination in (specific cases), 153–57; Global Fund projects in, 67, 120, 134; history of city, 47; HIV/AIDS epidemic and internal armed conflict (tension between in), 32–33; HIV/AIDS in (specific cases), 92–93; Huayco (neighborhood), 43–44, 157; nightlife in, 109–11; organizations, 92, 93; *peches* in, 39; photographs of, *41*; postconflict period and, 40–47; Pride march, 12, *13*; recreation in, 72; scandalous storytelling in, 29; sexual positions in, 57–58; social relations, 33, 37; stories (circulation of) in, 91; terrorism era in, 37; volleyball games, 26

Tenth Round (funding): coordination of, 138; implementation, 176; legacy of, 166, 170, 171; limitations, 142; memories of informants on, 141–42; NGOs and, 133–37, 139; peer community health promoters and, 132–33; in Pucallpa, 131; scandalous storytelling and, 137–41; social relationships and, 130; System of Community Protection and, 126, 201n2; in Tarapoto, 134; termination and freezing of, 128, 129, 130, 133, 134–35, 141, 143, 153, 154, 160, 161, 166, 173, 207n10

*terruco/a* ("terrorist"), 191n14

theater, political, 41

Thomann, Matthew, 24

Thomas, Rebekah, 200n1

transactional sex: overview, 38–39, 56; HIV prevention and, 56, 59, 212n1; morality and, 60–61; *peches* and, 33, 39, 47, 52, 53, 61; Peru and, 56–57, 58–59; problematization of, 59–62

transgender women: use of term, 10–12, 179n2, 180n6, 186n28; beauty contests, 28; community-based organizations for, 94, 134; discrimination and violence against, 44, 101–7, 113, 114, 115–16, 125–26, 157–58, 205n20, 210n9; feminized labor, 193n24; Global Fund's Tenth Round and, 180n6; HIV rates, 22, 168; medical care (access to), 210n9; nightlife and, 101–7, 111; Pride march in Tarapoto, 12, *13*; salons as work for, 36, 42–43, 73; scandal wielded against, 118; scholarship on, 186n28; violence towards, 190n11. *See also* Las Amazonas (community-based organization); community-based organizations (CBOS); *travesti*

trauma and humor, 46–47

*travesti*: use of term, 12–13, 180n3; community-based organizations for, 134; deaths of, 41–42; discrimination against, 104; HIV experiences, 64–65; scholarship on, 181n11; violence toward, 190n11. *See also* transgender women treatment: access to, 19, 60; alternative, 64–65; funding for, 6, 20–22; as prevention, 6, 21, 23; universal access, 19; vertical approaches to, 24, 25. *See also* PrEP (pre-exposure prophylaxis)

Treichler, Paula, 211n18

*triunfo en el exterior* (success abroad), 101

Truth and Reconciliation Commission (Comisión de la Verdad y Reconciliación, CVR), 40–42, 50, 148–49, 192n19

Tupac Amaru Revolutionary Movement (MRTA) (insurgency group), 19

Uganda, 186n25

UNAIDS (United Nations Programme on HIV/AIDS), 145, 175, 202n7, 208n15

undetectable status, 24, 145, 185n22

United Nations Programme on HIV/AIDS (UNAIDS), 145, 175, 202n7, 208n15

Valdez, Natali, 209n1

Vargas, Deborah, 192n18

Vaso de Leche (social support program), 86, 198n13

Vasquez del Aguila, Ernesto, 181n10, 204n19

Venezuela, 168–69

Veronica, 73, 77, 80, 81, 83, 84, 200n20

vertical approaches to treatment, 24, 25

victim blaming, 48

violence: against gay men, 45; heteronormative, 42; quantifying in research, 147–48; sexual violence, 126; state-sanctioned, 125–26; against transgender women, 44, 101–7, 113, 114, 115–16, 125–26, 157–58, 205n20, 210n9

#VisibleWeAreStronger, 163–64

Vista Alegre (Peru), 64

volleyball games and playing: Anderson and author at, 154–56; *la colaboración* and, 197n10; collaboration (ethos of) and, 147; descriptions of games, 154; as fundraisers, 161, 166; gay and trans community and, 3, 26; gender categories and, 79; locations of games, 209n5; Martín's story about, 44–46; other references to, 50, 156, 171; photographs of games, 68; scandalous stories about, 29; Tiffany Abreu, 79, 200n19

"vulnerable populations," 155, 159, 165

Walter, 53

Wardlow, Holly, 56, 193n27

War of the Salons, 80–84, 82, 85

Weismantel, Mary, 188n36, 203n13

Wentzell, Emily, 193n26

western terminology for sexuality, 56

Weston, Kath, 180n5

Whyte, Susan Reynolds, 121

Wilmer: author and, 83; life, 43–44, 72–73; *peches* and, 47–48; soccer tournament and, 73, 76, 77, 80–81, 83, 198n14

"winning one's name," 196n8

workshops. *See* capacity-building workshops

World AIDS Day, 167

world-making, 7

Yesika: culture of denouncement and, 116, 204n18, 205n20; discrimination against, 101–5, 106–9, 113, 118; scandalous storytelling and, 92, 106; War of the Salons and, 81, 84

Yezer, Caroline, 192n19

Yogyakarta Principles, 209n4

www.ingramcontent.com/pod-product-compliance
Lightning Source LLC
Chambersburg PA
CBHW020849270326
41928CB00006B/620